UCLA Symposia on Molecular and Cellular Biology, New Series

Series Editor, C. Fred Fox

Please contact the publisher for information about previous titles in this series.

Liposomes in the Therapy of Infectious Diseases and Cancer

Liposomes in the Therapy of Infectious Diseases and Cancer

Proceedings of a Ciba-Geigy-Squibb-UCLA Colloquium
Held at Lake Tahoe, California
February 16–20, 1988

Editors

Gabriel Lopez-Berestein
Clinical Immunology/Biological Therapy
M.D. Anderson Hospital
Houston, Texas

Isaiah J. Fidler
Department of Cell Biology
M.D. Anderson Hospital
Houston, Texas

Alan R. Liss, Inc. • **New York**

Address all Inquiries to the Publisher
Alan R. Liss, Inc., 41 East 11th Street, New York, NY 10003

While the authors, editors, and publisher believe that drug selection and dosage and the specifications and usage of equipment and devices, as set forth in this book, are in accord with current recommendations and practice at the time of publication, they accept no legal responsibility for any errors or omissions, and make no warranty, express or implied, with respect to material contained herein. In view of ongoing research, equipment modifications, changes in governmental regulations and the constant flow of information relating to drug therapy, drug reactions and the use of equipment and devices, the reader is urged to review and evaluate the information provided in the package insert or instructions for each drug, piece of equipment or device for, among other things, any changes in the instructions or indications of dosage or usage and for added warnings and precautions.

Library of Congress Cataloging-in-Publication Data

Liposomes in the therapy of infectious diseases and cancer :
  proceedings of a Ciba-Geigy-Squibb-UCLA Symposium, held at Lake
  Tahoe, California, February 16–20, 1988 / editors, Gabriel Lopez-
  Berestein, Isaiah J. Fidler.
      p. cm.—(UCLA) symposia on molecular and cellular biology :
  new ser., v. 89)
    Includes bibliographies and index.
      1. Communicable diseases—Chemotherapy—Evaluation—Congresses.
  2. Cancer—Chemotherapy—Evaluation—Congresses. 3. Liposomes—
  Testing—Congresses. 4. Drugs—Vehicles—Testing—Congresses.
  5. Clinical trials—Congresses. I. Lopez-Berestein, Gabriel.
  II. Fidler, Isaiah J., 1936–. III. CIBA-GEIGY Corporation.
  IV. E.R. Squibb & Sons. V. University of California, Los Angeles.
  VI. Series.
      [DNLM: 1. Communicable Diseases—drug therapy—congresses.
  2. Liposomes—congresses. 3. Neoplasms—drug therapy—congresses.
  W3 U17N new ser. v. 89 / QU 93 L7655 1988]
  RC112.L57 1988   616.9'0461—dc19   DNLM/DLC
  for Library of Congress   88–8516
  ISBN 0-8451-2688-1   CIP

Contents

VI. NOVEL APPROACHES IN LIPOSOME DEVELOPMENT

Contributors

Jill P. Adler, Department of Biological Sciences, California State Polytechnic University, Pomona, CA 91768 **[249]**

J. Alexander, Immunology Division, University of Strathcylde, Glasgow, Scotland, United Kingdom **[215]**

T.M. Allen, Department of Pharmacology, University of Alberta, Edmonton, Alberta T6G 2H7, Canada **[405]**

Carl R. Alving, Departments of Immunology and Membrane Biochemistry, Walter Reed Army Institute of Research, Washington, DC 20307-5100 **[167]**

S. Amselem, Departments of Oncology and Membrane Biochemistry, Hadassah Medical Center and Hebrew University, Hadassah Medical School, Jerusalem, Israel **[391]**

Kathe Andrejcio, Ciba-Geigy Corporation, Pharmaceuticals Division, Summit, NJ 07901; present address: CIBA-GEIGY Ltd., Basel, Switzerland **[297,305,329]**

G. Atassi, Service de Médecine Interne et Laboratoire d'Investigation Clinique H.J. Tagnon, Institut J. Bordet, Centre des Tumeurs de l'Université Libre de Bruxelles, 1000 Brussels, Belgium **[343]**

A.J. Baillie, Pharmacy Department, University of Strathcylde, Glasgow, Scotland, United Kingdom **[215]**

Malcolm Baines, Department of Microbiology and Immunology, McGill University, Montreal, Quebec H3G 1A4, Canada **[15]**

Irma A.J.M. Bakker-Woudenberg, Department of Clinical Microbiology, Erasmus University, 3000 DR Rotterdam, The Netherlands **[275]**

Y. Barenholz, Departments of Oncology and Membrane Biochemistry, Hadassah Medical Center and Hebrew University, Hadassah Medical School, Jerusalem, Israel **[391]**

S. Berger, Zürich Institute of Pharmacology, University of Zürich, Zürich, Switzerland **[95]**

C. Brassinne, Service de Médecine Interne et Laboratoire d'Investigation Clinique H.J. Tagnon, Institut J. Bordet, Centre des Tumeurs de l'Université Libre de Bruxelles, 1000 Brussels, Belgium **[343]**

Dean E. Brenner, Departments of Clinical Pharmacology and Therapeutics, Roswell Park Memorial Institute, New York State Department of Health, Buffalo, NY 14263 **[297]**

The numbers in brackets are the opening page numbers of the contributors' articles.

E.N. Brunette, Cancer Research Institute, University of California, San Francisco, CA 94143-0128 **[287]**

K.C. Carter, Pharmacy Department, Immunology Division, University of Strathcylde, Glasgow, Scotland, United Kingdom **[215]**

M.L. Corvo, Departamento de Tecnologia de Industrias Químicas (LNETI), 2745 Queluz, Portugal **[417]**

André Coune, Service de Médecine Interne et Laboratoire, d'Investigation Clinique H.J. Tagnon, Institut J. Bordet, Centre des Tumeurs de l'Université Libre de Bruxelles, 1000 Brussels, Belgium **[343]**

M. Court, Research and Development Laboratories, Pharmaceuticals Division, CIBA-GEIGY Limited, Basel, Switzerland **[191]**

J. Wayne Cowens, Departments of Clinical Pharmacology and Therapeutics and Experimental Therapeutics, Roswell Park Memorial Institute, New York State Department of Health, Buffalo, NY 14263 **[297]**

Patrick J. Creaven, Departments of Clinical Pharmacology and Therapeutics, Roswell Park Memorial Institute, New York State Department of Health, Buffalo, NY 14263 **[297]**

D.J.A. Crommelin, Department of Pharmaceutics, University of Utrecht, 3522 AD Utrecht, The Netherlands **[105]**

M.E. Cruz, Departamento de Tecnologia de Industrias Químicas (LNETI) 2745 Queluz, Portugal **[417]**

Joan E. Cunningham, Departments of Clinical Immunology and Biological Therapy, M.D. Anderson Hospital and Tumor Institute, Houston, TX 77030 **[329]**

M. Kelli Cushman, Department of Clinical Pharmacology and Therapeutics, Roswell Park Memorial Institute, New York State Department of Health, Buffalo, NY 14263 **[297]**

Barbara Dadey, Department of Medical Oncology, Roswell Park Memorial Institute, New York State Department of Health, Buffalo, NY 14263 **[297]**

Toos Daemen, Laboratory of Physiological Chemistry, State University Groningen, Medical School, 9712 KZ Groningen, The Netherlands **[81]**

David Davis, Medical Research Council Group, Academic Department of Medicine, Royal Free Hospital School of Medicine, London NW3 2QG, United Kingdom **[35]**

Robert J. Debs, Mycobacteriology Research Laboratory, National Jewish Center for Immunology and Respiratory Medicine, Denver, CO 80206; present address: Cancer Research Institute, University of California, San Francisco, CA 94143–0128 **[177, 287]**

W.H. de Jong, Department of Pathology, National Institute of Public Health and Environmental Hygiene, 3720 BA Bilthoven, The Netherlands **[105]**

Jan Dijkstra, Infectious Disease Unit, Veterans Adminstration Medical Center, West Haven, CT 06516 **[81]**

T.F. Dolan, Pharmacy Department, University of Strathcylde, Glasgow, Scotland, United Kingdom **[215]**

S. Druckmann, Departments of Oncology and Membrane Biochemistry, Hadassah Medical Center and Hebrew University, Hadassah Medical School, Jerusalem, Israel **[391]**

Nejat Düzgüneş, Cancer Research Institute and the Department of Pharmaceutical Chemistry, University of California, San Francisco, CA 94143-0128 **[177, 287]**

Daniel Estrella, Liposome Technology Inc., Menlo Park, CA 94025 **[239]**

P. Fankhauser, Research and Development Laboratories, Pharmaceuticals Division, CIBA-GEIGY Limited, Basel, Switzerland **[191,435]**

Isaiah J. Fidler, Department of Cell Biology, M.D. Anderson Hospital and Tumor Institute, Houston, TX 77030 **[xix,3,329]**

Joshua Fierer, U.C. San Diego School of Medicine, V.A. Medical Center, San Diego, CA 92161 **[239]**

M. Fischer, Research and Development Laboratories, Pharmaceuticals Division, CIBA-GEIGY Limited, Basel, Switzerland **[191]**

H. Frost, CIBA-GEIGY Corp., Summit, NJ 07901; present address: CIBA-GEIGY Ltd., Basel, Switzerland **[305]**

A. Gabizon, Cancer Research Institute and Liposome Technology Inc., Menlo Park, CA 94025; present address: Departments of Oncology and Membrane Biochemistry, Hadassah Medical Center and Hebrew University, Hadassah Medical School, Jerusalem, Israel **[135,391]**

P.R.J. Gangadharam, Mycobacteriology Research Laboratory, National Jewish Center for Immunology and Respiratory Medicine, Denver, CO 80206 **[177,287]**

Nathalie Garcon, Medical Research Council Group, Academic Department of Medicine, Royal Free Hospital School of Medicine, London NW3 2QG, United Kingdom **[35]**

Brian E. Gilbert, Department of Microbiology and Immunology, Baylor College of Medicine, Houston, TX 77030 **[229]**

Micheal J. Gilbreath, Departments of Immunology and Membrane Biochemistry, Walter Reed Army Institute of Research, Washington, DC 20307-5100 **[167]**

Richard S. Ginsberg, The Liposome Company, Inc., Princeton, NJ 08540 **[205]**

Jayne Goldstein, Cancer Research Institute, University of California, San Francisco, San Francisco, CA 94143 **[177]**

D. Goren, Departments of Oncology and Membrane Biochemistry, Hadassah Medical Center and Hebrew University, Hadassah Medical School, Jerusalem, Israel **[391]**

P. Graepel, Research and Development Laboratories, Pharmaceuticals Division, CIBA-GEIGY Limited, Basel, Switzerland **[191]**

Andrew R. Greenspan, Division of Medical Oncology, Lombardi Cancer Research Center, Georgetown University Hospital, Washington, DC 20007 **[353]**

Gregory Gregoriadis, Medical Research Council Group, Academic Department of Medicine, Royal Free Hospital School of Medicine, London NW3 2QG, United Kingdom **[35]**

Daniel A. Guerra, Department of Biological Sciences, California State Polytechnic University, Pomona, CA 91768 **[249]**

Jordan U. Gutterman, Departments of Clinical Immunology and Biological Therapy, M.D. Anderson Hospital and Tumor Institute, Houston, TX 77030 **[329]**

Tin Han, Department of Medical Oncology, Roswell Park Memorial Institute, New York State Department of Health, Buffalo, NY 14263 **[297]**

J.R. Hanagan, CIBA-GEIGY Corp., Summit, NJ 07901; present address: CIBA-GEIGY Ltd., Basel, Switzerland **[305]**

Machiel Hardonk, Laboratory of Pathology, State University Groningen, Medical School, 9713 EZ Groningen, The Netherlands **[81]**

Loren Hatlin, U.C. San Diego School of Medicine, V.A. Medical Center, San Diego, CA 92161 **[239]**

H. Hengartner, Department of Experimental Pathology, University Hospital, University of Tübingen, Federal Republic of Germany **[95]**

C. Hollaert, Service de Médecine Interne et Laboratoire d'Investigation Clinique H.J. Tagnon, Institut J. Bordet, Centre des Tumeurs de l'Université Libre de Bruxelles, 1000 Brussels, Belgium **[343]**

Eric G. Holmberg, Department of Biochemistry, University of Tennessee, Knoxville, TN 37996-0840 **[25]**

Rick Hogue, Liposome Technology Inc., Menlo Park, CA 94025 **[239]**

Leaf Huang, Department of Biochemistry, University of Tennessee, Knoxville, TN 37996-0840 **[25]**

Robert Huben, Department of Urologic Oncology, Roswell Park Memorial Institute, New York State Department of Health, Buffalo, NY 14263 **[297]**

Melissa M. Hudson, Department of Cell Biology and Pediatrics, University of Texas System Cancer Center, M.D. Anderson Hospital and Tumor Institute, Houston, TX 77030 **[71]**

Jo-Ann Jedrusiak, The Liposome Company, Inc., Princeton, NJ 08540 **[205]**

Gordon Jendrasiak, Department of Pathology, East Carolina University School of Medicine, Greenville, NC 27858 **[441]**

J.S. Jorge, Departamento de Tecnologia de Industrias Quimicas (LNETI), 2745 Queluz, Portugal **[417]**

Constantine Karakousis, Department of Soft Tissue Melanoma Service, Roswell Park Memorial Institute, New York State Department of Health, Buffalo, NY 14263 **[297]**

Majeed Kareem, Department of Surgery, McGill University, Montreal, Quebec, Canada H3G 1A4 **[15]**

L. Kesavalu, Mycobacteriology Research Laboratories, National Jewish Center for Immunology and Respiratory Medicine, Denver, CO 80206 **[177]**

A.R. Khokhar, Departments of Clinical Immunology, Biological Therapy, and Medical Oncology, The University of Texas System Cancer Center, M.D. Anderson Hospital and Tumor Institute, Houston, TX 77030 **[59]**

Eugenie S. Kleinerman, Department of Cell Biology, M.D. Anderson Hospital and Tumor Institute, Houston, TX 77030 **[71,329]**

Vernon Knight, Department of Microbiology and Immunology, Baylor College of Medicine, Houston, TX 77030 [229]

Jan Koudstaal, Laboratory of Pathology, State University Groningen, Medical School, 9713 EZ Groningen, The Netherlands [81]

Irwin H. Krakoff, Division of Medicine, M.D. Anderson Hospital and Tumor Institute, Houston, TX 77030 [329]

Ilene D. Kurzman, Department of Medical Sciences, School of Veterinary Medicine, University of Wisconsin, Madison, WI 53706 [117]

C. Laduron, Service de Médecine Interne et Laboratoire d'Investigation Clinique H.J. Tagnon, Institut J. Bordet, Centre des Tumeurs de l'Université Libre de Bruxelles, 1000 Brussels, Belgium [343]

Robert P. Lenk, The Liposome Company, Inc., Princeton, NJ 08540 [205]

Jose Lepe-Zuniga, Departments of Clinical Immunology and Biological Therapy, M.D. Anderson Hospital and Tumor Institute, Houston, TX 77030 [329]

D. LeSher, CIBA-GEIGY Corp., Summit, NJ 07901; present address: CIBA-GEIGY Ltd., Basel, Switzerland [305]

Jan-Ping Lin, Liposome Technology Inc., Menlo Park, CA 94025 [239]

A.F. Lokerse, Department of Clinical Microbiology, Erasmus University, 3000 DR Rotterdam, The Netherlands [275]

F. Lopes, Departamento de Tecnologia de Industrias Quimicas (LNETI), 2745 Queluz, Portugal [417]

Gabriel Lopez-Berestein, Section of Immunobiology and Drug Carriers, The University of Texas System Cancer Center, M.D. Anderson Hospital and Tumor Institute, Houston, TX 77030 [xix, 59, 263, 317]

N. Lopez, Department of Pharmacology, University of California, San Francisco, CA 94143 [135]

Antoine Loutfi, Department of Microbiology and Immunology, McGill University, Montreal, Quebec H3G 1A4, Canada [15]

E. Gregory MacEwen, Department of Medical Sciences, School of Veterinary Medicine, University of Wisconsin, Madison, WI 53706 [117]

Reeta Taneja Mehta, Section of Immunobiology and Drug Carriers, The University of Texas, M.D. Anderson Cancer Center, Houston, TX 77030 [263]

Monte S, Meltzer, Departments of Immunology and Membrane Biochemistry, Walter Reed Army Institute of Research, Washington, DC 20307-5100 [167]

George M. Mitilenes, The Liposome Company, Inc., Princeton, NJ 08540 [205]

Page S. Morahan, Department of Microbiology and Immunology, The Medical College of Pennsylvania, Philadelphia, PA 19129 [441]

J. Lee Murray, Department of Clinical Immunology and Biological Therapy, M.D. Anderson Hospital and Tumor Institute, Houston, TX 77030 [329]

Carol A. Nacy, Departments of Immunology and Membrane Biochemistry, Walter Reed Army Institute of Research, Washington, DC 20307-5100 [167]

U.K. Nässander, Department of Pharmaceutics, University of Utrecht, 3522 AD Utrecht, The Netherlands [105]

Rajiv Nayar, The Canadian Liposome Co., V7M 1A5 North Vancouver, British Columbia, Canada [427]

Wolter Oosterhuis, Laboratory of Pathology, State University Groningen, Medical School, 9713 EZ Groningen, The Netherlands [81]

Marc J. Ostro, The Liposome Company, Inc, Princeton, NJ 08540 [155]

Bijay K. Pal, Department of Biological Sciences, California State Polytechnic University, Pomona, CA 91768 [249]

D. Papahadjopoulos, Cancer Research Institute, University of California, San Francisco, CA 94143 [135]

A. Peil, Research and Development Laboratories, Pharmaceuticals Division, CIBA-GEIGY Limited, Basel, Switzerland [191]

T. Peretz, Departments of Oncology and Membrane Biochemistry, Hadassah Medical Center and Hebrew University, Hadassah Medical School, Jerusalem, Israel [391]

R. Perez-Soler, Immunobiology and Drug Carriers Section, The University of Texas System Cancer Center, M.D. Anderson Hospital and Tumor Institute, Houston, TX 77030 [35]

V.K. Perumal, Mycobacteriology Research Laboratory, National Jewish Center for Immunology and Respiratory Medicine, Denver, CO 80206 [177, 287]

B. Pestalozzi, Departments of Experimental Pathology and Medicine, University Hospital, University of Tübingen, Federal Republic of Germany [95]

Nigel C. Phillips, McGill Centre for Host Resistance and Department of Medicine, Montreal General Hospital Research Institute, Montreal, Quebec, Canada H3G 1A4 [15]

Jim S. Pieratos, Department of Biological Sciences, California State Polytechnic University, Pomona, CA 91768 [249]

Angelo J. Pinto, Department of Microbiology and Immunology, The Medical College of Pennsylvania, Philadelphia, PA 19129 [441]

A. Probst, Research and Development Laboratories, Pharmaceutical Division, CIBA-GEIGY Limited, Basel, Switzerland [191]

Aquilur Rahman, Division of Medical Oncology, Lombardi Cancer Research Center, Georgetown University, Washington, DC 20007 [353,367]

F.H. Roerdink, Laboratory of Physiological Chemistry, University of Groningen, 9712 KZ Groningen, The Netherlands [105, 275]

Jae-Kyung Roh, Division of Medical Oncology, Georgetown University, Washington, DC 20007 [367]

Robert C. Rosenthal, Department of Medical Sciences, School of Veterinary Medicine, University of Wisconsin, Madison, WI 53706 [117]

C. Sauter, Department of Medicine, University Hospital, University of Tübingen, Federal Republic of Germany [95]

Kathy Savage, The Liposome Company, Inc., Princeton, NJ 08540 [205]

J.-C. Schaffner, Research and Development Laboratories, Pharmaceuticals Division, CIBA-GEIGY Limited, Basel, Switzerland **[191]**

Gerrit Scherphof, Laboratory of Physiological Chemistry, State University, 9712 KZ Groningen, The Netherlands **[81]**

H. Schott, University of Zürich and Institute of Organic Chemistry, University of Tübingen, Federal Republic of Germany **[95]**

Alan J. Schroit, M.D. Anderson Hospital and Tumor Institute, Houston, TX 77030 **[427]**

G. Schumann, Research and Development Laboratories, Pharmaceuticals Division, CIBA-GEIGY Limited, Basel, Switzerland **[191]**

R. Schwendener, Department of Experimental Pathology, University Hospital, University of Tübingen, Federal Republic of Germany **[95]**

Jean-Paul Sculier, Service de Médecine Interne et Laboratoire d'Investigation Clinique H.J. Tagnon, Institut J. Bordet, Centre des Tumeurs de l'Université Libre de Bruxelles, 1000 Brussels, Belgium **[343]**

Henry Shibata, McGill Centre for Host Resistance and Department of Medicine, Montreal General Hospital Research Institute, Montreal, Quebec, Canada H3G 1A4 **[15]**

Howard R. Six, Department of Microbiology and Immunology, Baylor College of Medicine, Houston, TX 77030 **[229]**

T. Skripsky, Research and Development Laboratories, Pharmaceuticals Division, CIBA-GEIGY Limited, Basel, Switzerland **[191]**

Bernard W. Smith, Department of Medical Sciences, School of Veterinary Medicine, University of Wisconsin, Madison, WI 53706 **[117]**

Saburo Sone, Third Department of Internal Medicine, The University of Tokushima School of Medicine, Tokushima 770, Japan **[125]**

P.A. Steerenberg, Department of Pathology, National Institute of Public Health and Environmental Hygiene, 3720 BA Bilthoven, The Netherlands **[105]**

Deneen Stewart, Department of Microbiology and Immunology, The Medical College of Pennsylvania, Philadelphia, PA 19129 **[441]**

G. Storm, Department of Pharmaceutics, University of Utrecht, 3522 AD Utrecht, The Netherlands **[105]**

A. Sulkes, Departments of Oncology and Membrane Biochemistry, Hadassah Medical Center and Hebrew University, Hadassah Medical School, Jerusalem, Israel **[391]**

Glenn M. Swartz, Departments of Immunology and Membrane Biochemistry, Walter Reed Army Institute of Research, Washington, DC 20307-5100 **[167]**

Christine E. Swenson, The Liposome Company, Inc., Princeton, NJ 08540 **[205]**

Lloyd Tan, Medical Research Council Group, Academic Department of Medicine, Royal Free Hospital School of Medicine, London NW3 2QG, United Kingdom [35]

Janet R. Tatom, Departments of Clinical Immunology and Biological Therapy, M.D. Anderson Hospital and Tumor Institute, Houston, TX 77030 [329]

Joseph Treat, Division of Medical Oncology, Lombardi Cancer Research Center, Georgetown University Hospital, Washington, DC 20007 [353,367]

P. Trunet, CIBA-GEIGY Corp., Summit, NJ 07901; present address: CIBA-GEIGY Ltd., Basel, Switzerland [305]

P. van Hoogevest, Research and Development Laboratories, Pharmaceuticals Division, CIBA-GEIGY Limited, Basel, Switzerland [191,453]

Nico van Rooijen, Department of Histology, Free University, Amsterdam, The Netherlands [441]

J.C. Vink, Department of Clinical Microbiology, Erasmus University, 3000 DR Rotterdam, The Netherlands [275]

Alvin Volkman, Department of Pathology, East Carolina University School of Medicine, Greenville, NC 27858 [441]

Volkmar Weissig, Medical Research Council Group, Academic Department of Medicine, Royal Free Hospital School of Medicine, London NW3 2QG, United Kingdom [35]

Sam Z. Wilson, Department of Microbiology and Immunology, Baylor College of Medicine, Houston, TX 77030 [229]

Philip R. Wyde, Department of Microbiology and Immunology, Baylor College of Medicine, Houston, TX 77030 [229]

Qifu Xiao, Medical Research Council Group, Academic Department of Medicine, Royal Free Hospital School of Medicine, London NW3 2QG, United Kingdom [35]

Annie Yau-Young, Liposome Technology Inc., Menlo Park, CA 94025 [239]

Preface

The ability to target therapeutic agents selectively to different tissues has long been a goal in medicine. During the last few years, considerable attention has been focused on the use of synthetic phospholipid vesicles known as liposomes to accomplish this task. Recent clinical trials of liposomes that contain anticancer drugs, antifungal agents, or immunomodulators have carried these synthetic agents from laboratory concept to clinical reality.

To evaluate these new and exciting developments, a UCLA Colloquium, **Liposomes in the Therapy of Infectious Diseases and Cancer,** cosponsored by Ciba-Geigy, Ltd., and E.R. Squibb & Sons, was held at Lake Tahoe, California, February 16–20, 1988. The conference attracted basic researchers from academia and industry, as well as clinicians whose expertise spans a broad spectrum of medical specialties. The focus of the conference was on the development of the liposomal-drug carrier concept from physicochemistry to clinical application.

The volume is organized along the lines of the meeting. It begins with presentations about liposomes in immunobiology, proceeds to the clinical trials with liposomes in immunobiology, then to the clinical trials with liposomes as drug carriers, and ends with contributions on novel approaches in liposome development.

Considerable interest was generated by new biotechnological processes for the industrial scale-up and pharmaceutical development of liposomes. These new production techniques will have an enormous impact on availability of liposomes for general use and on commercialization of liposomal carriers.

The design of drug carrier-dependent drugs with optimal attributes of the drug and drug carrier was also discussed extensively and proved provocative. Several meeting participants examined the preclinical evaluation and development of liposomal drugs. It was the consensus that liposomal drugs be treated as new entities, in part because of the modified bioavailability and distribution of the entrapped drug.

Selective targeting of therapeutic agents to appropriate sites of action while avoiding the reticuloendothelial system is still a challenging and unresolved issue. New approaches to selective targeting as well as elaborate methods for prolonging drug availability and improving targeting to intracellular sites were presented. The design of liposome-dependent drugs also was discussed.

Phase I clinical trials with anti-infective liposomes, antineoplastic liposomes, and liposomal immunomodulators are underway in several centers. Although those studies are in an early stage of clinical development, some of the early reports are encouraging; it is these types of clinical data that encourage further development of liposomes as drug carriers.

Special thanks are due to Ciba-Geigy, Ltd., and E.R. Squibb & Sons for generous sponsorship of this meeting. We also acknowledge additional support from Liposome Technology, Inc., Smith Kline & French Laboratories, the Canadian Liposome Company, and Syntex Research. We wish to thank the UCLA Symposia staff for excellent organization.

G. Lopez-Berestein
Isaiah J. Fidler

I. LIPOSOMES IN IMMUNOBIOLOGY

Liposomes in the Therapy of Infectious Diseases and Cancer, pages 3–13
© **1989 Alan R. Liss, Inc.**

THE BIOLOGY OF CANCER METASTASIS AND ITS
CHANGE FOR THERAPY[1]

Isaiah J. Fidler, D.V.M., Ph.D.

University of Texas System Cancer Center
M. D. Anderson Hospital and Tumor Institute
Department of Cell Biology
Houston, Texas 77030

During the last decade, we have witnessed remarkable advances in surgical treatment of primary neoplasms and aggressive adjuvant therapies. Although these developments have increased the success rate for treatment of primary neoplasms, the lethality of most cancers can still be attributed to the propensity of cells from malignant neoplasms to disseminate from their primary site to distant organs and develop into metastases.

There are several reasons for the lack of success in eradication of metastases. First, by the time of diagnosis and initial treatment in the majority of patients with malignant tumor, excluding those with some skin cancers, metastasis has probably occurred (1). Second, many metastases are located in organs which are difficult to saturate with therapeutic agents sufficiently selective to destroy tumor cells and not also destroy normal host cells. The third and most formidable barrier to therapy of metastasis may well be the fact that cells populating a primary neoplasm, as well as those in various metastases, are not uniform, but are biologically heterogeneous.

This heterogeneity is exhibited in a wide range of genetic, biochemical, immunological and biological characteristics, such as cell surface receptors, enzymes, karyotypes, cell morphologies, growth properties, sensitivities to various therapeutic agents, and abilities to invade and produce metastasis (1-5). At present, metastases can not be detected before cellular diversification into heterogeneous cell subpopulations has occurred. Moreover,

---

[1] This work was supported in part by funds from the National Institutes of Health, National Cancer Institute, Grant R35-CA42107.

biological diversity can be generated rapidly in tumors that are either of unicellular or multicellular origin (1, 4). The evolvement of highly metastatic cells is sufficiently rapid to provide a mechanism for modulation escape from selection pressures, such as therapeutic agents.

The implications of tumor cell diversity for the outcome of treatment of cancer metastasis cannot be overemphasized. For example, by the time of clinical diagnosis, many metastases are fairly large. A lesion at the lower limit of detection by radiography could well measure 1 cm^3, and thus contain in excess of one billion cells. Even the remarkable 99.9% destruction of this lesion would leave one million cells to proliferate and provide a base population for generating new and diverse variants which are likely to be resistant to the modality used to destroy the majority of the tumor cells in the neoplasm (3, 6).

A heterogeneous disease cannot be treated by a homogeneous therapy, nor can we continue to treat cancer by empiricism. Understanding the mechanisms responsible for the process of cancer metastasis, for the origin of metastases, and for the development of biological heterogeneity in metastases should allow for rational design of more effective therapy for malignant disease and in the way physicians deal with cancer metastasis. This brief review concerns recent data that provide some answers to these difficult questions.

Biologic Heterogeneity of Malignant Neoplasms.

There is now overwhelming evidence that clinically apparent malignant neoplasms are heterogeneous. Cells obtained from individual tumors have been shown to differ with respect to all biologic characteristics important to the outcome of therapy, such as antigenicity or immunogenicity, growth rate, cell surface receptors, enzyme markers, hormone receptors, and sensitivity to cytotoxic drugs (1-6). Whether this heterogeneity of cells exists is not controversial; what has been controversial is whether neoplasms are also heterogeneous for metastatic properties. The first experimental proof of metastatic heterogeneity of neoplasms was provided by Fidler and Kripke in 1977 working with the murine B16 melanoma (7). Using the modified fluctuation assay of Luria and Delbruck (8), we showed that different tumor cell clones, each derived from an individual cell isolated from the parent tumor, varied dramatically in their ability to produce pulmonary nodules after intravenous inoculation into syngeneic recipient mice. Control subcloning procedures demonstrated that the observed diversity was not a consequence of the cloning procedure (7). The finding that preexisting tumor cell subpopulations proliferating in the same tumor exhibit heterogeneous metastatic potential has since been confirmed in many laboratories with a wide range of experimental animal tumors of different histories and histologic origins (Review 1-3). In addition, studies using young nude mice as models for metastasis of human neoplasms have shown that several human tumor lines and freshly isolated tumors such as colon carcinoma and renal carcinoma also contain subpopulations of cells with widely differing metastatic properties (9).

Selective Factors which Influence the Outcome of Metastasis.

To produce a metastasis, a tumor cell must complete a series of steps that are potentially lethal to the cells. The outcome of this process is therefore dependent on both the responses of the host and the intrinsic properties of the tumor cells (10-12). Metastasis begins with the detachment of tumor cells from the primary lesion. After they invade the blood vessels and/or the lymphatics, single tumor cells or multicell emboli circulate and eventually reach the capillary bed of distant organs, where they are arrested. After tumor cells extravasate into the organ parenchyma, they must proliferate in order to give rise to secondary lesions (10-12). Multiple metastases, even those within the same organ, often exhibit a diversity in their various biological properties, such as antigenicity, immunogenicity, hormone receptors, metastatic potential, or response to various chemotherapeutic agents (1-3). This diversity could result from the process of tumor progression-evolution or the nature of the metastatic process or both.

The pathogenesis of metastasis involves a series of steps that eliminate the majority of tumor cells. In other words, few cells survive the process of metastasis. In the B16 melanoma, less then 0.1% of circulating cells are the progenitors of metastatic lesions (13). This finding has prompted us to examine whether the process of metastasis is due to the chance survival of a few tumor cells or to the selective survival of preexisting metastatic cells (7).

Two distinct mechanisms are probably responsible for the death of most tumor emboli. To some extent, natural host immunity is able to destroy blood-borne malignant cells (14). However, nonspecific immunity by macrophages, natural killer cells, neutrophils, and specific immunity (15) by

cytotoxic T cells and antibodies, even under optimal circum-
stances, cannot account for the rapid destruction of almost
all circulating tumor cells. Instead, passive mechanical
processes such as turbulence probably are more likely to be
responsible.   Unlike blood cells, tumor cells are not
sufficiently deformable to survive the high shear forces
imposed on them by the microcirculation (16). The few cells
that do survive circulatory transport may do so because they
possess enhanced deformability (17) or form an embolus.

A circulating tumor cell can form an embolus by
attaching to other tumor cells (18) or by attaching to host
cells such as platelets (19) or lymphocytes (20). In either
case, tumor cells within the central zone of the embolus are
protected from the hostile environment of the vasculature by
the surrounding outer cells, thus gaining a potential
survival advantage. The ability of tumor cells to aggregate
is dependent upon their unique surface properties, and thus
this property can be a positive selective advantage in
metastases. However, whether a tumor cell is located on the
periphery of an embolus or in its central zone is probably
random.

Tumor cell entrapment in distant capillary beds can
occur by a nonspecific mechanical trapping caused by the
relatively large size of tumor emboli compared to individual
cells (21).   Alternatively, specific interactions between
the components of the embolus and the vascular lining
contribute to tumor cell arrest. For example, tumor cells
coated by platelets can adhere preferentially to the exposed
basement membrane of blood vessels. If the vascular
endothelium covering the basement membrane is intact in the
region where an embolus lodges, the tumor cells can extravasate from the circulation by invading the intercellular
junction between adjacent endothelial cells or by
penetrating the endothelial cell cytoplasm with tumor cell
pseudopodia (22). By secreting degradative enzymes in a
manner similar to that by which it originally gained access
to the circulation, tumor cells invade the basement membrane
into the parenchyma where the metastasis becomes established. Collectively, these data support the concept that
metastasis, as a whole, is a selective process, but also
contains stochastic elements (23).

Further evidence that the process of metastasis selects
for metastatic cells which preexist within the parental
neoplasm comes from data comparing cells populating
metastases with those in parental tumors. Most lines
derived from metastatic deposits produce significantly more
metastases than cells of the parent line. Studies with

heterogeneous, unselected neoplasms have therefore led us to conclude that metastasis is a highly selective process regulated by a number of different mechanisms. This is a more optimistic view in terms of cancer therapy than one that postulates that tumor dissemination is an entirely random event. Belief that certain rules govern the spread of neoplastic disease implies that understanding of these rules will lead to better therapeutic interventions.

The Origin of Cancer Metastasis

Multiple metastases are heterogeneous for a large number of different properties. In part, this may be due to whether metastases originate from the expansion of one (clonal) or more (polyclonal) cells.

To determine whether individual metastases are clonal in their origin and whether different metastases can be produced by different progenitor cells, Talmadge et al. (24) performed a series of experiments using the fact that x-irradiation of tumor cells induces random chromosome breaks and rearrangements. Analysis of the karyotype composition of different melanoma lung metastases revealed unique karyotypic patterns of abnormal, marker chromosomes in most of the lines established from solitary metastases. This finding suggested that each metastasis originated from a single and different progenitor cell. Similar results have been obtained in other rodent tumor systems using drug markers (25), cytogenetic analysis (26), unique insertion sites of plasmid vectors (27,28) and isoenzyme profile (29). All these studies with mouse melanomas, fibrosarcoma and different mammary carcinomas concluded that the majority of metastases are of clonal origin.

Taken together, these observations indicate that different metastases arise from different progenitor cells and account for the well-documented differences in behavior of different metastases. Among individual metastases of proved clonal origins, however, heterogeneity can develop rapidly to create significant intralesional heterogeneity (6,30).

Role of the Organ Environment in the Pathogenesis of Metastasis

Clinical observations of cancer patients and studies with experimental rodent tumors show that some tumors have a marked preference for metastasis to specific organs independent of vascular anatomy, rate of blood flow, and number of tumor cells delivered to these organs (1). While the frequent occurrence of metastases in the liver from carcinomas arising in the gastrointestinal tract can be readily explained as cells draining into the portal venous system and arresting in the first capillary bed, the frequent dissemination of lung bronchial carcinoma to the cerebellum and adrenal glands cannot be explained in terms of vascular anatomy alone.

The search for the mechanisms that regulate the pattern of metastasis began a long time ago. In 1889, Paget questioned whether the distribution of metastases was due to chance and therefore analyzed 735 autopsy records of women with breast cancer (3). The nonrandom pattern of visceral metastases suggested to Paget that the process was not due to chance but, rather, that certain tumor cells (the "seed") had a specific affinity for the milieu provided by certain organs (the "soil"). Metastases resulted only when the seed and soil were matched (31). These observations, and those from case histories of other cancers (1), pose the question of whether the normal organs differ in their ability to support, or conversely suppress, the growth of cancer metastases.

Recent studies provide direct evidence for the validity of the "seed and soil" hypothesis. The introduction of peritoneovenous shunts for palliation of malignant ascites has provided an opportunity to study some of the factors affecting metastatic spread in humans. Tarin and colleagues (32, 33) described the outcome of ascitic fluids of patients with malignant ascites draining into the circulation, with the resulting entry of viable tumor cells into the jugular veins. Good palliation with minimal complications was reported for 29 patients with different neoplasms. The autopsy findings in 15 patients substantiated the clinical observations that the shunts do not increase the risk of metastasis. In fact, despite the continuous entry into the circulation of millions of tumor cells, metastases in the lung (the first capillary bed encountered) were rare (33). In eight of the patients, small metastases were found in extra-abdominal organs, and in seven, no evidence of metastasis was found (33). These results suggested that even though the tumor cells were spread systemically in the circulation, micrometastases formed only in some organs or not at all.

Challenges for Therapy of Cancer Metastases

Two main areas where the biologic heterogeneity of metastases is likely to prove of practical importance are in the detection of tumor deposits using cell-produced markers and in therapeutic regimens other than surgical resection. We have recently determined whether the expression of 40 isozymes by tumor cells was heterogeneous among 56 cell lines, from nine different murine and human tumors (34). We set out to determine whether the expression of one or another isozyme correlated with metastatic potential of tumor cells. The enzymes chosen for study are involved in nucleotide, carbohydrate, and pentose phosphate metabolism, and as such are indicators of the general metabolic and differentiative status of the cell. Different patterns of isozyme expression were observed among different tumor types as well as between tumors of the same type; however, there were no differences in isozyme expression for any enzyme tested that correlated with metastatic ability of tumor cells. Findings such as these cast doubt on the feasibility of using any one product of tumor cells in which diversity in synthesis and/or secretion occurs for the quantitation of disseminated disease.

Similar difficulties exist with the use of monoclonal antibodies directed against one or another antigen specific to a particular tumor. The antigenic heterogeneity of cancer cells is well documented (35-37). Even within one organ, different metastases can exhibit intra- and interlesional antigenic heterogeneity (35, 36).

Equally important, the existence of heterogeneous subpopulations of cells within neoplasms presents a dilemma for the therapist. The emergence of drug-resistant variants during or subsequent to chemotherapy has been documented extensively in the clinical literature, and differences in the response of primary and metastatic tumors to therapeutic agents are also well documented (38-39). These differences may be exacerbated by the anatomic location of the secondary tumor deposits, since it is not an infrequent finding that metastases in one organ are susceptible to chemotherapy, whereas metastases in other organs are resistant (1-3). The obstacle to therapy that heterogeneity imposes upon treatment modalities can also affect the likelihood of success of immunotherapy.

The cure of metastasis requires the total destruction of all tumor cells. Anything short of that can produce only long-term remissions. For example, if a therapeutic modality can eradicate as many as 99.9% of a 1 cubic centimeter tumor, 10^6 cells remain to undergo rapid proliferation and diversification.

As stated previously, a multifactorial disease cannot be treated by a single modality. Cancer is a collection of heterogeneous diseases. The successful therapy of cancer metastasis requires combined modalities which include an approach to circumvent the problems of neoplastic hetero-geneity and the development of resistance to therapy by tumor cells.

This realization has stimulated us to examine the possibility that appropriately activated macrophages can fulfill these demanding criteria. Macrophages can be activated to become tumoricidal by interaction with phospholipid vesicles (liposomes) containing various immunomodulators (40). Tumoricidal macrophages can recognize and destroy neoplastic cells in vitro and in vivo, while leaving non-neoplastic tumorigenic and normal cells unharmed. Although the exact mechanism(s) by which macrophages discriminate between tumorigenic and normal cells is unknown, it is independent of tumor cell character-istics, such as immunogenicity, metastatic potential, and sensitivity to cytotoxic drugs. Moreover, macrophage destruction of tumor cells apparently is not associated with the development of tumor cell resistance. Intravenously administered liposomes are cleared from the circulation by phagocytic macrophages in situ, and the multiple administrations of such liposomes have been shown to bring about eradication of cancer metastases. Macrophage destruction of metastases in vivo is significant, provided that the total tumor burden at start of treatment is small. For this reason, we have been investigating various methods to reduce the tumor burden in metastases by modalities such as chemotherapy or radiotherapy. The ability of tumoricidal macrophages to distinguish neoplastic from bystander non-neoplastic cells presents an attractive possibility for treatment of these few tumor cells which escape destruction by conventional therapeutics (41).

REFERENCES

1. Fidler IJ, Balch CM (1987). The biology of cancer metastasis and implications for therapy. Curr Probl Surg 24:137.
2. Fidler IJ, Hart IR (1982). Biological diversity in metastatic neoplasms: Origins and implications. Science 217:998.

3. Fidler IJ, Poste G (1985). The cellular heterogeneity of malignant neoplasms: Implications for adjuvant chemotherapy. Semin Oncol 12:207.

4. Nicolson GL (1984). Generation of phenotypic diversity and progression in metastatic tumors. Cancer Metastasis Rev 3:25.

5. Nicolson GL, Poste G (1982). Tumor cell diversity and host responses in cancer metastasis. I. Properties of metastatic cell. Curr Probl Cancer 6:4.

6. Poste G (1986). Pathogenesis of metastatic disease: Implications for current therapy and for the development of new therapeutic strategies. Cancer Treat Rep 70:1223.

7. Fidler IJ, Kripke M (1977). Metastasis results from pre-existing variant cells within a malignant tumor. Science 197:893.

8. Luria SE, Delbruck M (1943). Mutations of bacteria from virus sensitivity to virus resistance. Genetics 28:491.

9. Fidler IJ (1986). Rationale and methods for the use of nude mice to study the biology and therapy of human cancer metastasis. Cancer Metastasis Rev, 5:29.

10. Poste G, Fidler IJ (1979). The pathogenesis of cancer metastasis. Nature 283:139.

11. Weiss L (1985). "Principles of metastasis." Orlando: Academic Press.

12. Talmadge JE, Fidler IJ (1982). Cancer metastasis is selective or random depending on the parent tumor population. Nature 27:593.

13. Fidler IJ (1970). Metastasis: Quantitative analysis of distribution and fate of tumor emboli labeled with ^{125}I-5-iodo-2'-deoxyuridine. JNCI 45:773.

14. Hanna N (1982). Role of natural killer cells in control of cancer metastasis. Cancer Metastasis Rev 1:45.

15. Fidler IJ, Kripke ML (1980). Tumor cell antigenicity, host immunity and cancer metastasis. Cancer Immunol Immunother 7:201.

16. Weiss L, Dimitrov DS (1986). Mechanical aspects of the lungs as cancer cell-killing organs during hematogenous metastasis. J Theor Biol 121:307.

17. Waller CA, Braun M, Schirrmacher V (1986). Quantitative analysis of cancer invasion in vitro: Comparison of two new assays and of tumor sublines with different metastatic capacity. Clin Exp Metastasis 2:78.

18. Nicolson GL (1982). Organ colonization and the cell surface properties of malignant cells. Biochim Biophys Acta 695:113.

19. Gasic GJ (1984).   Role of plasma, platelets, and endothelial cells in tumor metastasis.   Cancer Metastasis Rev 3:99.
20. Fidler IJ, Bucana C (1977).   Mechanism of tumor cell resistance to lysis by syngeneic lymphocytes.   Cancer Res 37:3945.
21. Fidler IJ (1973).   The relationship of embolic homogeneity, number, size, and viability to the incidence of experimental metastasis.   Eur J Cancer 9:223.
22. Nicolson GL (1982).   Metastatic tumor cell attachment and invasion assay utilizing vascular endothelial cell monolayer. J Histochem Cytochem 30:214.
23. Price JE, Aukerman SL, Fidler IJ (1986).   Evidence that the process of murine melanoma metastases is sequential and selective and contains stochastic elements. Cancer Res 46:5172.
24. Talmadge JE, Wolman SR, Fidler IJ (1982).   Evidence for the clonal origin of spontaneous metastasis.   Science 217:361.
25. Poste G, Tzeng J, Doll J, Greig JR (1982).   Evolution of tumor cell heterogeneity during progressive growth of individual lung metastases.   Proc Natl Acad Sci USA 79:6574.
26. Hu F, Wang RY, Hsu TC (1987).   Clonal origin of metastasis in B-16 murine melanoma: A cytogenetic study. JNCI 78:155.
27. Talmadge JE, Zbar B (1987).   Clonality of pulmonary metastases from the bladder 6 subline of the B16 melanoma studied by Southern hybridization.   JNCI 78:315.
28. Kerbel RS, Waghorne C, Man MS, Elliot B, Breitman ML (1987).   Alteration of the tumorigenic and metastatic properties of neoplastic cells is associated with the process of calcium phosphate-mediated DNA transfection. Proc Natl Acad Sci USA 84:1263.
29. Ootsuyama A, Tanaka K, Tanooka H (1987).   Evidence by cellular mosaicism for monoclonal metastasis of spontaneous mouse mammary tumors. JNCI 78:1223.
30. Talmadge JE, Benedict K, Madsen J, Fidler IJ (1984). Development of biological diversity and susceptibility to chemotherapy in murine cancer metastases. Cancer Res 44:3801.
31. Paget S (1889).   The distribution of secondary growths in cancer of the breast. Lancet, 1:571.
32. Tarin D, Price JE, Kettlewell MGW, Souter RG, Vass ACR, Crossley B (1984). Mechanisms of human tumor metastasis

studied in patients with peritoneovenous shunts. Cancer Res 44:3584.
33. Souter RG, Tarin D, Kettlewell MGW (1983). Peritoneovenous shunts in the management of malignant ascites. Br J Surg 70:478.
34. Aukerman SL, Siciliano MJ, Fidler IJ (1986). Heterogeneity of isozyme expression in tumor cells does not correlate with metastatic potential. Clin Exp Metastasis 4:177.
35. Miller FR (1982). Intratumor immunologic heterogeneity. Cancer Metastasis Rev 1:319.
36. Kerbel RS (1979). Implications of immunological heterogeneity of tumors. Nature 280:358.
37. Albino AP, Lloyd KO, Houghton AN, Oettgen HF, Old LJ (1981). Heterogeneity in surface antigen and glycoprotein expression of cell lines derived from different melanoma metastases of the same patient. J Exp Med 154:1764.
38. Tsuruo T, Fidler IJ (1981). Differences in drug sensitivity among tumor cells from parental tumors, selected variants, and spontaneous metastases. Cancer Res 41:3058.
39. Fugman RA, Anderson JC, Stoli R, Martin DS (1977). Comparison of adjuvant chemotherapeutic activity against primary and metastatic spontaneous murine tumors. Cancer Res 37:496.
40. Fidler IJ, Poste G (1982). Macrophage-mediated destruction of malignant tumor cells and new strategies for the therapy of metastatic disease. Springer Semin Immunopathol 5:161.
41. Fidler IJ (1985). Macrophages and metastasis: A biological approach to cancer therapy. Cancer Res 45:4714.

Liposomes in the Therapy of Infectious Diseases and Cancer, pages 15–24
© 1989 Alan R. Liss, Inc.

EXPERIMENTAL AND CLINICAL EVALUATION OF LIPOSOME-TUMOR ANTIGEN IMMUNOTHERAPY[1]

Nigel C. Phillips, Antoine Loutfi[2], Majeed Kareem[2], Henry Shibata and Malcolm Baines[3]

McGill Centre for Host Resistance and Department of Medicine, Montreal General Hospital Research Institute, Montreal, Quebec, Canada H3G 1A4

ABSTRACT   The results of active-specific immunotherapy using autologous tumor-associated antigens (TAA) incorporated within liposomal carriers has been evaluated in an experimental model of melanoma and in a phase I study in patients with metastatic malignant melanoma. Immunization of mice with liposomes containing melanoma TAA gave significant protection against subsequent tumor cell challenge, especially when a synthetic immunoadjuvant - MDP-GDP - was incorporated within the liposomal carrier. Irradiated tumor cells or free antigen were ineffective. Ten patients were entered on a phase I study and given sc injections of liposome-TAA preparations at 2-4 week intervals. Clinical monitoring did not reveal any short or long-term systemic or local toxicity. Two patients had a mixed response, one patient had a partial response and one patient remains stable. The remaining 6 patients had no response with disease progression. The TAA preparation stimulated peripheral blood lymphocyte proliferation (PBL) in vitro in patients exhibiting a clinical response: no responses were observed in the non-responder patients. NK activity did not correlate with PBL proliferation or clinical response status. Liposomal immunotherapy appears to be a feasible candidate for a much larger phase I/II study.

---

[1]This work was supported in part by the Cancer Research Society Inc., Montreal, Canada.
[2]Department of Surgery, McGill University
[3]Department of Microbiology and Immunology, McGill University

INTRODUCTION

Early surgery is the only effective method of treating malignant melanoma in man. The need for an effective treatment is compelling because of the rapidly increasing incidence and poor prognosis associated with currently available treatments (1). The progression of melanoma is influenced by two factors: the intrinsic malignant potential of the tumor cells and the immunological response of the host (2,3). The latter has encouraged many investigators to explore immunotherapy as a treatment modality using specific or non-specific immunizations (2,4-6). Specific-active immunization with melanoma cells or tumor-associated antigens (TAA) has given positive results in animal studies (7,8) and in clinical trials (9-11).

The extraction of TAA's using n-butanol results in preparations which do not possess allogeneic activity and which are not contaminated with cytoplasmic or transmembrane components (12). These antigens are capable of inducing prophylactic immunity against subsequent tumor cell challenge in animal models (13). n-Butanol-extracted TAA's have also been isolated from human malignant melanoma (14) and other human tumors (15,16).

Liposomes, small phospholipid vesicles, possess immunoadjuvant activity (17). Their immunoadjuvanticity may be due in part to their ability to stimulate T-helper lymphocyte activity (18). It has also been shown that liposomes containing n-butanol-extracted TAA's are therapeutically active in increasing long-term survivors after resection of the primary tumor in a metastatic rat colon cancer model (19). Liposomes have been extensively used to target immunomodulators to the reticuloendothelial system, leading to the eradication of metastases in animal models (20-23) via macrophage activation (24). Liposomes are taken up by the lymphatic system after sc administration (25): the potential for a sustained and directed delivery of liposome-TAA to sites of antigen processing and presentation (ie, the lymph node) is particularly attractive and relatively unexplored as a treatment for cancer.

The above considerations led us to conduct experimental and phase I clinical studies of sc administered liposomes containing autologous TAA's in an animal model of melanoma and in patients with metastatic malignant melanoma.

MATERIALS AND METHODS

Tumor-Associated Antigen Preparations

TAA's were made from B16-BL6 melanoma tumor cells in
culture or from freshly excised tumor samples. Single cell
preparations were resuspended in PBS containing 3% v/v n-
butanol (10 ml/gm tissue). After 4-5 min incubation at room
temperature, the cell suspension was centrifuged at 1000 x g
for 15 min at 4°C, and the supernatant collected. The
supernatant was dialysed against 5 x 1000 ml PBS, filtered
(0.2 u) and stored in aliquots at -30°C. All manipulations
were carried out with sterile, pyrogen-free materials and
equipment.

Liposomal Tumor-Antigen Preparation

DPPC (30-120 mg) and DMPG (5-20 mg) in 5 ml chloroform
were placed in 250 ml round-bottomed flasks and rotary-
evaporated to dryness under vacuum at 50°C. One to 2 ml TAA
was added to the flask, and the lipid layer allowed to
hydrate for 30 min at room temperature. Liposomes were
prepared by agitation of the flask at 45°C followed by
standing at room temperature for a further 30 min. The
liposomes were washed by centrifugation at 12,000 x g for 15
min at 4°C to eliminate unincorporated material. The final
pellet was resuspended in 1.0 ml 0.9% saline.

Experimental Studies.

Male C57BL/6 mice were immunized with 2 injections of 5
x 10^6 irradiated (18,000 rad) tumor cells, 40 ug TAA or 1
injection of 0.1 ug TAA incorporated within liposomes
followed by a boost with 40 ug TAA on days 0 and +21. The
mice were challenged with a lethal inoculum of 5 x 10^5 tumor
cells sc on day +28, and tumor size and survival monitored
at daily intervals.

Clinical Studies.

Patient selection and follow-up. Ten patients with
histologically confirmed advanced malignant melanoma (stage

III, WHO classification) were entered into the study. All patients had an ECOG performance status of 2 or less (0 or 1) on entry. Immunotherapy or chemotherapy had been stopped at least 2 months prior to entry. All patients were monitored regularly by physical examination, hematological profile, liver and renal function tests, and radiological examination when necessary. Liposomal TAA preparations were given sc every 2-4 weeks, with a starting dose of 35 mg phospholipid and dose escalation (50%) every 4 weeks.

NK activity. NK activity of PBL was determined as previously described (26) using [^{51}Cr]-labeled K562 or Raji tumor cells and a lymphocyte:tumor ratio of 20:1.

Mitogen responsiveness. Ficoll-Paque purified PBL's (5 x 10^5 cells in 200 ul) in RPMI 1640 medium containing 5% heat-inactivated fetal calf serum were placed in the wells of microtiter plates. Concanavalin A (4 ug/ml final concentration) or TAA (2-10 ug) were added to the cells, and incubation was carried out for 72 hr at 37°C / 5% CO$_2$. [^{3}H]-thymidine (0.1 uCi) was added to the cultures for the last 18 hr of incubation. The cells were harvested, and radioactivity determined in a beta-counter.

Tumor stasis activity. HTB-71 human melanoma tumor cell line (American Type Culture Collection, Rockville, Md) was maintained in monolayer culture using MEM with Earle's salts containing 10% heat-inactivated fetal calf serum, non-essential amino acids, pyruvate, glutamine and vitamins (MEM-FCS). PBL's in MEM-FCS (1 x 10^5) were added to adherent tumor cells (5 x 10^3) in the wells of microtiter plates in a final volume of 200 ul, and incubated for 72 hr. A minimum of 6 replicates was carried out for each determination. [^{3}H]-thymidine (0.1 uCi) was added for the last 18 hr of culture, after which the nonadherent lymphocytes were removed by washing with warm MEM-FCS. The adherent tumor cells were lysed by the addition of 200 ul of 0.5 M NaOH, and the radioactivity determined in a beta-counter. Tumor stasis was calculated using the equation:

$$\frac{[CPM\ tumor\ cells] - [CPM\ tumor\ cells + lymphocytes]}{[CPM\ tumor\ cells]} \times 100$$

RESULTS

Experimental studies.
    Immunization of C57BL/6 mice with irradiated tumor
cells, TAA or control liposomes failed to affect the growth
of sc tumors or increase survival time when compared to
non-immunized mice. Immunization with liposomes containing
TAA resulted in a significant decrease in tumor growth rate
and a significant increase in the number of survivors. This
was especially true for the liposomal antigen preparation
containing the synthetic immunoadjuvant MDP-GDP (Table 1).

TABLE 1

IMMUNIZATION OF C57/BL6 MICE WITH B16 MELANOMA TAA

Immunization	Tumor diameter, mm Mean ± SD (n=15)	% Survival at 6 weeks
Control	14.8 ± 2.4	0
Tumor cells	15.9 ± 3.3	0
Antigen 40 ug	14.1 ± 3.1	0
Liposomal antigen 0.1 ug	10.1 ± 2.1[a]	27[b]
Liposomal antigen containing 10 ug MDP-GDP	5.2 ± 2.8[a]	60[b]

[a]Significantly different from control immunization
(Student's t-test for unpaired data, $p < 0.05$).
[b]Significantly different from control immunization (Chi^2
with Yate's correction, $p < 0.05$).

Phase I Clinical Trial

    Tolerance. No local or systemic reactions were noted in
any of the ten patients (follow-up 9-66 weeks). Monitoring
of hematological and biochemical parameters revealed no
evidence of systemic toxicity.
    Responses. Of the ten patients, one had a partial
response, 2 had mixed responses, and one had disease
stabilization (Table 2). The remaining 6 patients showed no
evidence of response and continued to have progressive
disease.
    PBL proliferative responses. Significant enhancement of
the ability of the TAA preparations to stimulate PBL
proliferation in vitro occurred in those patients showing
clinical stabilization or reduction in tumor mass. No
proliferative responses to autologous TAA's were seen in
those patients who did not respond to the liposomal TAA
therapy (Table 3).

TABLE 2

PATIENT CHARACTERISTICS AND SUMMARY OF THERAPY

No.	Age/sex	Metastatic distribution[a]	Injections	Period (weeks)	Response
1.	42 M	Sc, Li, Lu, Sb	3	11	Mixed
2.	66 M	Sc, Li, Lu, B[c]	3	36	None
3.	52 F[b]	Sc	20	64	Partial
4.	22 M	Sc, Lu	4	14	None
5.	36 F	Sc, Sk Lu, B[c]	7	32	Mixed
6.	61 M	Sc, Li, Lu[c]	6	27	None
7.	66 F[b]	Sc	15	44	Stable
8.	46 M	Sc, Li, Lu	3	12	None
9.	34 F	Sc, Sk, Rp	4	9	None
10.	42 F	Sc, Lu[c]	4	15	None

[a]B, bone; Li, liver; Lu, lung, Rp, retroperitoneum; Sb, small bowel; Sc, subcutaneous; Sk, skin.
[b]Alive.
[c]Brain metastasis developed during treatment.

NK activity. All patients with normal NK activity before entry showed a progressive decrease in activity during the course of therapy. This group included patients 1, 3 and 7. The second group had a low initial activity and had variable (but still low) activity at the end of therapy.

TABLE 3

PBL RESPONSES AGAINST AUTOLOGOUS TAA

Patient	Stimulation index[a]	
	Pre-immunization	Maximal post-immunization
1	1.0	15.1 CR[c]
3	1.0	16.8[b] CR
4	1.5	1.6
5	1.0	11.8 CR
6	1.0	1.9
7	1.0	15.0[b] S
2, 8-10	1.0	1.0

[a]Stimulation index is proliferative response in the

presence of TAA's divided by the control proliferative
response.
[b]Alive.
[c]CR, clinical response; S, stable

   Tumor _cell_ _stasis_. PBL's from patients 1,3,5 and 7
demonstrated an enhanced ability to inhibit the growth of a
human melanoma tumor cell line during the course of the
therapy. All the other patients (clinical non-responders)
demonstrated a decline in their ability to inhibit tumor
cell growth (Table 4).
   Immunological _function._ A common characteristic in
those patients who failed to respond to liposomal TAA
therapy was the development of anergy. Six out of 10
patients became unresponsiveness to common recall antigens,
showed diminished T-cell responses (as demonstrated by
Concanavalin A mitogenesis) and falling NK activity.
   Dose _Responsiveness._ Objective clinical responses were
obtained using a liposome dose of 52.5 mg. The maximal
tolerated dose has yet to be reached. This phase I trial
indicates that doses in excess of 150 mg phospholipid are
well tolerated.

TABLE 4
TUMOR STASIS ACTIVITY OF PBL's

Patient	Tumor stasis activity (% inhibition)[a]	
	Pre-immunization	Maximal post-immunization[b]
1	5.0	78.8 CR[c]
2	45.2	7.7
3	51.1	85.9 CR
4	70.0	44.8
5	11.3	26.6 CR
6	94.1	42.8
7	55.0	84.2 S
8	43.0	26.7
9	29.3	7.0
10	12.6	3.5

[a]Activity determined at an effector:target ratio of 20:1.
[b]Maximal inhibition observed during immunization.
[c]CR, clinical response; S, stable.

DISCUSSION

The reality of obtaining sufficient autologous tumor-associated antigenic material for the evaluation of immunization procedures is perhaps the major challenge facing immunotherapeutic intervention. In addition, such intervention in those cancers where there is no well defined or readily available tumor antigen will require the formulation and exploitation of procedures designed to maximize any impact on the immune system (27)

The experimental data obtained with the B16 melanoma clearly shows that liposomal administration of TAA results in a significant degree of protection against subsequent tumor cell challenge. That the incorporation of an adjuvant-active muramyl dipeptide derivative within such liposomes results in enhanced protective activity compared with liposomes alone suggests that liposomal TAA alone may not be an optimal formulation.

Our data obtained from this phase I clinical trial indicates that the sc administration of liposomes containing autologous tumor-antigen preparations does not result in any acute or chronic toxicity. The clinical and immunological responses (PBL proliferation to TAA's, tumor stasis activity) observed in 4/10 patients indicates that liposomal tumor antigen therapy may be of use in an immunoadjuvant setting. These responses are encouraging, and indicate a stimulated anti-tumor immunity in those patients showing a clinical response. The deterioration of NK activity in those patients showing clinical responses suggests that immunotherapy using liposomal encapsulated TAA's occurs independently of such cytotoxic activity. These observations will, however, have to be confirmed with a larger population group. That immunotherapy will have minimal impact against metastatic diseases with a high tumor bulk has been demonstrated in animal studies and clinical trials (2).

This study has clearly demonstrated that the sc administration of liposomes containing TAA's is safe and feasible. The observation that some clinical responsiveness can be obtained in patients with significant tumor burdens is of considerable interest, and indicates that such liposome preparations can be used in an immunoadjuvant setting for the treatment of malignant melanoma.

REFERENCES

1. Seegar J, Richman SP, Allegra JC (1986). Systemic therapy of malignant melanoma. Med Clin North Amer 70:89.
2. Bystryn J-C (1985). Immunology and immunotherapy of human malignant melanoma. Derm Clin 3:327.
3. Carey TE (1982). Immunological aspects of melanoma. Crit Rev Clin Lab Sci 18:141.
4. Creagen ET, Cupps RE, Ivins JC et al (1978). Adjuvant radiation therapy for regional nodal metastasis from malignant melanoma. A randomized, prospective study. Cancer 42:2206.
5. Morten DL, Goodnight JE, Jr (1978). Clinical trials of immunotherapy. Present status. Cancer 42:2224.
6. Seigler MD, Cox E, Mutzner F, et al (1979). Specific active immunotherapy for melanoma. Ann Surg 190:366.
7. Bystryn J-C (1978). Antibody response and tumor growth in syngeneic mice immunized to partially purified B16 melanoma-associated antigen. J Immunol 120:96.
8. Avent J, Vervaert C, Siegler HF (1979). Nonspecific and specific active immunotherapy in a B16 melanoma system. J Surg Oncol 12:87.
9. Hollinshead A, Arlen M, Yonemoto R, et al (1982). Pilot study using melanoma tumor-associated antigens (TAA) in specific-active immunotherapy of malignant melanoma. Cancer 49:1387.
10. Cassel WA, Murray DR, Phillips HS (1983). A phase II study on the postsurgical management of stage II melanoma with a Newcastle disease virus oncolysate. Cancer 52:856.
11. Humphrey LJ, Taschler-Collins S, Goldfarb PM, et al (1984). Adjuvant immunotherapy for melanoma. J Surg Oncol 25:303.
12. Legrue SJ, Allison JP, Macek CM, et al (1981). Immunobiological properties of 1-butanol-extracted cell surface antigens. Cancer Res 41: 3956.
13. Legrue SJ (1985). Noncytolytic extraction of cell surface antigen using butanol. Cancer and Metastasis Rev 4:209.
14. Liao SK, Smith JW, Kwong PC (1984). Selective extraction by 1-butanol of surface glycoprotein antigens from human melanoma cells. Cancer Immunol Immunother 17:95.
15. Roth JA, Wesley RA (1982). Human tumor-associated antigens detected by serological techniques: analysis of

autologous humoral immune responses to primary and
metastatic human sarcomas by an enzyme-linked
immunoabsorbant solid phase asay (ELISA). Cancer Res
42:3978.
16. Legrue SJ, Rustky LR, Kahan BD (1980). Noncytolytic
extraction of cell surface antigens. In vitro 16:208.
17. Allison AC, Gregoriadis G (1974). Liposomes as
immunological adjuvants. Nature 252:252.
18. Beatty DV, Beatty BG, Paraskevas F, et al (1984).
Liposomes as immune adjuvants: T cell dependence.
Surgery 96:345.
19. Steele G, Ravikumar T, Ross D, et al (1984). Specific
active immunotherapy with butanol-extracted, tumor-
associated antigens incorporated into liposomes.
Surgery 96:352.
20. Fidler IJ (1980). Therapy of spontaneous metastasis by
intravenous injection of liposomes
containing lymphokine. Science 208:1469.
21. Fidler IJ, Sone S, Fogler WE, Barnes ZL (1981).
Eradication of spontaneous metastasis and activation of
alveolar macrophages by intravenous injection of
liposomes containing muramyl dipeptide. Proc Natl Acad
Sci USA 78:1680.
22. Phillips NC, Moras ML, Chedid L, Lefrancier P, et al
(1985). Activation of alveolar macrophage tumoricidal
activity and eradication of experimental metastases by
freeze-dried liposomes containing a new lipophilic
muramyl dipeptide. Cancer Res 45:128.
23. Phillips NC, Chedid L, Bernard JM, et al (1987).
Induction of murine macrophage tumoricidal activity and
treatment of experimental metastases by liposomes
containing lipophilic muramyl dipeptide analogs. J Biol
Resp Modif 6:678.
24. Deodhar SD, Barna BP (1986). Macrophage activation:
Potential for cancer therapy. Clev Clin Q 53:223
25. Perez-Soler R, Lopez-Berestein G, Johns M, et al (1985).
Distribution of radio-labelled multilamellar liposomes
injected intralymphatically and subcutaneously. Int J
Nucl Med Biol 12:261.
26. Pross HF, Baines MG, Rubin P, et al (1981). Spontaneous
human lymphocyte mediated cytotoxicity against tumor
target cells. IX. The quantitation of natural killer
cell activity. J Clin Immunol 1:51.
27. Phillips NC, Major PP, Sikorska H (1988). Tumor-
associated antigens as immunotherapy targets. Cancer
Detect Prevent (in press).

Liposomes in the Therapy of Infectious Diseases and Cancer, pages 25–34
© **1989 Alan R. Liss, Inc.**

pH-SENSITIVE AND TARGET SENSITIVE IMMUNOLIPOSOMES
FOR DRUG TARGETING

Eric G. Holmberg and Leaf Huang

Department of Biochemistry, University of Tennessee
Knoxville, Tennessee 37996-0840

ABSTRACT   We have designed pH-sensitive and target-
sensitive immunoliposomes, taking advantage of the
polymorphic structure of phosphatidylethanolamine (PE).
Unsaturated PE by itself forms hexagonal (H_{II})
physiologic conditions, but the bilayer phase of PE can
be stablized by the addition of a second lipid or an
amphipathic protein (1). pH-sensitive liposomes were
prepared by using a weakly acidic amphiphile such as
fatty acid or fatty acyl amino acid as a bilayer
stablizer. These liposomes, bearing monoclonal
antibody for target cell specificity, rapidly
destablize and become fusion competent when they
encounter the acidic environment of the endosome, after
endocytosis by the target cell. Enhanced cytoplasmic
delivery by these liposomes was demonstrated for
antitumor drugs (cytosine arabinoside and methotrexate)
(2), toxin (diptheria toxin, fragment A) (3), and
plasmid DNA (4). Futhermore, we have used an athymic
nude mouse model to test the target-specific delivery
of a foreign gene in vivo (4). These liposomes are
very promising as an effective delivery system. The
target-sensitive immunoliposome is a drug delivery
vehicle which is independent of cellular endocytosis.
The bilayer phase of PE is directly stablized with
fatty acylated antibody. These immunoliposomes rapidly
lyse (few min.) at the cell surface when they bind to
the cell surface antigen (5). Since drugs can be
entrapped in these liposomes at high concentrations,
significant drug uptake by the target cells, but not by
the control cells, can be readily achieved. We have
used mouse L-929 cells infected with Herpes Simplex
Virus as a model system and demonstrated superior

efficacy and greatly reduced toxicity with cytosine
arabinoside and acylovir (6). Work supported by NIH
grant CA24553 and a contract from LipoGen, Inc.

INTRODUCTION

     Encapsulation of therapeutic pharmaceutical products by
a targetable vehicle will greatly increase the efficiency,
while reducing many of the adverse side effects, of drug
therapy. The natural occurence of the components of a
liposome make it an ideal candidate for drug encapsulation
and targeting. We have designed two types of lipososmes for
a potential drug delivery system. Both types of liposomes
take advantage of the polymorphic properties of
phosphatidylethanolamine (PE) in that unsaturated PE, by
itself, forms a hexagonal phase (H_{II}) at physiological
conditions, but a shift from H_{II} phase to bilayer phase
occurs with the addition of a second lipid or amphipathic
protein.(1) These liposomes also contain a fatty acylated
antibody or target ligand that makes them cell specific.
The first type of liposome is the pH-sensitive liposome.
These liposomes are stablized by a fatty acid or fatty acyl
amino acid. Upon protonation in the low pH prelysosomal
compartment they become fusion competent and destabilize,
thereby, delivering their contents prior to lysosomal
degradation. A variety of antitumor drugs (2), toxin (3),
and plasmid DNA (4) have been successfully delivered to
target cells using pH-sensitive liposomes developed in our
lab. Furthermore, a foreign gene, chloramphenicol
acetyltransferase (CAT) from Escherichia Coli, has been
specifically targeted and expressed in the tumor cells in an
athymic nude mouse model (4). The second type of liposome is
the target-sensitive immunoliposome. These liposomes are
stabilized directly by the acylated monoclonal antibody
rather than the fatty acid or fatty acyl amino acid present
in the pH-sensitive liposome. The binding event between the
acylated antibody and the cell surface antigen causes a
destabilization in the PE bilayer; subsequent disruption of
the liposome bilayer causes its contents to be released at
the target cell surface. We have delivered cytosine
arabinoside and acyclovir to mouse L-929 cells infected with
Herpes Simplex Virus with greatly enhanced efficacy and
reduced toxicity (6).
     In this review we will discuss the development of the
pH-sensitive and target-sensitive immunoliposome in our lab
while focusing on the rapidly developing field of DNA
delivery as it relates to pH-sensitive immunoliposomes.

pH- AND TARGET-SENSITIVE LIPOSOMES

A major obstacle that exists with the encapsulation of drugs in liposomes is the prevention of degradation of the liposomal contents by the cellular lysosomes after delivery to the cell. Specific targeting of the liposome has been successfully demonstrated by the addition of a covalently attatched monoclonal antibody to the liposome, an immunoliposome (7). These immunoliposomes are taken up via a mechanism of receptor mediated endocytosis and become products of cellular degradation in the lysosomes. In such a case, only drugs that are spared of this degradation may be delivered to the cellular cytoplasm. Delivery of methotrexate using immunoliposomes has been shown to be effective in cultured cells but cytosine arabinoside, ara-C, and plasmid DNA containing immunoliposomes have been shown to be ineffective (2,4). In order to circumvent the cellular lysosomal degradation the liposomal contents must be delivered to the cellular cytoplasm prior to reaching the lysosomal stage of degradation. It is well known that the pH of the cellular endosomes are mildly acidic (8). We have utilized this natural phenomenon to construct a liposome, a pH-sensitive immunoliposome, that will deliver its contents in response to this endosomal acidification.

Immunoliposomes composed of dioleoylphophatidylethanol-amine (DOPE) and oleic acid (OA) (8:2 molar ratio) have been shown to become unstable and fusion competent at a weakly acidic pH of 5-6.5 (9,10). These liposomes demonstrated a significant enhancement of the cytotoxicity of the chemotherapeutic drug ara-C when delivered to target L-929 cells (2). The effectiveness of pH-sensitive immunoliposome delivery of ara-C to L-929 cells was measured by the inhibition of [^{3}H]dT incorporation when compared to an untreated control cell population. pH-sensitive immunoliposomes exhibited nearly a 5-fold enhancement in cell cytotoxicity over that of free ara-C. pH-insensitive immunoliposomes, composed of dioleoylphosphatidylcholine (DOPC), demonstrated a cell cytotoxicity that was less than that of free ara-C. pH-sensitive and pH-insensitive liposomes (containing no monoclonal antibody for target cell specificity) showed very little inhibition of [^{3}H]dT incorporation. DOPE:OA immunoliposomes containing no drug were completely non-toxic to L-929 cells. The cytotoxicity of ara-C containing DOPE:OA immunoliposomes was completely inhibitable in the presence of excess underivitized free .pa antibody. The cytotoxicity of pH-sensitive immunoliposomes was reduced by the pretreatment of the L-929 cells with the weak bases chloroquine or ammonium chloride. Both chloroquine and ammonium chloride effectively raise the pH of the intacellular acidic organelles. Studies with the drug methotrexate show that there is a slight increase in the cellular toxicity when using pH-sensitive immunoliposomes over pH-insensitive immunoliposomes for drug delivery. Both these methods are more efficient than exposure to the free drug.

These results clearly indicate that drug delivery by a pH-sensitive immunoliposome is superior to drug encapsulated in a pH-insensitive immunoliposome, pH-sensitive liposome, or free drug. Drug delivery with pH-sensitive immunoliposomes has the advantage of both increased efficiency and reduced toxicity.

We have used pH-sensitive immunoliposomes to deliver the cytotoxic fragment A of diptheria toxin (DTA) to L-929 cells (3). DTA cannot cross the cellular endosomal membrane without the translocating B fragment. In murine cells a translocation block occurs between the endosome and the cytoplasm. To effectively target this toxic fragment to cells an intracellular delivery mechanism was needed. pH-sensitive immunoliposomes were prepared (DOPE:OA=8:2) containing the DTA fragment and successfully delivered to L-929 cells. As previously described (2) pH-insensitive, non-targeted pH-sensitive liposomes were not able to deliver the DTA fragment. Delivery was also blocked by the addition of chloroquine and ammonium chloride and no delivery was found to non-target cells. Target-specific delivery of a toxin such as DTA by pH-sensitive immunoliposomes offers a possible alternative to the traditional treatment of cancer. pH-sensitive immunoliposomes are a very effective delivery vehicle for drugs to target cells that exhibit a substantial amount of endocytic activity. If the endocytic activity of the target cells is naturally low, or is affected by disease, the use of a pH-sensitive immunoliposome will not be an effective form of drug delivery. We have developed an immunoliposome that will circumvent the problem of reduced cellular uptake (5). Target-sensitive immunoliposomes have been show to deliver their contents to a cell with a high local concentration at the target cell surface. The acylated monoclonal antibody, present for cell specificity, acts as the bilayer stablizer for a liposome composed of PE. This antibody stabilized immunoliposome becomes unstable upon binding to the target cell antigen presumably by the mechanism of "contact capping". The antibody/antigen binding causes an aggregation of the stabilizer in the contact region with the cell, effectively removing the stabilizers from the rest of the immunoliposome. The phase-separated liposome membrane, upon collision with other liposomes, rapidly destabilizes and releases the contents at the cell surface. Subsequently a high local concentration of the drug is transiently present at the target cell surface (5).

Target-sensitive immunoliposomes were used to deliver antiviral drugs to cells that were infected by the herpes simplex virus I (HSV). The liposomes were targeted with a monoclonal antibody to the glycoprotein D of HSV (6). PE, transphosphaditylated from egg PC (TPE), was found to be the most effective lipid for these liposomes due to the increased stability and lifetime in the presence of serum and divalent cations present in growth media.

The antiviral efficacy and cellular toxicity of the nucleosides ara-C and acycloguanosine (acyclovir, ACV) were tested on mouse fibroblast L-929 cells by a comparison of drug delivery by target-sensitive immunoliposomes, target-insensitive immunoliposomes, and free drug. L-929 cells were infected with HSV at a low multiplicity and exposed to free drug or drug containing target-sensitive immunoliposomes. Target-sensitive immunoliposomes, composed of TPE showed effective virus inhibition at a dose at least 1000 fold lower than free drug and reduced cell cytotoxicity, at least four orders of magnitude lower, as compared to the free drug. Drug containing targeted phosphatidylcholine vesicles showed very little effect on the virus production and a corresponding reduced cellular cytotoxicity. Non-targeted phosphatidylcholine liposomes and target-sensitive immunoliposomes containing no drug had no effect on the viral production or cellular cytotoxicity in infected or uninfected control cell populations. Identical experiments performed with ACV yeilded similar, but less dramatic, results to experiments with ara-C.

In a comparison of target-sensitive immunoliposome components, TPE was found to be superior to egg PC by approximately four orders of magnitude with respect to the therapeutic effect. Delivery by target-sensitive immunoliposomes composed of egg PC was still superior to delivery by free drug. The most effective target-sensitve immunoliposome composition remains the antibody and TPE formulation. Addition of a nucleoside transport inhibitor, such as p-nitrothiobenzylinosine or dipryridamole, caused a reduction in the therapeutic effect of ara-C encapsulated target-sensitive immunoliposomes. This result indicates that drug delivery to the cellular cytoplasm is accomplished via nucleoside tranporters and that drug release, from the targeted immunoliposome, was at the cell surface. The developement of target-sensitive immunoliposomes has created another method to utilize the liposome to carry drugs to diseased cells. The target-sensitive

immunoliposome has the advantages of reducing the effective
dosages of cytotoxic drugs and reducing the cytotoxic
effects to healthy, non-diseased cells. Although much more
investigation is needed to elucidate the physical mechanism
of delivery and a "fine tuning" of liposome composition is
needed, the utilization of target-sensitive immunoliposomes
can be accomplished.

DNA DELIVERY

    Correction of genetic disorders by modification of
endogenous genes with the introduction of a foreign
exogenous gene is currently a rapidly developing area in the
treatment of disease. Gene therapy has been marginally
successful to date due to problems such as low efficiency of
delivery, instability of the foreign gene, introduction of
undesireable genetic information, and poor target
specificity. We have addressed the problems of low
efficiency and target specificity by using pH-sensitive
immunoliposomes to deliver foreign plasmid DNA to cultured
cells and an athymic nude mouse model.
    We have used the Escherichia coli chloramphenical
acetyltransferase (CAT) gene as a marker to observe gene
transfer in an athymic nude mouse (4). CAT was placed under
the control of a promoter that contained the cAMP regulatory
element to test whether the expression of the foreign gene
could be controlled by an exogenous signal mechanism. DNA
plasmid, containing cAMP controlled CAT, was entrapped in
antibody coated liposomes containing DOPE, cholesterol, and
OA (4:4:2). The targeting antibody was $H-2K^k$, the mouse
major histocompatability antigen. Entrapped DNA or free DNA
was injected intraperitoneally into immunodeficient (nude)
BALB/c mice that possesed ascites tumors generated by $H-2K^k$
positive RDM-4 lymphoma cells. Figure 1 shows the result of
experiments where CAT activity was assayed in ascites and
different organs of injected nude mice. pH-sensitive
immunoliposomes, containing DNA, were injected into the
peritoneum of mice with a corresponding injection of 8-
bromo-cAMP and 3-isobutyl-1-methylxanthine (iBuMeXan) (+) or
without 8-Br-cAMP and iBuMeXan (-). Ascites cells and
organs were removed and assayed for CAT activity. Adherent
ascites cells (macrophages), heart cells, and lung cells
showed no detectable activity when assayed for CAT with or

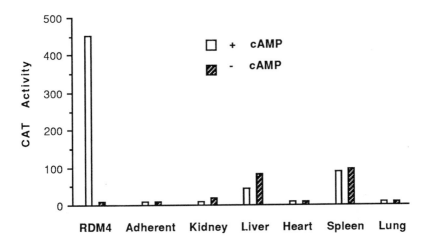

FIGURE 1. CAT activity in ascites cells and organs.

without a corresponding cAMP injection. As shown, nonadherent lymphoma cells demonstrated an elevated CAT activity in the presence of cAMP and no detectable activity in the absence of cAMP. This result indicates the exogenous cAMP controlled trigger mechanism existing on the CAT gene is sensitive after in vivo gene delivery and gene expression can be controlled. The target specificity of the pH-sensitive immunoliposome is demonstated in the increased CAT activity expressed in the target nonadherent lymphoma cells over the other organs that were tested. CAT activity was significantly lower in the liver and spleen cells when compared to the nonadherent lymphoma cells and activity was independent of cAMP. This result shows the selective delivery of the gene to the target cells and will increase the efficiency of delivery and reduce the normal uptake by the organs of the reticuloendothelial system.

Figure 2 shows the effect of lipid composition on the delivery of the foreign gene to the mouse lymphoma cells. Antibody coated liposomes were prepared from DOPE:ch:OA and DOPC:ch:OA. The replacement of DOPE with DOPC resulted in an immunoliposome that was pH-insensitive, therefore, resulting in the delivery of DNA largely to the lysosomes for destruction. CAT activity in the pH-sensitive immunoliposome was four fold greater in the targeted pH-sensitive immunoliposome over the pH-insensitive immunoliposome. This shows that the delivery of the DNA plasmid to the target cell cytoplasm prior to lysosomal

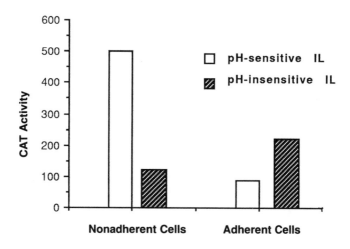

FIGURE 2.   CAT activity in ascites cells.

degradation will greatly increase the amount of gene
expression. pH-insensitive immunoliposomes deliver their
contents to the cell, but lysosomal degradation renders the
gene inactive. Gene expression in adherent cells was much
lower than in nonadherent cells using delivery by pH-
sensitive immunoliposomes indicating the target specificity
of that particular liposome was very high.
      The potential advantages of high transfer efficiency and
target cell specificity (safe delivery) for gene delivery by
pH-sensitive immunoliposomes has been demonstrated by this
work. Delivery of a protected gene to the cellular
cytoplasm, prior to lysosomal degradation, along with the
ability to control the gene expression is one key to
successful gene therapy.
      We have also used pH-sensitive immunoliposomes to
deliver the plasmid pPCTK-6A into mouse Ltk⁻ cultured cells
(11). The pPCTK-6A plasmid contains the Herpes Simplex virus
thymidine kinase gene (HSV-TK). To allow for regulatory
control of the gene during therapy the endogenous promotor of
HSV-TK gene was replaced by the promotor of the rat
phosphoenolpyruvate carboxykinase gene. This promotor
contains the same cAMP regulatory element that allows control
of the TK expression by exogenous or endogenous cAMP (12).
Short term expression of the exogenous gene was
measured by the relative TK activity and by autoradiography
of experimental cells labled with [³H] thymidine. The

optimal concentration of entrapped plasmid was 2 ug/10^5
cells and the optimal incubation time, for short term gene
expression, was 24 hours. Non-targeted liposomes
(containing no antibody) and liposomes that were not pH-
sensitive (containing DOPC rather than DOPE) were found to
be less effective with respect to gene expression in treated
cells by factors of 6 and 8, respectively.

Long term transformation efficiency was determined by
limiting dilutions of DNA-contaning liposome treated cells.
This method was compared to cells treated by Ca^{2+}-phosphate
precipitated DNA. Southern blot analysis showed that
exogenous gene expression was present in the host chromosome
in long term transformed cells. The efficiency of long term
transformation from liposome treated cells was 9% as compared
to the 1% efficiency of Ca^{2+}-phosphate treated cells.

It is clear that because of the increased short term
gene expression and the increased expression of the long term
transformants, pH-sensitive immunoliposomes are the preferred
vehicle for the introduction of a foreign gene into mammalian
cells. Other methods have been developed to transfect cells
with foreign genes, but these methods involve the use of
retroviruses that can be potentially harmful (13). The
advantages liposomes possses range from their natural
occurence, that is nontoxic and biodegradable, to their
relative ease of preparation. For these reasons, we feel
that liposomes are a potentially effective, and preferred,
vehicle for gene therapy.

FUTURE

Clinical applications of liposomes for the treatment of
cancer and infectious diseases is still in the early stages
of developement. Approximately seventeen liposome products
will be in clinical trials in the United States in 1988 (14).
These clinical trials include cancer and fungal therapy to
hair growth and post-surgical healing therapy. We have shown
that liposomes are very effective for delivery of
chemotherapeutic drugs, anti-viral drugs, and foreign genes
in a variety of in vivo and in vitro models. Future problems
that need to be investigated include the stability of
liposomes in physiological environments, the transport of
drug-containing liposomes to target sites that are not
directly exposed to the routes of liposome administration,
and a rigorous characterization of the physical interactions
between the components of pH-sensitive and target-sensitive
immunoliposomes.

REFERENCES

1. Cullis, P.R. and DeKruijff, B. (1979). Lipid Polymorphism and the Functional Roles of Lipids in Biological Membranes. Biochim. Biophys. Acta 559, 339.
2. Connor, J. and Huang, L. (1986). pH-Sensitive Immunoliposomes as an Efficient and Target-Specific Carrier for Antitumor Drugs. Cancer Res. 46, 3431.
3. Collins, D. and Huang, L. (1987). Cytotoxicity of DTA Fragment to Toxin Resistant Murine Cells Delivered by pH-Sensitive Immunoliposomes. Cancer Res. 47, 735.
4. Wang, C.Y. and Huang, L. (1987). pH-Sensitive Immunoliposomes Mediate Target-Cell-Specific Delivery and Controlled Expression of a Foreign Gene in Mouse. Proc. Natl. Acad. Sci. USA 84, 7851.
5. Ho, R.J.Y., Rouse, B.T. and Huang, L. (1986). Target-Sensitive Immunoliposomes: Preparation and Characterization. Biochem. 25, 5500.
6. Ho, R.J.Y., Rouse, B.T. and Huang L. (1987). Target-Sensitive Immunuliposomes as a Efficient Drug Carrier for Antiviral Activity. J. Biol. Chem. 262(29), 13973.
7. Huang, A., Tsao, Y.S., Kennel, S.J., and Huang, L. (1982). Characterization of Antibody Covalently Coupled to Liposomes. Biochim. Biophys. Acta 716, 140.
8. Tycko, B. and Maxfield, F.R. (1982). Rapid Acidification of Endocytic Vesicles Containing β 2 Macroglobulin. Cell 28, 643.
9. Shen, D.F., Huang, A., and Huang, L. (1982). An Improved Method for Covalent Attatchment of Antibody to Liposomes. Biochim. Biophys. Acta 689, 31.
10. Huang, L., and Liu S.S. (1984). Acid Induced Fusion of Liposomes with Inner Membranes of Mitochondria. Biophys. J. 45, 72a.
11. Wang, C.Y. (1987). Cytoplasmic Delivery of Macromolecules Via pH-sensitive Liposomes. Dissertation, University of Tennessee, Knoxville, Tennessee.
12. Wynshaw-Boris, A., Lugo, T.G., Short, J.M., Fournier, R.E.K., and Hanson, R.W. (1984). Identification of a cAMP Regulatory Region in the Gene for Rat Cytosolic Phosphoenolpyruvate Carboxykinase (GTP). J. Biol. Chem. 259, 12161.
13. Bishop, J.M. (1987). The Molecular Genetics of Cancer. Science 235, 305.
14. Klausner, A. (1988). Will 1988 be 'The Year of the Liposome'?. Biotech 6(1), 20.

Liposomes in the Therapy of Infectious Diseases and Cancer, pages 35–56
© **1989 Alan R. Liss, Inc.**

THE IMMUNOADJUVANT ACTION OF LIPOSOMES

Gregory Gregoriadis, David Davis, Nathalie Garcon, Lloyd Tan, Volkmar Weissig and Qifu Xiao

Medical Research Council Group, Academic Department of Medicine, Royal Free Hospital School of Medicine, Pond Street, London NW3 2QG, UK.

ABSTRACT   The immunological adjuvant properties of cholesterol-rich liposomes prepared by the dehydration-rehydration method have been investigated using tetanus toxoid as a model antigen. Immunization studies in Balb/c mice have dealt with (a) the nature of immune responses to a liposomal antigen, (b) the role of a variety of structural characteristics of liposomes (eg. membrane fluidity, liposomal lipid to antigen mass ratio and antigen localization) on immune responses, (c) the effect of a macrophage targeting ligand (ie. mannosylated albumin) incorporated onto the surface of liposomes, on their adjuvanticity, (d) the influence of physiological (eg. IL-2 and interferon-γ) or non-physiological (eg. threonyl muramyl dipeptide) mediators co-entrapped with the toxoid in the same liposomes or separately entrapped, on liposomal adjuvanticity and (e) comparison of liposomal adjuvanticity with that of alum and Syntex adjuvant formulation (SAF-1).

INTRODUCTION

The immunoadjuvant action of liposomes was first established in 1974. This initial

observation (1,2) was subsequently confirmed and
extended using a multitude of antigens relevant to
human and veterinary immunization (3). The list
includes Streptococcus pneumonia serotype 3 (4),
Salmonella typhimurium lipopolysaccharide (5),
cholera toxin (6,7), adenovirus type 5 hexon (8),
Simplex virus type 1 antigens (9), hepatitis B
virus surface antigen (10), Epstein-Barr virus gp
340 protein (11), tetanus toxoid (12,13),
synthetic peptides of foot-and-mouth disease virus
(14) and rat spermatozoal polypeptide (15).
     The great variability of liposomes in terms
of structural characteristics and mode of antigen
accommodation as well as the possible use of co-
adjuvants or mediators in association with
liposomes warrant versatility in immunoadjuvant
action and vaccine design (16). However, although
considerable amount of work has been already
carried out in this area, the nature or mechanisms
of liposomal immunoadjuvant action are essentially
unknown (3,17). Moreover, opposing views have
been aired regarding liposomal characteristics
(eg. liposomal membrane fluidity and antigen
localization) deemed optimal for such action
(3,17-20). Added to these, are problems with the
procedures used for antigen entrapment, which must
be resolved if liposomal vaccines are to compete
with alum and other (proposed) adjuvants in human
and veterinary immunization programmes. For
instance, some procedures are complicated or give
low antigen entrapment values and may thus be
uneconomical. With others, the use of organic
solvents, sonication and detergents is required in
the presence of antigen (21) all of which could
lead to the masking or modification of antigenic
sites. Some of these questions and problems have
been recently investigated in this laboratory and
findings are discussed below.

INCORPORATION OF ANTIGENS INTO LIPOSOMES

     A recently reported method (22) for liposome
preparation is based on the fusion of preformed
phospholipid vesicles by dehydration followed by
rehydration in the presence of solute destined for

entrapment. This leads to the formation of multilamellar liposomes (dehydration-rehydration vesicles, DRV) entrapping up to 80% of the solute without the involvement of conditions (eg. organic solvents, sonication and detergents) potentially damaging to the solute. Such features of the procedure and its amenability to scale-up for industrial use (22), render it particularly suitable for liposomal vaccines (13,23). We have therefore adopted multilamellar DRV in our studies of liposomal immunoadjuvant action, mostly using aggregate-free immunopurified tetanus toxoid as the model antigen. The toxoid was also entrapped in DRV coated with a mannosylated ligand which is expected to facilitate interaction of liposomes with macrophages known to express the mannose receptor. In addition, toxoid has been covalently coupled to the surface of preformed multilamellar vesicles, so as to provide us with an alternative means of antigen presentation (3,12,19,20,24).

Entrapment of Tetanus Toxoid in DRV Liposomes.

In agreement with previous data obtained for a variety of solutes (eg. drugs, proteins etc.) (22,25,26), entrapment of tetanus toxoid in DRV liposomes made of equimolar egg phosphatidylcholine (PC) and cholesterol and generated from preformed small unilamellar vesicles (SUV) was substantial (47.5 $\pm$ 7.4% of the amount used) (13). The use of other unsaturated or saturated phospholipids with varying acyl chain lengths to prepare DRV also gave similar entrapment values. However, when distearoyl phosphatidylcholine (DSPC) was used, entrapment values were nearly twice as great (82.3 $\pm$ 3.4%) (13), possibly because the antigen, in addition to being passively entrapped, also interacts in some way with DSPC, perhaps hydrophobically. Higher entrapment values (61-76%) were also achieved with PC liposomes when charged negatively or positively, probably because of the increased (27) width of the aqueous spaces between the charged bilayers. More recently, work with other antigens, namely polio type 3-VP2 and 1-VP2 peptides (28) and reconstituted influenza virus envelopes (RIVE) (29) has also shown similarly high entrapment values.

Covalent Coupling of Tetanus Toxoid to MLV Liposomes.

Recent reports (eg. ref.19) have claimed that adjuvanticity of liposomes for proteins located on the surface of liposomes is not as great as when proteins are secluded within the aqueous phase of the vesicles. This claim was further tested (see later) by covalently linking the toxoid to the surface of multilamellar liposomes via diazotization (24). We found (13) that coupling of the antigen to such liposomes was efficient (63.1 $\pm$ 8.3%) and, in terms of amount of antigen bound, comparable to that seen with passive entrapment.

Freeze-Dried Liposomes

There are situations where a freeze-dried form of liposomal vaccines would be preferable provided that, on addition of physiological saline prior to injection, re-formed vesicles still retain entrapped all, or at least most, of the originally incorporated antigen. Multilamellar liposomes made of equimolar phospholipid and cholesterol with the toxoid passively entrapped or covalently linked to their surface, were therefore freeze-dried and then reconstituted in saline. In some experiments freeze-drying was carried out in the presence of trehalose, known to act as a cryoprotectant. Our results (13) show that after dehydration in the absence of trehalose, DRV PC liposomes retained on rehydration most (78.3%) of the entrapped toxoid. Interestingly, retention of the toxoid by DSPC DRV was quantitative (93.5%). It seems that quantitative retention of the protein on freeze-drying is not peculiar to the toxoid since DRV PC liposomes containing bovine serum albumin (BSA) retained the protein similarly (73.2%) when subjected to freeze-drying (13). The

presence of trehalose during dehydration improved
(to 86.9%) the retention of toxoid entrapped in
DRV PC liposomes and a small increase in the
already high retention values was noted for DRV
DSPC liposomes. PC liposomes with covalently
linked toxoid and dehydrated in the absence (or
presence) of trehalose, also retained much of the
toxoid (13). These studies were taken a step
further to see whether structural alterations in
the liposomal membrane during freeze-drying and
rehydration, lead to the relocation of the
covalently linked toxoid from the surface of the
multilamellar liposomes to inner lamellae. We
found (13) no obvious changes in antigen localization in freeze-dried liposomes compared to
untreated preparations.

IMMUNE RESPONSES TO DRV LIPOSOMAL TETANUS TOXOID

In immunization experiments (30) using Balb/c
mice, the adjuvant activity of toxoid-containing
liposomes was reflected in various IgG
immunoglobulin subclasses: For instance, IgG_1
response to high doses (2 and 10 µg) of tetanus
toxoid were similar for free and liposome-
entrapped antigen. At a lower dose (0.1 µg),
however, there was a significant increase in the
titre of IgG_1 antibody following stimulation by
liposomal antigen in comparison to free antigen
(30). Further, there was a significant increase
in the level of IgG_{2b} antibody at all antigen
doses in comparison to free antigen, when
liposomal antigen was used to induce immune
responses. Less consistent adjuvant effect was
obtained in terms of IgG_{2a} and IgG_3 responses
although significant differences between the
responses to the liposomal and free antigen were
observed when tetanus toxoid was injected in
higher doses (30). There was no increase in IgG_1,
IgG_{2a} or IgG_{2b} levels of anti-tetanus toxoid
antibodies following a third injection of toxoid
into mice (30). Analysis of the secondary
response revealed that no liposomal adjuvant
effect which could be ascribed solely to events
following the second injection could be observed

(30). In conclusion, therefore, results (30) indicate that liposomes increase the antibody response within an individual IgG subclass, independently of their effect on other subclasses. On comparing the responses of mice injected with high and low doses of tetanus toxoid, it appears that as the dose of antigen increases, there is an increase both in the antibody response within an individual subclass (whether the antigen is associated with liposomes or not) and the number of subclasses involved in the response.

INFLUENCE OF LIPOSOMAL CHARACTERISTICS ON THE IMMUNE RESPONSES TO INCORPORATED ANTIGEN

As already stated, liposomes are uniquely versatile in structural charateristics and mode of antigen accommodation. Such properties should allow, in turn, for a wide range of options in designing effective vaccines. They may also account for the variability of data obtained with regard to the role of a number of liposomal parameters in adjuvanticity (16). Recently, some of these parameters were examined (23) using DRV liposomes with tetanus toxoid either entrapped or covalently linked to their surface. The choice of the dehydration-rehydration procedure for liposome preparation was based, as alluded to earlier, on findings (13,22) of realistically and reproducibly high antigen entrapment values. The method of diazotization on the other hand, has provided us with a rapid and efficient means for the coupling of antigen to the liposomal surface (12,13,24).

The Effect of Liposomal Phospholipid to Tetanus Toxoid Mass Ratio on Antibody Response.

It was originally assumed that liposomal immunoadjuvant action would be favoured by an increased concentration of antigen in individual vesicles as this would allow presentation of sufficient quantities of antigen to immunocompetent cells. However, three separate experiments (each with a variety of liposomal

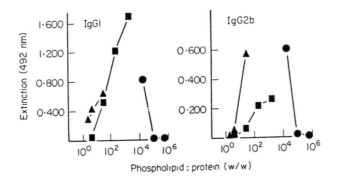

FIGURE 1. Immune responses to tetanus toxoid given in liposomes of varying phospholipid to toxoid mass ratio. In three separate experiments Balb/c mice (in groups of five) were injected with 0.1 (▲), 0.025 (■) or 0.005 (●) µg of tetanus toxoid per mouse, free or entrapped in DRV liposomes composed of equimolar PC and cholesterol and with phospholipid to protein ratios shown in the Figure. Animals were bled 9-10 days after an identical booster injection and sera analysed for IgG_1 and IgG_{2b} by the ELISA immunosorbent assay. Results are expressed as median readings for each of the treated groups. Phospholipid to toxoid ratios are plotted on a logarithmic scale. Readings (not shown) for sera of control mice injected with free toxoid in one of the exper- iments (▲) were below 0.1 or nil. Results from statistical analysis (carried out by the Kruskal- Wallis non-parametric test) of differences between the various phospholipid to toxoid mass ratios in each of the experiments were: ▲, H=4.16, p > 0.1 (IgG_1) and H=8.93, p < 0.01 (IgG_{2b}); ■, H=15.61, p < 0.01 (IgG_1) and H=11.30, p < 0.01 (IgG_{2b}); ●, H=12.02, p < 0.01 (IgG_1) and H=11.18, p < 0.01 (IgG_{2b}) (23).

phospholipid to toxoid mass ratios ranging from 2:1 to 5 x 10^5:1) suggested the opposite, namely that the higher the phospholipid to toxoid mass ratio, the higher the immune response (IgG_1 and IgG_{2b})(Fig.1 and legend). Although a ratio of about 30:1 was considered (23) sufficiently high

for the purpose of the present studies, it is
clear that adjuvanticity is improved to a much
greater extent when higher (about 2×10^3:1)
ratios are used. At much higher ratios (e.g. 9×10^4:1 or above), however, adjuvanticity is
drastically reduced. It thus, appears that
liposomal adjuvanticity is related (up to a
certain level) to the lipid dose, possibly in
conjunction with a slow rate of degradation/
removal of liposomes injected in large amounts,
from the site of injection. We are unable to
explain at present the reduction in adjuvanticity
at very high phospholipid to toxoid mass ratios
although, it could be tentatively attributed to an
immunosuppressive effect of excessive PC. For
instance, interaction of T lymphocytes with both
MHC and antigen (or antigenic fragments) on the
surface of macrophages (31) may require a certain
degree of fluidity of the domains surrounding the
two antigens. If there is excessive incorporation
of PC (from liposomal toxoid of a very high
phospholipid to protein mass ratio) into the
macrophage membrane, then its fluidity could be
altered to an extent that T lymphocyte effect is
inhibited. Alternatively or concurrently, it may
be that as the phospholipid to antigen mass ratio
increases, a state is reached where the number of
vesicles in the preparation is so great that only
a small proportion of them contain antigen,
probably at a concentration too low for induction
of immune responses.

Antibody Responses to Entrapped and Surface-Linked
Tetanus Toxoid.

    Comparison of dose-related immune responses
in Balb/c mice using entrapped and surface-linked
toxoid, revealed no significant difference in
responses between the two liposomal preparations
for either anti-toxoid IgG_1 or IgG_{2b} (23). These
results contrast findings by Shek and Sabiston
(19) that a liposomal surface-linked antigen
(albumin) is less efficient in stimulating
indirect plaque forming cells than the entrapped
protein. Similarly, our results are in

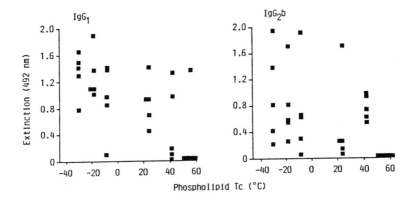

FIGURE 2. Effect of the liposomal
phospholipid Tc on liposome adjuvanticity. Balb/c
mice in groups of five were injected twice with
0.25 µg of tetanus toxoid entrapped in DRV
liposomes composed of equimolar phospholipid and
cholesterol. Animals were bled 9-10 days after
the booster injection and analysed for IgG_1 and
IgG_{2b} by the ELISA immunosorbent assay. The
phospholipid to toxoid mass ratios are given in
the text. Readings for individual mice are
plotted against the liquid-crystalline phase
transition temperatures (TC) ($^{\circ}$C in parentheses)
of the DLPC (-32), DOPC (-20), PC (-10) DMPC (23),
DPPC (41.5) and DSPC (54.0) components of DRV.
Differences in response between DSPC DRV and the
other DRV preparations were significant: (IgG_1),
H=15.37, p $\langle$0.01; (IgG_{2b}), H=11.23, p $\langle$0.05, as
determined by the Kruskall-Wallis non parametric
test (23).

(dimyristoyl phosphatidylcholine; DMPC), 29.0:1
(dipalmitoyl phosphatidylcholine; DPPC) and 14.3:1
(DSPC). Results of reduced or no antibody
response with the water soluble toxoid entrapped
in DSPC liposomes contrast those obtained by other
workers (18,33,34) who, however, used membrane
antigens. For instance, Kinsky and colleagues
(18,33) reported that liposomes incorporating a

hapten-phospholipid complex (20:1 estimated lipid to complex ratio) promote immune response to the hapten if beef sphingomyelin (Tc 37-39°C), but not egg phosphatidylcholine, were the phospholipid component. A broad correlation between increasing phospholipid Tc and increasing antibody response to liposomal Gross virus cell surface antigen (estimated phospholipid to protein ratio 7.8:1; see ref.35) has been similarly reported by Bakouche and Gerlier (34). Interestingly however, recent findings in this laboratory (29) with reconstituted influenza virus envelopes (RIVE) incorporated in PC or DSPC DRV liposomes suggest that both primary and secondary immune responses (IgG_1) to the RIVE in Balb/c mice, are similar for the two compositions. It thus seems that even for membrane antigens, high melting phospholipids alone will not necessarily give a stronger response and that other parameters such as lipid to antigen ratios may play a role (see below).

It is conceivable that differences in the nature of the antigens studied in the present experiments and those quoted above may account for the opposite effects of phospholipids with high Tc on liposomal adjuvanticity. Membrane antigens may pass into the plasma membrane of the antigen-presenting cells without being first processed and indeed, albumin-coated dipalmitoyl phosphatidylethanolamine (Tc 63.5°C) liposomes incorporating MHC antigens were found to stimulate T-cell clones in vitro in the absence of antigen presenting cells (36). Soluble antigens on the other hand, must be taken into such cells and processed before they can be exposed on their surface (31,37). It is possible that membrane antigen transfer into the plasma cell membranes depend on the mobility and/or distribution of the antigen within the liposomal bilayers and also on its accessibility. These could, in turn, be influenced by a reduced bilayer fluidity (in liposomes composed of "high-melting" phospholipids) in a manner that promotes antigen transfer to antigen presenting cells (23). On the other hand, liposomal DSPC or other "high melting" phospholipids may inhibit the processing of soluble antigens. In recent work (23,32) however,

using a much greater DSPC to toxoid mass ratio
(about $4.2 \times 10^3 : 1$), anti-toxoid antibody (IgG_1
and IgG_{2b}) responses to DSPC DRV were as high as
those obtained with PC liposomes of a similar
ratio. A mixture of low ratio (12:1) PC DRV and
"empty" (toxoid free) PC liposomes giving a high
(about $2.7 \times 10^3 : 1$) overall ratio, also improved
immune responses to levels approaching those
obtained with toxoid entrapped in PC DRV of an
identical (about $2.7 \times 10^3 : 1$) ratio.

The way by which liposomes exert their
immunoadjuvant action is unclear. However, it is
probable that such action is promoted in at least
two ways, one related to the rate of antigen
release from the vesicles at the site of injection
and the other to the mode of vesicle interaction
with antigen presenting cells. Both ways are
likely to depend on liposomal fluidity. With
regard to the rate of antigen release, it is known
(3) that "solid" DSPC liposomes become unstable in
vivo at a much slower rate than "fluid" ones. On
the other hand, liposomal fluidity is thought (38)
to influence the extent to which liposomes fuse
with or are endocytosed and processed by cells.
The enhancement of immune responses by excess DSPC
may, as suggested above in the case of excess PC
liposomes, result from a prolonged release of the
antigen at the site of injection, which could
conceivably override any inhibitory action that
DSPC may have on such responses at the level of
liposome-cell interaction.

Targeted Adjuvanticity of Liposomes.

Antigen presenting cells such as phagocytes
take up conventional liposomes avidly and, in
terms of immunoadjuvant action, modification of
the liposomal surface leading to selective uptake
by the cells would seem unnecessary. However, it
has been shown (39) that certain invading
microorganisms interact via mannose-terminating
ligands on their surface with the mannose receptors on phagocytes and it may be that this event
relates to natural immunization. It was thought
that, on this basis, liposomes coated with a

mannose-terminating ligand might show improved
adjuvanticity (32,40). Experiments were therefore, carried out (40) to initially confirm that
DRV liposomes incorporating tetanus toxoid and
coated with mannosylated albumin (by a method (41)
which allows linking of the ligand to the
liposomal surface prior to toxoid entrapment),
bind to the relevant receptors on (mouse
peritoneal) macrophages. As expected, such
liposomes exhibited greater affinity for the cells
than mannose-free DRV of the same composition and
content (40). Furthermore, the specificity of
interaction with macrophages was demonstrated
when, in the presence of excess   methyl-D-
mannoside, binding was reduced to levels seen with
mannose-free DRV.

Immunization experiments (40) were carried
out to investigate the effect, if any, of mannose
residues linked to the surface of tetanus toxoid-
containing DRV on liposome adjuvanticity. Fig.3
shows serum titres (IgG_1) from groups of mice
injected with tetanus toxoid entrapped in DRV
which were either uncoated or coated with albumin
only or with mannosylated albumin. It is apparent
that mannosylated DRV mediate greater (eight-fold)
immune response than the two control preparations.
In other experiments, Balb/c mice were immunized
with (a) DRV preparations bearing two different
amounts of mannosylated albumin (ie. different
number of protein chains) which, however, had the
same number (ie. 36) of mannose moles per mole
albumin; (b) DRV preparations bearing
approximately the same amount of mannosylated
albumin (ie. the same number of protein chains)
which had either 8 or 36 moles mannose per mole
albumin. Results (40) suggest that, under the
conditions of experimentation, immune response
(IgG_1 and IgG_{2b}) to tetanus toxoid-containing DRV,
is dependent on the number of mannosylated albumin
molecules exposed on the vesicle surface rather
than the number of mannose residues available. If
targeted adjuvanticity (as determined here) is
related to the extent (or firmness) of vesicle
binding to phagocytes, it is conceivable that a
certain number of mannose moles per mole albumin
(8 in the present experiment) promotes binding

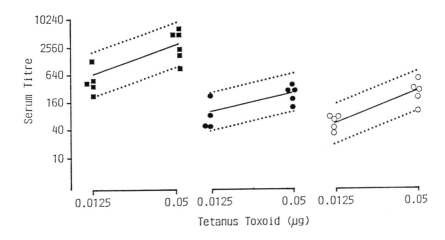

FIGURE 3. Anti-tetanus toxoid IgG$_1$ titres in
mice immunized with toxoid-containing DRV coated
with mannosylated albumin. Balb/c mice (in groups
of five) were immunized intramuscularly with
tetanus toxoid (0.0125 or 0.05 µg) entrapped DRV
composed of equimolar PC and cholesterol (90 ug
lipid per 1 µg toxoid) (o) in similar DRV coated
with albumin (1 µg toxoid per 120 µg lipid per 2.4
µg albumin) (●) or in similar DRV coated with
mannosylated (36 mannose moles per mole albumin (1
µg toxoid per 67 µg lipid per 1.36 µg albumin)
(■). Three weeks after primary immunization,
mice received identical injections of the same
preparations and bled nine days later. The least
squares estimate of the regression line of IgG$_1$
antibody titre against antigen dose was derived
separately for the three groups. Regression lines
(■ versus ● or o) were significantly different
(p < 0.05). Dotted lines denote 95 percent confidence interval of the regression lines (32,40).

which cannot be improved upon by the presence of a
larger number (ie. 36) of mannose moles. On the
other hand it may be that binding is substantially
augmented (or becomes firmer) by increasing the
number of mannosylated albumin molecules on the
surface of vesicles.

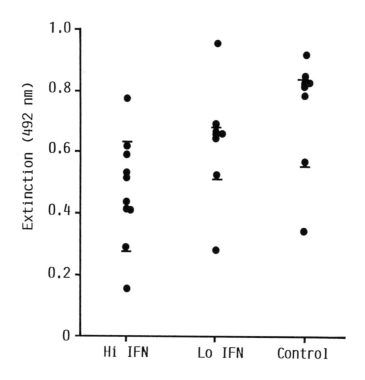

FIGURE 4. The effect of IFN-γ co-entrapped with tetanus toxoid in liposomes on the primary immune response to the antigen. Balb/c mice were injected intramuscularly with tetanus toxoid (0.75 μg) entrapped in DRV composed of equimolar PC and cholesterol (control; phospholipid to toxoid mass ratio 342:1) or in similar DRV also co-entrapping 5533 (Hi) or 585 (Lo) units IFN-γ (phosphilipid to toxoid mass ratios: 201:1 and 324:1 respectively). Mice were bled 28 days later and sera analysed (23) by ELISA for IgG$_1$. Statistical analysis by the Kruskall-Wallis test revealed a significant (H=11.65, p$\langle$0.01) reduction of response when IFN-γ was co-entrapped with the antigen.

THE EFFECT OF PHYSIOLOGICAL AND NON-PHYSIOLOGICAL
MEDIATORS AND OTHER CO-ADJUVANTS ON THE PRIMARY
IMMUNE RESPONSE TO LIPOSOMAL TETANUS TOXOID

Recently, we have studied liposomal
adjuvanticity in terms of primary immune response
and possible modulation of such response by
interleukin-2 (IL-2), interferon-γ (IFN-γ), the
water soluble N-acetylmuramyl-L-threonyl-D-
isoglutamine (Thr-MDP) and its liposoluble 6-O-
stearoyl derivative (St. Thr. MDP). These agents
were administered in cholesterol-rich PC DRV
together with tetanus toxoid using a variety of
protocols (D. Davis, D. Eppstein and G. Gregoriadis, in preparation). Liposomal adjuvanticity
was also compared with that of alum and Syntex
Adjuvant Formulation (SAF-1). Results suggest
that primary immune response (IgG_1) to the toxoid
is augmented by liposomes of phospholipid to
antigen mass ratios, of up to about $2.8 \times 10^3:1$
and reduced with liposomes of a higher ratio (eg.
$1.7 \times 10^4:1$). The level of response using optimal
ratios peaks at 4 weeks and declines slowly
thereafter. By 24 weeks ELISA readings attain
levels seen 2 weeks after injection. IL-2,
IFN-γ and Thr. MDP co-entrapped with the toxoid
in the same liposomes, generally reduced primary
response to levels below those obtained with
control liposomes containing the antigen alone
(Figs.4,5). However, IL-2 in separate liposomes
mixed with the liposomal toxoid significantly
improved immune resonse (results not shown). On
the other hand, the liposoluble St. Thr. MDP (co-
entrapped with the toxoid or incorporated in
separate liposomes and then mixed with the
liposomal toxoid) gave significantly higher immune
response than those observed with the water
soluble Thr. MDP in similar forms. The significance of these findings is now under investigation. Further, there was no difference in
responses when liposomes and alum were compared as
adjuvants although alum appeared a stronger
adjuvant than SAF-1 (D. Davis, D. Eppstein and G.
Gregoriadis, in preparation).

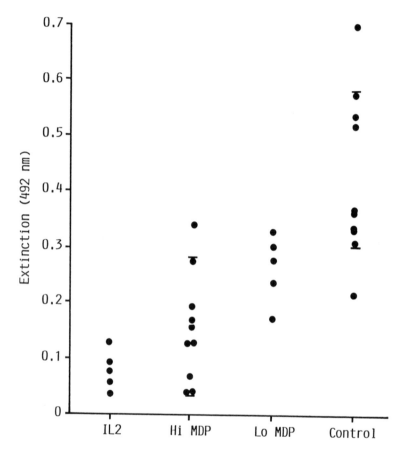

FIGURE 5. The effect of IL-2 and Thr. MDP co-entrapped with tetanus toxoid in liposomes on the primary response to the antigen. Balb/c mice were injected intramuscularly with tetanus toxoid (1.0 µg) entrapped in DRV liposomes composed of equimolar PC and cholesterol (control; phospholipid to toxoid mass ratio 318:1) or in similar DRV also co-entrapping 350 units IL2 or 50.3 µg Thr. MDP (Hi) or 25.2 µg Thr. MDP (Lo) (phospholipid to toxoid mass ratios: 794:1, 221:1 and 226:1 respectively). Mice were bled 28 days later and sera analysed (23) by ELISA for IgG_1. As in Fig. 4, there was a statistically

significant (Kruskall-Wallis test) reduction of
response when IL-2 or Thr. MDP (either dose) were
co-entrapped with the antigen. Bars show 95%
confidence limits.

CONCLUSIONS

Current evidence strongly supports further
evaluation of DRV liposomes as carriers of
vaccines. From the practical point of view, DRV
are easy to prepare and entrap antigens
quantitatively in the absence of conditions
damaging to the antigen. Coupling procedures can
also be employed for the attachment of antigens
(or ligands) to the surface of DRV liposomes.
When antigens or ligands are sensitive to the
coupling procedures, they can be firstly linked to
SUV which can then be used to generate DRV bearing
much of the antigen or ligand on their surface
(41). Preparations with entrapped or surface-
linked antigen can be freeze-dried with most of
the antigen being recovered within or on intact
vesicles after reconstitution in saline.

Data from immunization experiments in Balb/c
mice injected with DRV-incorporated tetanus
toxoid, suggest that liposomal adjuvanticity is
reflected in most IgG subclasses. It appears that
there is no shift in subclasses when compared to
the response obtained with the free antigen and
that adjuvanticity is the outcome of events
following primary immunization. Our studies also
indicate that liposomal structural characteristics
such as membrane fluidity, amount of liposomal
lipid relative to the antigen (but not mode of
antigen localization in the vesicles) influence
adjuvanticity. In addition, a number of
physiological and non-physiological mediators
appear to modulate (primary) immune response
depending on whether the mediator is given in the
same or separate liposomes with the antigen.

Vaccines based on synthetic peptides and
recombinant subunit antigens will, in many cases,
require a new generation of immunological
adjuvants. In contrast to other adjuvants
presently under investigation (42), liposomes

exhibit unique structural versatility which allows
freedom in vaccine design. Liposomes of
appropriate lipid composition produce no side
effects and are known to elicit both humoural and
cell-mediated immunity. Most significantly, many
of the earlier technological difficulties have
been resolved and production on industrial scale
is feasible. At least one commercial liposome
preparation is now available. More recently,
several large scale phase one and phase two
clinical trials on the use of liposomes in
antimicrobial and cancer therapy have been
initiated (43; also this volume), a development
which should facilitate similar trials of
liposomal vaccines. It remains to be seen whether
liposomes will prove sufficiently superior to
other adjuvants (both technologically and in terms
of immunoadjuvant action) so as to warrant their
development in vaccine formulation. In terms of
their use as carriers of synthetic peptide
vaccines, evidence (28) with polio type 1-VP2 and
3-VP2 indicates that both primary and secondary
responses (IgG_1) of Balb/c mice to the peptides
can be elicited when these are administered in PC
DRV liposomes.

ACKNOWLEDGEMENTS

Work reported here was supported by a Medical
Research Council project grant and grants from the
the British Council, Wellcome Biotechnology Ltd.,
Government of Peoples Republic of Germany and the
University of Singapore. The authors thank Mr. A.
Davies for technical assistance and Mrs. Angela
Massaro for immaculate secretarial assistance.

REFERENCES

1.   Allison AC, Gregoriadis G (1974). Liposomes as
     immunological adjuvants. Nature (Lond.)
     252:252.
2.   Gregoriadis G, Allison AC (1974). Entrapment
     of proteins in liposomes prevents allergic
     reactions in preimmunized mice. FEBS Lett
     45:71.

3. Gregoriadis G (1985). Liposomes as carriers for drugs and vaccines. Trends Biotechnol 3:235.

4. Snippe H, van Dam JEG, van Houte AJ, Williers JMN, Kamerling JP, Vliegenthart JFG (1983). Preparation of a semisynthetic vaccine to Streptococcus pneumoniae Type 3. Inf Immun 42:842.

5. Desiderio JV, Campbell SG (1985). Immunisation against experimental murine salmonellosis with liposome-associated O-antigen. Inf Immun 48:658.

6. Alving CR, Banerji B, Shiba T, Kotani S, Clements JD, Richards RL (1980). Liposomes as vehicles for vaccines. In "New Developments with Human and Veterinary Vaccines," New York: Alan R. Liss, p.339.

7. Pierce NF, Sacci Jr JB (1984). Enhancement by Lipid A of Mucosal Immunogenicity of Liposome-Associated Cholera Toxin. Rev Inf Dis 6:563.

8. Kramp WJ, Six HR, Kasel JA (1982). Postimmunization clearance of liposome-entrapped adenovirus type 5 hexon. Proc Soc Exp Bioc Med 169:135.

9. Naylor PT, Larsen HS, Huang L, Rouse BT (1982). In-vivo induction of anti-herpes simplex virus immune response by type 1 antigens and lipid A incorporated into liposomes. Inf Immun 36: 1209.

10. Manesis EK, Cameron CH, Gregoriadis G (1979). Hepatitis B surface antigen-containing liposomes enhance humoral and cell-mediated immunity to the antigen. FEBS Lett 102:107.

11. Epstein MA, Morgan AJ, Finerty S, Randle BJ, Kirkwood JK(1985). Protection of cottontop tamarins against Epstein-Barr virus-induced malignant lymphoma by a prototype subunit vaccine. Nature (Lond.) 318:287.

12. Davis D, Davies A, Gregoriadis G (1986). Liposomes as immunological adjuvants in vaccines: Studies with entrapped and surface-linked antigen. Biochem Soc Trans 14:1036.

13. Gregoriadis G, Davis D, Davies A (1987). Liposomes as immunological adjuvants in vaccines: Antigen incorporation studies. Vaccine 5:145.

14. Francis MJ, Fry CM, Rowlands DJ, Brown F, Bittle JL, Houghten RA, Lernerr RA (1985). Immunological priming with synthetic peptides of foot-and-mouth disease virus. J Gen Virol 66:2347.

15. Mettler L, Czuppon AB, Buchheim W, Baukloh V, Ghyczy M, Etschenberg J, Holstein AF (1983). Induction of high titre mouse-antihuman spermatozoal antibodies by liposome incorporation of spermatozoal membrane antigens. Am J Reprod Immunol 4:127.

16. Gregoriadis G (1986). Liposomal subunit vaccine against Epstein-Barr virus-induced malignant lymphoma. Nature (Lond.) 320:87.

17. Hedlund G, Jansson B, Sjogren HO (1984). Comparison of immune responses induced by rat RT-1 antigens presented as inserts into liposomes, as protein micelles and as intact cells. Immunology 53:69.

18. Kinsky SC (1978). Immunogenicity of liposomal model membranes. Ann NY Acad Sci 308:111.

19. Shek PN, Sabiston BH (1982). Immune response mediated by liposome-associated protein antigens. II. Comparison of the effectiveness of vesicle-entrapped and surface-associated antigen in immunopotentiation. Immunology 47:627.

20. van Rooijen N, van Nieuwmegen R (1980). Liposomes in immunology: Evidence that their adjuvant effect results form surface exposition of the antigens. Cell Immunol 49:402.

21. Gregoriadis G (ed) (1984). "Liposome Technology" Boca Raton: CRC Press Inc. Vol. 1.

22. Kirby C, Gregoriadis G (1984). Dehydration-rehydration vesicles (DRV): A new method for high yield drug entrapment in liposomes. Biotechnology 2:979.

23. Davis D, Gregoriadis G (1987). Liposomes as adjuvants with immunopurified tetanus toxoid: Influence of liposomal characteristics. Immunology 61:229.

24. Snyder SL, Vannier WE (1984). Immunologic response to protein immobilised on the surface of liposomes via covalent azo-bonding, Biochim Biophys Acta 772:288.

25. Norley SG, Huang L, Rouse BT (1986). Targeting of drug-loaded immunoliposomes to herpes simplex virus infected corneal cells. An effective means of inhibiting virus replication in vitro. J Immunol 136:681.

26. Seltzer S, Gregoriadis G, Dick R (1988). DRV liposomes in contrast imaging. Invest Radiol 23:131

27. Sessa G, Weissmann G (1968). Phospholipid spherules (liposomes) as a model for biological membranes. J Lipid Res 9: 310.

28. Gregoriadis G, Weissig V, Tan L, Xiao Q, Lasch J (1988). A novel method for the covalent coupling of peptides and sugars to liposomes. Biochem Soc Trans. (In press).

29. Tan L, Gregoriadis G, Loyter A (1988). Incorporation of reconstituted influenza virus envelopes into liposomes: Studies of immune response in mice. Biochem Soc Trans (In press).

30. Davis D, Davies A, Gregoriadis G (1987). Liposomes as adjuvants with immunopurified tetanus toxoid: The immune response. Immunology Letters 14:341.

31. Unanue ER, Beller DI, Lu CY, Allen PM (1984). Antigen presentation: Comments on its regulation and mechanism. J Immunol 132:1.

32. Gregoriadis G, Garcon N, Senior J, Davis D (1988). The immunoadjuvant action of liposomes: Nature of immune response and influence of liposomal characteristics. In Gregoriadis G (ed): "Liposomes as Drug Carriers: Trends and Progress", Chichester: John Wiley, p 279.

33. Dancey GF, Yasuda T, Kinsky SC (1978). Effect of liposomal model membrane composition on immunogenicity. J Immunol 120: 1109.

34. Bakouche O, Gerlier D (1986). Enhancement of Immunogenicity of tumour virus antigen by liposomes. The effect of lipid composition. Immunology 57:219.

35. Gerlier D, Sakai F, Dore JF (1978). Inclusion d'un antigene de surface cellulaire associe au virus de Gross dans des liposomes, CR Acad Sc Paris, 286, Serie D:439.

36. Walden P, Nagy ZA, Klein J (1985). Induction of regulatory T- lymphocyte responses of liposomes carrying major histocompatibility complex molecules and foreign antigen. Nature (Lond.) 315:327.

37. Mills KHG (1986). Processing of viral antigens and presentation to class II-restricted T cells. Immunology Today 7: 260.

38. Poste G (1980). The interaction of lipid vesicles with cultured cells and their use as carriers for drugs and macromolecules. In Gregoriadis G, Allison AC (eds): "Liposomes in Biological Systems," Chichester: John Wiley p.101.

39. Perry A, Ofek I (1984). Inhibition of blood clearance and hepatic tissue binding of Escherichia coli by liver lectin- specific sugars and glycoproteins. Inf Imm 43:257.

40. Garcon N, Gregoriadis G, Taylor M, Summerfield J (1988). Mannose-mediated targeted immuno-adjuvant action of liposomes. Immunology (In press).

41. Garcon N, Senior J, Gregoriadis G (1986). Coupling of ligands to liposomes before entrapment of agents sensitive to coupling procedures. Biochem Soc Trans 14:1038.

42. Allison AC, Byars NE (1986). An adjuvant formulation that selectively elicits the formation of antibodies of protective isotypes and of cell-mediated immunity. J Immunol Meth 95:157.

43. Gregoriadis G (1988) (ed) "Liposomes as Carriers of Drugs: Recent Trends and Progress," Chichester: John Wiley and Sons.

II. LIPOSOMES IN CANCER

Liposomes in the Therapy of Infectious Diseases and Cancer, pages 59–69
© 1989 Alan R. Liss, Inc.

DESIGN AND DEVELOPMENT OF LIPOSOME-DEPENDENT ANTITUMOR AGENTS[1]

R. Perez-Soler, G. Lopez-Berestein, and A.R. Khokhar[2]

Immunobiology and Drug Carriers Section, Departments of Clinical Immunology and Biological Therapy, and Medical Oncology[2], The University of Texas System Cancer Center, M. D. Anderson Hospital and Tumor Institute, Houston, TX 77030

ABSTRACT   The formulation and preclinical development of a lipophilic cisplatin analogue entrapped in multilamellar liposomes (L-NDDP) is summarized. L-NDDP is manufactured as a lyophilized powder that forms a liposome suspension upon reconstitution with normal saline. L-NDDP meets reproducibility and stability criteria for clinical use. L-NDDP was shown to have antitumor activity comparable to that of cisplatin against L1210 leukemia, was not cross resistant with cisplatin against a murine tumor model (L1210/PDD), and was significantly more effective than cisplatin against liver metastases of M5076 reticulosarcoma. In toxicity studies, L-NDDP was devoid of significant nephrotoxicity both in mice and dogs. Myelosuppression was profound in mice at the LD50 dose but mild at the maximum tolerated dose in dogs. No significant cumulative or chronic toxicites were observed in dogs. Clinical studies with L-NDDP are in progress.

INTRODUCTION

Successful therapy for a limited number of disseminated human malignancies, mainly of hematologic origin, has become

[1]This work was supported by NIH grant CA 41581 to A.R.K., and a grant from The Liposome Company, Inc., Princeton, NJ

available during the last two decades in the form of systemic combination chemotherapy. However, most chemotherapeutic
agents are extremely toxic and their administration may
result in acute or chronic life-threatening side effects.
Anticancer chemotherapy was developed as an in-hospital type
of treatment, with drugs being administered intravenously to
optimize their bioavailability and the patients being
closely monitored to treat the side-effects. As a result,
the most effective antitumor agents are highly hydrosoluble
compounds that are administered dissolved in water solutions. Compounds with poor solubility traditionally did not
have an opportunity of reaching advanced stages of development in spite of promising biological activity.

For the past 10 years, liposomes have been explored as
carriers of antitumor agents as a potential way of reducing
certain drug related toxicities and of increasing the
antitumor activity against selected tumors (1-5). Most
investigations concentrated their effort on the use of
standard hydrosoluble anticancer agents entrapped in small
unilamellar liposomes (size 0.1-0.2 μm in diameter) for the
following reasons: 1) the assumption that the use of new
chemical entities designed for liposome entrapment would
delay FDA approval and increase the cost of drug development, 2) the hope that by exploring different vesicle lipid
compositions, optimal formulations could be obtained, 3)
small unilamellar vesicles (SUV's) are better suited for the
entrapment of hydrophilic molecules because they have a
larger aqueous space compared with large multilamellar
vesicles (MLV's), 4) the theoretical principle that SUV's
should permeate the tumor better than MLV's for obvious
mechanical reasons.

Obtaining an optimal formulation is a sine qua non step
for the development of liposome entrapped drugs. It is our
intention to illustrate here that an adequate combination of
simple chemistry (drug design) and simple liposomology
(freeze-drying techniques) may be the best way to overcome
the problem.

In July 1985, our laboratories started to explore the use
of newly designed lipophilic cisplatin analogues for liposome entrapment. The goals of such effort were to obtain
more active and less toxic platinum complexes that would be
suitable for liposome entrapment. We felt that the following characteristics should be pursued for drug/liposome
selection: 1. decreased target organ toxicity, 2. enhanced
activity, 3. non-cross resistance and 4. lipophilicity.
These liposome entrapped compounds could then be used for

those uses or tumors for which liposome entrapment may offer definite therapeutic advantages. The research program has so far resulted in several different liposomal-platinum preparations with a high entrapment and stability. We present here the formulation characteristics and biological activity of the liposomal-platinum preparation that was selected for further development (liposomal-NDDP, L-NDDP). Clinical studies with L-NDDP are at present in progress under an FDA appoved IND at M. D. Anderson Hospital.

Chemical Structure of Platinum Compounds Designed for Liposome Entrapment

The main guideline for the synthesis of these molecules is shown in Table 1. Essentially, two types of structural changes were incorporated: changes that increase the therapeutic index of the drug and changes that make the molecule lipophilic and hopefully suited for liposome entrapment. Among the structural changes that increase the therapeutic index of the drug, the attachment of a cyclohexane group to the 2 amino groups was a logical choice since it has been previously shown to decrease the nephrotoxicity of the drug and make the complex not cross resistant with cisplatin (6). Among the structural changes that make the complex lipophilic, different aliphatic leaving groups were attached substituting the chloride groups, in general with very good results.

Following these guidelines, several platinum derivatives were synthesized and formulated in liposomes (7-9). Cis-bis-neodecanoato trans R,R,- 1,2-diaminocyclohexane (DACH) platinum (II) (NDDP) was selected for further preclinical development based on its high antitumor activity and satisfactory liposome formulation in a lyophilized form. Chemical structure of NDDP is shown below:

R,R',R" can be an aliphatic group comprising 2 to 6 carbons.

TABLE 1
DESIGN OF PLATINUM COMPOUNDS FOR LIPOSOME ENTRAPMENT

Chemical Structure	Properties
Cisplatin	Nephrotoxic Liposome formulation: Not possible
1,2-DACH-dichloro Platinum	Less nephrotoxic Not cross resistant Liposome formulation: Not possible[a]
Dicarboxylato-1,2-DACH Platinum R=R'=aliphatic leaving group	Less nephrotoxic Not cross resistant Satisfactory liposome Formulation

[a]Compound is insoluble in common organic solvents

Preparation and Characterization of Liposomal-NDDP (L-NDDP) for Clinical Use

Dimyristoylphosphatidyl choline (DMPC) and dimyristoyl-phosphatidyl glycerol (DMPG) (Avanti Polar Lipids,

Birmingham, AL) (in a 7:3 molar ratio) are mixed with NDDP
in a ratio of 15:1 (lipid:drug) in chloroform. The
chloroform is evaporated using a rotary evaporator. The
lipid bilayer containing the phospholipids and NDDP is
redissolved in t-butanol (1 mg NDDP:1 ml t-butanol) with
mild hand-shaking, the solution is frozen and lyophilized
overnight. A white flaky powder is obtained with the
characteristics shown in Table 2.

TABLE 2
CHARACTERIZATION OF LYOPHILIZED L-NDDP

Characteristics	Batch #1	Batch #2
1. Appearance	White, flaky powder	White, flaky powder
2. Purity by TLC	No impurities	No impurities
3. Sterility	Sterile	Sterile
4. Endotoxin content (ng/mg NDDP)	<.025	<.025
5. Platinum (weight%)	1.31	1.25
6. Phospholipid (weight%)	85.9	85.1
7. Residual organic solvent (weight%) t-butyl alcohol chloroform	0.004 0.059	0.013 0.057

Lyophilized L-NDDP is stable at 4°C for at least 28 days.

Liposomes containing NDDP are obtained by reconstituting
the lyophilized L-NDDP with sodium chloride solution (0.9%)
in water (1 ml/mg NDDP) and mild hand shaking for 1 minute.
The liposomes obtained are multilamellar vesicles with the
characteristics shown in Table 3.

In Vivo Antitumor Activity of L-NDDP

The antitumor activity of L-NDDP was tested in 3 mouse tumor models using different schedules and routes of administration and compared with those of free NDDP (in suspension in 2% ethanol and Tween 20), cisplatin (Platinol, Bristol Lab), and carboplatin (Bristol Lab).

TABLE 3
CHARACTERIZATION OF RECONSTITUTED L-NDDP

Characteristics	Batch #1	Batch #2
1. Appearance	White, milky suspension	White, milky suspension
2. Purity by TLC	no detectable impurities	no detectable impurities
3. Entrapment (%)	100	99.6
4. Osmolality (mosm/l)	292	293
5. Ph	5.53	5.53
6. Size (% vesicles 1-5 μm)	>95	>95

Reconstituted L-NDDP is stable at least for 6 hours at room temperature.

Initially, the activity against intraperitoneal L1210 leukemia was assessed. Drugs were administered intraperitoneally on day 1 or days 1, 5, and 9. Results were expressed in %T/C (median survival of treated animals:median survival of control animals x 100) and are shown below. Results presented are the mean of several different experiments.

Subsequently, the antitumor activity against intraperitoneal L1210/PDD leukemia, a tumor resistant to cisplatin was tested. Drugs were administered intraperitoneally on days 1, 5, and 9. Mean results of different experiments are shown in Table 5.

TABLE 4
ANTITUMOR ACTIVITY OF L-NDDP AGAINST L1210 LEUKEMIA

Drug	Optimal Dose mg/kg	Schedule Day	%T/C
Cisplatin	10	1	175
Carboplatin	125	1	133
L-NDDP	25	1	187
Free NDDP	50	1	128
Cisplatin	6	1,5,9	225
Free NDDP	25	1,5,9	133
L-NDDP	12.5	1,5,9	300

TABLE 5
ANTITUMOR ACTIVITY OF L-NDDP AGAINST L1210/PDD LEUKEMIA

Drug	Optimal Dose mg/kg	Schedule Day	%T/C
Cisplatin	6	1,5,9	112
L-NDDP	12.5	1,5,9	200
Free NDDP	50	1,5,9	128

Finally, the antitumor activity of L-NDDP administered intravenously against established experimental liver metastases of a phagocytic tumor, M5076 reticulosarcoma, was assessed (10). Tumor cells (2 x 10^4) were inoculated intravenously on day 0. Treatment at the maximum tolerated dose was administered intravenously on days 4, 8, and 12. Control animals usually die between days 21 and 28 after tumor inoculation. Treated animals were divided in 2 groups. Some animals were sacrificed approximately 1 week after the death of the control animals, the livers were ressected, fixed in Bouin's fixative and the number of liver metastases counted.

The remaining animals were used for recording the survival times. A summary of the results obtained is shown in Table 6.

TABLE 6
ANTITUMOR ACTIVITY OF L–NDDP AGAINST LIVER METASTASES OF
M5076 RETICULOSARCOMA

Drug	Optimal Dose mg/kg	Median N^o Liver Metastases	Mean Survival Days
Cisplatin	7.5	>200	39 ± 3
L–NDDP	12.5	0	57 ± 9^a
Free NDDP	25	–	23 ± 3
Control	–	–	21 ± 2

[a] p <.05 compared with animals treated with cisplatin and free NDDP.

Similar survival experiments were also performed comparing equimolar doses of cisplatin and L–NDDP instead of maximum tolerated doses. At a dose of 20 μmol/kg on days 4, 8, 12, and 16, survival of animals treated with L–NDDP was significantly longer than that of animals treated with cisplatin (mean survival 48 ± 5 vs 36 ± 2 days, p=<.05).

These studies show that L–NDDP has comparable antitumor activity against L1210 leukemia, is not cross resistant with cisplatin against the L1210/PDD cell line, and is more effective than cisplatin in the treatment of established liver metastases of M5076 reticulosarcoma.

Toxicity of L–NDDP

Nephrotoxicity and neurotoxicity are the acute and chronic dose–limiting toxicities of cisplatin, respectively. Toxicity studies were carried out in mice and dogs to ascertain the safety and spectrum of toxicity of L–NDDP. In CD1 mice, the single dose intravenous LD50 of different batches of L–NDDP ranged from 46 to 64 mg/kg depending on the weight of the animals used. In the same experiments,

cisplatin (Platinol, Bristol) had an LD50 of 21 to 23 mg/kg.
For both drugs, all deaths occurred within 2 weeks of drug
administration.

The renal dysfunction and myelosuppression secondary to
L-NDDP and cisplatin were studied at the LD50 dose. Blood
was drawn 96 hours after intravenous drug administration.
Results of BUN, granulocyte count, and platelet count are
shown in Table 7.

TABLE 7
ACUTE TOXIC EFFECTS OF L-NDDP

Drug	BUN mg%	Granulocytes $10^3/mm^3$	Platelets $10^6/mm^3$
Cisplatin	255 $\pm$ 86	2.1 $\pm$ 0.6	1.3 $\pm$ 0.3
L-NDDP	30 $\pm$ 2	0.2 $\pm$ 0.1	0.2 $\pm$ 0.1
Control	31 $\pm$ 5	1.9 $\pm$ 1.0	1.3 $\pm$ 0.0

These studies demonstrate that the spectrum of toxicity
of cisplatin and L-NDDP in mice are different. Cisplatin at
the LD50 dose is markedly nephrotoxic but does not produce
significant myelosuppression while at an equitoxic dose
L-NDDP does not affect the renal function but produces
profound myelosuppression. Pathology studies in mice treated
with the LD50 dose of L-NDDP did not show significant
changes in major organs.

Toxicity studies in dogs were designed to establish the
maximum tolerated dose of L-NDDP administered intravenously
in a rapid infusion (4mg/NDDP per minute), to assess the
spectrum of toxicity of L-NDDP at the maximum tolerated
dose, to establish the dose-limiting toxicity of L-NDDP, and
to assess the cumulative toxicity of L-NDDP administered
monthly for 4 to 6 months.

The maximum tolerated dose was above 150 mg/m^2. This
dose was well tolerated repeatedly by 3 different animals
and resulted in short-lasting side effects with vomiting
starting 2 hours after the completion of drug infusion and
lasting for 2 hours, transient elevation of liver enzymes
for 48 hours, mild and short-lived granulocytopenia and
thrombocytopenia occurring 7-10 days after drug infusion,

and mild and transient BUN elevation. No significant weight
loss was observed.
The lethal dose was established at 225 mg/m². This dose
was given to 2 animals. One animal had protracted diarrhea
for 2-3 weeks, requiring intravenous fluids, 30-40% weight
loss, transient elevation of liver enzymes, and mild granulocytopenia, thrombocytopenia, and BUN elevation. The animal
was sacrificed 5 weeks after drug administration. Autopsy
did not show significant changes apart from mild enteritis.
The second animal died with gastrointestinal bleeding 48
hours after drug infusion. Autopsy showed diffuse hemorrhagic enteritis and acute renal tubular damage. A third
animal received 300 mg/m². This animal also died with
gastrointestinal bleeding 48 hours after drug infusion.
Autopsy showed diffuse hemorrhages, mainly in the gastrointestinal tract, and acute renal tubular damage. These
studies suggest that the dose limiting toxicity of L-NDDP in
dogs is not myelosuppression but gastrointestinal toxicity
and a diffuse hemorrhagic syndrome, probably related to
endothelial damage.
   In chronic toxicity studies, 3 dogs were treated at the
maximum tolerated dose monthly up to a cumulative dose of
600 to 700 mg/m² of L-NDDP. No weight loss was recorded.
The side effects after each dose administration were as
described above. Cumulative effects on the bone marrow and
kidney function were minor. Findings at autopsy were limited
to mild gastrointestinal, liver and kidney changes.

Conclusions and Remarks

   We have presented here a summary of the preclinical
development (liposomal formulation, antitumor activity, and
toxicity) of an antineoplastic agent formulated in a
liposomal carrier (L-NDDP). The drug was specifically
selected among several promising compounds of similar
structure because its formulation in liposomes was simple,
reproducible, and amenable to scaling up procedures. The
antitumor activity studies showed that the liposomal
formulation of the drug was more active than the parent
compound (cisplatin) against 2 in vivo murine tumor models.
The non-entrapped drug was not active, either because it
could not be delivered appropriately, or because it degrades
fastly in aqueous milieu. NDDP is a liposome-dependent drug.
We are, at present, applying this concept to the development
of other liposome entrapped antitumor agents.

REFERENCES

1. Weinstein JN, Leserman LD (1984). Liposomes as drug
    carriers in cancer chemotherapy. Pharmacol Ther
    24:207-232.
2. Mayhew E, Papahadjopoulos D (1983). Therapeutic
    applications of liposomes. In Ostro MJ (ed):
    "Liposomes," New York: Marcel Dekker, p 289-338.
3. Herman EH, Rahman A, Ferrans VJ, Vick JA, Schein PS
    (1983). Prevention of chronic doxorubicin cardiotoxicity
    in beagles by liposomal encapsulation. Cancer Res
    43:5427-5432.
4. Gabizon A, Goren D, Fuks Z, Barenholz Y, Dagan A,
    Meshorer A (1983). Enhancement of adriamycin delivery to
    liver metastatic cells with increased tumoricidal effect
    using liposomes as drug carriers. Cancer Res
    43:4730-4735.
5. Mayhew E, Goldrosen M, Vaage J, Rustum Y (1986).
    Liposomal-adriamycin and survival of mice bearing liver
    metastases of colon carcinomas 26 and 38. Proc Am Assoc
    Cancer Res 27:403.
6. Burchenal JH, Kalaher K, O'Toole T, Chisholm J (1977).
    Lack of cross-resistance between certain platinum
    coordination compounds in mouse leukemia. Cancer Res
    37:3455-3457.
7. Perez-Soler R, Khokhar AR, Lopez-Berestein G (1986).
    Toxicity and antitumor activity of cis-bis-
    cyclopentenecarboxylato-1,2-diaminocyclohexane platinum
    (II) encapsulated in multilamellar vesicles. Cancer Res
    46:6269-6273.
8. Lautersztain J, Perez-Soler R, Khokhar AR, Newman RA,
    Lopez-Berestein G (1986). Pharmacokinetics and tissue
    distribution of liposome-encapsulated cis-bis-N-
    decyliminodiacetato-1,2- diaminocyclohexane platinum
    (II). Cancer Chemother Pharmacol 18:93-97.
9. Perez-Soler R, Khokhar AR, Lopez-Berestein G (1987).
    Treatment and prophylaxis of experimental liver
    metastases of M5076 reticulosarcoma with cis-bis-
    neodecanoato- trans-R,R- 1,2-diaminocyclohexane platinum
    (II) encapsulated in multilamellar vesicles. Cancer Res
    47:6462-6466.
10. Talmadge JE, Key ME, Hart IR (1981). Characterization of
    a murine ovarian reticulum cell sarcoma of histiocytic
    origin. Cancer Res 41:1271-1280.

Liposomes in the Therapy of Infectious Diseases and Cancer, pages 71–80
© 1989 Alan R. Liss, Inc.

LIPOSOME THERAPY: A NOVEL APPROACH
TO THE TREATMENT OF CHILDHOOD OSTEOSARCOMA[1]

Eugenie S. Kleinerman, M.D. and Melissa M. Hudson, M.D.[2]

University of Texas System Cancer Center
M.D. Anderson Hospital and Tumor Institute
Department of Cell Biology and Pediatrics
Houston, Texas 77030

The majority of children who present with osteosarcoma have pulmonary micrometastasis at the time of diagnosis. However, these micrometastasis are not visible on X-ray, computerized tomography (CT) scan or pulmonary tomography. Following surgical resection alone, 80 to 90% of the patients develop pulmonary metastasis within 6 to 9 months of diagnosis (1). Adjuvant chemotherapy coupled with surgical resection of the primary tumor has improved survival from 20% at 2 years to approximately 60% at 5 years (1-3). Unfortunately, despite the use of effective adjuvant chemotherapy, about 40% of patients with osteosarcoma still develop pulmonary metastasis. In our experience 30% of the total patient population develop their pulmonary metastasis while receiving adjuvant chemotherapy suggesting resistant tumor cell clones. The remaining 10% develop metastasis after chemotherapy is discontinued. Our proposal is to use monocytes activated by liposomal MTP-PE in vivo to eradicate the residual micrometastasis that we know exists in the lungs of these children and thus prevent the development of pulmonary tumors.

Following in vitro incubation with liposomal MTP-PE human monocytes selectively kill malignant but not normal cells (4, 5). Eighty to 90% of liposomes injected intravenously into mice are taken up in the liver, spleen and peripheral blood monocytes; 8 to 10% are localized in the pulmonary microvasculature resulting in activation of pulmonary macrophages to the tumoricidal stage without

[1]This work was supported by National Institutes of Health Grants CA42992 (ESK) and CA09070 (Training Program in Pediatric Oncology)
[2]Fellow of the American Cancer Society

evidence of local or systemic toxicity (6). Liposomal MTP-PE (a lipophilic derivative of muramyl dipeptide) can thus be directed to pulmonary macrophages to activate the host defense against pulmonary metastasis.

We are suggesting the use of liposomal MTP-PE as an additional adjuvant in the treatment of osteosarcoma for two reasons. First, since only microscopic disease exists in these patients after removal of the primary tumor, the tumor burden (i.e. tumor-to-macrophage ratio) is favorable for the effective destruction by activated macrophages (8). Second, the natural history of osteosarcoma parallels that of the B16 melanoma tumor model developed and subsequently successfully treated with liposome therapy (9). In this model microscopic pulmonary metastases arise from a primary tumor of the extremity. Once the primary tumor is surgically removed, these pulmonary metastases can be eradicated following multiple intravenous injections of liposomal MTP-PE.

Seventy-five per cent of the patients that we are attempting "to cure" develop pulmonary metastases while on chemotherapy. Therefore, we believe that liposomal MTP-PE should be combined with the chemotherapy regimens early in therapy in order to eliminate the resistant tumor cells. Prior to designing such a protocol, we felt imperative to evaluate two factors: (1) the ability of monocytes from patients with osteosarcoma to be activated in vitro by liposomal MTP-PE. (2) the effect of chemotherapy on liposomal MTP-PE's ability to activate monocyte-mediated cytotoxicity. Armed with this data, reasonable treatment schedules can be proposed to maximize the ability of macrophages to erradicate pulmonary micrometastases in osteosarcoma.

RESULTS AND DISCUSSION

Activation Of Monocyte-Mediated Tumoricidal Function By Liposomal MTP-PE.

To determine whether monocytes from children with osteosarcoma were capable of being activated by liposomal MTP-PE, peripheral blood monocytes from 20 newly diagnosed osteosarcoma patients were isolated prior to therapy and incubated overnight with medium or liposomal MTP-PE (100 nM/2×10^5 cells). Cytotoxicity was then measured against [^{125}I]IUdR-labeled A375 cells as previously described (4).

After stimulation with liposomal MTP-PE, monocytes from each of the 20 patients lysed tumor target cells at levels equal to or greater than those expressed by normal controls (Fig. 1). The median cytotoxic value of the osteosarcoma group was 20% and was not significantly different from that of our control group (median = 17%, P>0.2 by the Wilcoxon Rank Summation Test). Thus monocytes from patients with osteosarcoma can respond to the activating stimulus MTP-PE encapsulated in liposomes and are capable of killing tumor cells once activated.

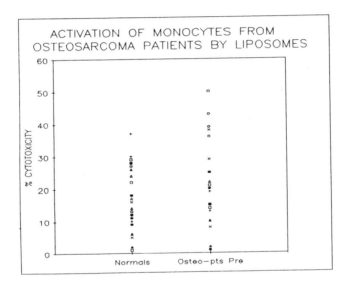

Fig 1.   Tumorilytic activity of liposomal MTP-PE activated monocytes from osteosarcoma patients vs. normal controls.   Peripheral blood monocytes were isolated separately from 20 newly diagnosed osteosarcoma patients and 24 normal controls, incubated with either control liposomes or liposomal MTP-PE for 24 hr, washed and then assayed for cytotoxicity against [^{125}IUdR-labeled A375 tumor target cells in a 72 hr assay. Effector-target ratio is 10:1. Each point represents the % generated cytotoxicity of the liposomal MTP-PE - activated monocytes minus control-treated monocytes.
    The monocytes from 2/20 osteosarcoma patients and 4/20 normal controls could not be activated by liposomal MTP-PE (Fig. 1, cytotoxic values < 10%). However, each of these individuals responded normally to free activators

(LPS 1 μg/ml; IFNγ+ MDP [1000 U/ml + 100 ng/ml]) making the likelihood of an intrinsic monocyte defect small. The failure of liposomal MTP-PE to activate tumorical function maybe secondary to an inability of these individuals to phagocytose the liposomes, although no data to support this hypothesis is available at this time. If liposomal uptake does not occur universally, liposome therapy may not be effective in every patient. An in vitro screening procedure may therefore provide a useful tool to assess which patients may respond to liposome-encapsulated activators such as MTP-PE.

Cisplatin (CDP) and Adriamycin (ADR) are two chemotherapeutic agents that are widely used as adjuvants in the treatment of osteosarcoma. We envision using liposomal MTP-PE in conjunction with other effective chemotherapy rather than as the sole agent for adjuvant treatment. If chemotherapy transiently depresses monocyte function, it would be important to know the time frame of the recovery phase before proposing in vivo treatment schedules with liposomal MTP-PE. We, therefore, wished to determine whether CDP or ADR administration would subsequently interfere with MTP-PE's ability to activate the tumoricidal properties of monocytes.

Effect of Cisplatin (CDP) Administration On Monocyte Activation By Liposomal MTP-PE.

To assess the effect of CDP therapy on the ability of liposomal MTP-PE to activate monocyte-mediated tumoricidal function, peripheral blood monocytes were isolated from 15 osteosarcoma patients immediately before and 2 weeks after the intra-arterial administration of CDP (150 mg/m^2). These monocytes were incubated with control liposomes or liposomal MTP-PE (100 nM/2x10^5 cells) overnight prior to the addition of [^{125}I]IUdR-labelled A375 cells. Cytotoxicity was determined 72 hours later as previously described (4). As shown in Figure 2, 5/15 patients showed a decrease in the level of cytotoxic activity generated by liposomal MTP-PE, 3/15 showed an increase and 7/15 demonstrated no changed. In this group there was no significant difference in mean cytotoxic values before (20%) and after (17%) CDP therapy. When 16 normal volunteers were tested on two separate occasions, 2/16 showed a decrease in the level of cytotoxic activity generated by liposomal MTP-PE, 4/16 showed an increase and 10/16 demonstrated no change. Therefore, we interpret these results to mean that CDP administration did not interfere with the ability of liposomal MTP-PE to activate monocyte tumoricidal function.

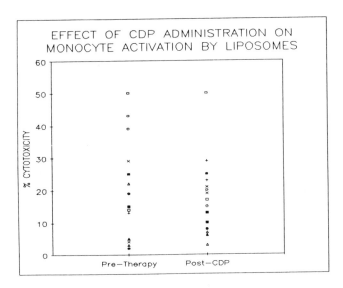

Fig. 2 Effect of CDP therapy on Monocyte Activation by Liposomal-MTP-PE. Ten milliliters of heparinized blood were drawn from 15 patients with osteosarcoma prior to and 2 weeks after intra-arterial CDP therapy (150 mg/m^2). Monocytes were isolated and incubated with control liposomes or liposomal MTP-PE for 24 hr, washed and then assayed for cytotoxicity against [^{125}I]IUdR-labeled A375 tumor targeted cells. Effector-target ratio is 10:1. Each point represents the % generated cytotoxicity as expressed in Fig 1.

Effect Of ADR on The Activation of Normal Monocytes by Liposomal MTP-PE.

To assess the effect of ADR on the ability of liposomal MTP-PE to activate monocyte-mediated cytotoxicity, normal monocytes were treated in the presence of ADR (0.5-500 ng/ml) with either control liposomes or liposomal MTP-PE (100 nM/2x10^5 cells). Monocytes incubated with liposomal MTP-PE demonstrated 39±3% cytotoxicity. The presence of ADR for 24 hours during the activation process of liposomal MTP-PE resulted in the generation of 31±9% cytotoxicity. Pretreatment of monocytes with ADR for 1 hour also failed to inhibit the ability of liposomal MTP-PE to activate normal monocytes.

Effect of ADR on Interleukin 1 (IL-1) Production by Monocytes.

Monocyte-mediated tumoricidal activity has recently been shown to be closely associated with the production of IL-1 by monocytes (10-12). Anything that interferes with the monocyte's ability to produce and secrete Il-1 may also interfere with its ability to kill tumor cells (12). We, therefore, studied the effect of ADR on monocyte-mediated IL-1 production. Monocyte cultures were incubated with medium alone, ADR (500 ng/ml), LPS (1 μg/ml) or ADR±LPS. All supernatants were collected 24 and 48 hours later, extensively dialyzed to remove ADR and then assayed for IL-1 activity using the D10G4.1 assay as previously described (12). Monocytes incubated with medium, or ADR alone did not release IL-1 at either 24 or 48 hours. Significant IL-1 activity was demonstrated in the supernatants of both LPS and LPS + ADR treated monocytes. The IL-1 activity was uneffected by the presence of ADR. Therefore, we found no evidence that ADR inactivates IL-1 release by tumoricidal monocytes. Furthermore, ADR by itself does not induce the secretion of IL-1 by monocytes.

Effect Of ADR Therapy On Monocyte Activation By Liposomal MTP-PE.

To determine if ADR therapy effects monocyte function in patients with osteosarcoma, peripheral blood monocytes were isolated from 9 patients at the time of referral prior to the initiation of any therapy and then one month after ADR therapy (75 mg/m^2). These monocytes were then incubated with control liposomes or liposomal MTP-PE overnight prior to the addition of radiolabelled A375 tumor cells. Cytotoxicity was determined 72 hours later. Table 1 shows the results of these studies. The peripheral blood monocytes from each patient isolated 1 month after ADR therapy could be activated in vitro by liposomal MTP-PE to kill tumor cells. In fact, the activated cytotoxic function was significantly increased in 7 of 9 patients (p<0.02). Similar results were obtained with peripheral blood monocytes from these patients 2 and 3 weeks after ADR therapy. Thus, ADR appeared to have no adverse effect on the ability of liposomal MTP-PE to activate monocytes.

There is even a suggestion of enhanced activation subsequent to ADR therapy (Table 1).

TABLE 1
EFFECT OF IN VIVO ADR THERAPY ON MONOCYTE
ACTIVATION BY LIPOSOMAL MTP-PE[a]

Patient No.	% Generated Cytotoxicity	
	Pre-ADR	Post-ADR
1	25	41
2	23	21
3	21	54
4	15	42
5	15	18
6	13	16
7	8	35
8	8	29
9	3	3

[a]Monocytes were isolated from patients before and one month after ADR therapy, then stimulated with control liposomes or liposomal MTP-PE for 24 h. Cytotoxicity against [^{125}I]IUdR-labeled A375 melanoma cells were quantified 72 hr later.

The monocytes from one patient (pt. #9) could not be activated by liposomal MTP-PE either pre or post ADR administration (Table 1). This same patient was one of the patients that failed to show activation to liposomal MTP-PE at the time of diagnosis, pre and post CDP therapy (See Figure 1, 2). Once again soluble agents were able to activate the cytotoxic function of this patients' monocytes (Table 2). The patient received ADR post surgical excision of the primary tumor and had no detectable metastasis at the time the blood samples were drawn. Therefore, the failure to respond to liposomal MTP-PE was not reversed by either tumor removal or chemotherapy.

To determine the immediate effect of ADR therapy on monocyte function, blood samples were obtained prior to ADR therapy and one day after ADR infusion in 4 patients. Liposomal MTP-PE activated the tumoricidal function of monocytes from 3 of 4 patients to levels equal to or even slightly greater than pre-ADR levels (Table 3). This suggestion of enhanced cytotoxicity after ADR therapy indicates that there may be a potential benefit to combining

ADR and liposomal MTP-PE in the adjuvant treatment setting. The monocytes from the one remaining patient could still be rendered tumoricidal by liposomal MTP-PE subsequent to ADR therapy, though the level of cytotoxic activity was markedly decreased (Table 3).

TABLE 2
TUMORILYTIC ACTIVITY OF ACTIVATED
MONOCYTES FROM ONE OSTEOSARCOMA PATIENT

| Treatment of Monocytes[a] | % Generated Cytotoxicity[b] | |
	Pre-ADR	Post ADR
LPS	36	58
IFNγ+ MDP	39	37
Liposomal MTP-PE	3	3

[a]Peripheral blood monocytes were isolated from one osteosarcoma patient prior to and one month after ADR therapy (75 mg/m^2) and incubated with free activators [LPS (1 µg/ml) or IFNγ(10^4 U/ml) plus MDP (100 ng/ml)] or liposomal MTP-PE for 24 hr. Cytotoxicity against [^{125}I]IUdR labeled A375 melanoma cells was quantified 72 hr later.

[b]% cytotoxicity as compared to monocytes treated with medium.

TABLE 3
EFFECT OF ADR ADMINISTRATION ON
MONOCYTE ACTIVATION BY LIPOSOMAL MTP-PE

| Patient | % Generated Cytotoxicity | |
	Pre ADR	Post ADR
A	17	34
B	56	79
C	70	29
D	17	40

[a]Monocytes were isolated from 4 patients with osteosarcoma before and one day after ADR therapy, then incubated with liposomal MTP-PE for 24 hr. Cytotoxicity against [^{125}I]IUdR-labeled A375 melanoma cells was quantified 72 hr later.

Based on the above data, we believe that liposomal MTP-PE may be effectively combined with either CDP or ADR therapy in the adjuvant treatment of osteosarcoma. All the results demonstrate that the administration of either CDP or ADR did not interfere with monocyte activation by liposomal MTP-PE or the subsequent lysis of tumor cells by the activated monocytes. There's even a suggestion of enhanced tumoricidal activity in patients' monocytes activated by liposomal MTP-PE after exposure to ADR. We would, therefore, like to propose that liposomal MTP-PE be coupled with ADR for the treatment of childhood osteosarcoma in the adjuvant setting.

REFERENCES

1. Jaffe, N (1985). Chemotherapy in osteosarcoma: Advances and controversies. In Muggia FH (ed): "Experimental and Clinical Progess in Cancer Chemotherapy", Boston: Martinus Nijhoff Publishers, p. 223.

2. Link MP, Goorin AM, Miser AW, Green AA, Pratt CB, Belasco JB, Pritchard J, Malpas JS, Baker AC, Kirkpatrick JA, Ayala AG, Shuster JJ, Abelson UT, Simone JV, Viehi TJ (1986). The effect of adjuvant chemotherapy on relapse-free survival in patients with osteosarcoma of the extremity. NEJM 314:1600.

3. Eilber F, Giulian A, Eckardt J, Patterson K, Moseley S, Goodnight J (1987). Adjuvant chemotherapy for osteosarcoma: A randomized prospective trial. J Clin Oncol 5:21.

4. Kleinerman ES, Schroit AJ, Fogler WE, Fidler IJ (1983). Tumoricidal activity of human monocytes activated in vitro by free and liposome-encapsulated human lymphokines. J Clin Invest 72:304.

5. Fidler IJ, Kleinerman ES (1984). Lymphokine-activated human blood monocytes destroy tumor but not normal cells under cocultivation conditions. J Clin Oncol 2:937.

6. Fidler IJ, Barnes Z, Fogler WE, Kirsh R, Bugelski P, Poste G (1982). Involvement of macrophages in the eradication of established metastases following intravenous injection of liposomes containing macrophage activators. Cancer Res 42:496.

7. Poste G, Bucana C, Raz A, Bugelski P, Kirsh E, Fidler IJ (1982). Analyses of the fate of systemically administered liposomes and implications for their use in drug delivery. Cancer Res 42:1412.

8. Fidler IJ, Poste G (1982). Macrophage-mediated destruction of malignant tumor cells and new strategies for the therapy of metastatic diseases. Springer Semin Immunopathol 5:161.

9. Fidler IJ (1980). Therapy of spontaneous metastases by intravenous injections of liposomes containing lymphokines. Science 208:1469.

10. Onozaki K, Matsushima K, Aggrawal BB, Oppenheim JJ (1985). Human interleukin 1 is a cytocidal factor for several tumor lines. J Immunol 135:3962.

11. Lachman LB, Dinarello CA, Llansa ND, Fidler IJ (1986). Natural and recombinant human interleukin 1-β is cytotoxic for human melanoma cells. J Immunol 136:3098.

12. Kleinerman ES, Lachman LB, Knowles RD, Snyderman R, Cianciola GJ (1987). A synthetic peptide homologous to the envelope proteins of retroviruses inhibits monocyte-mediated killing by inactivating interleukin 1. J Immunol 139:2329.

Liposomes in the Therapy of Infectious Diseases and Cancer, pages 81–94
© 1989 Alan R. Liss, Inc.

TUMORCYTOTOXICITY OF LIVER MACROPHAGES AS INDUCED BY LIPOSOME - ASSOCIATED IMMUNOMODULATORS[1]

Toos Daemen[2], Machiel Hardonk[3], Jan Koudstaal[3], Wolter Oosterhuis[3], Jan Dijkstra[4] and Gerrit Scherphof[2]

State University Groningen, Medical School

ABSTRACT   It is demonstrated that rat liver macrophages can be activated to a tumorcytotoxic state when incubated with muramyldipeptide(MDP)-containing liposomes. Liposome-encapsulation leads to a several hundred fold increase in the activating potency of the MDP, in contrast to lipopolysaccharide (LPS) or lipid A, which loose their activating potency as a result of liposome-encapsulation. It is shown that this may be due to intralysosomal inactivation since both LPS and lipid A, but not MDP, were shown to loose their immuno-modulating properties upon incubation with lysosomal enzymes. Liver macrophages isolated after intravenous administration of liposome-encapsulated MDP were also found to be cytotoxic, when assayed in vitro, and this cytotoxicity was shown to be evenly distributed among five subfractions of macrophages. Administration of liposome-encapsulated MDP effectively reduced the development of liver metastases in mice inoculated intrasplenically with colon adenocarcinoma cells and significantly extended the life span of the animals. The liver macrophage population was shown to double within 24 h after injection of liposomal MDP. This increase is transient and due to both influx of new cells and local proliferation of resident macrophages. Since,

[1] This work was supported by Grant no. GUKC 83-10 of the Netherlands Cancer Foundation, Koningin Wilhelmina Fonds
[2]Laboratory of Physiological Chemistry, Bloemsingel 10, 9712 KZ Groningen, The Netherlands
[3]Laboratory of Pathology, Oostersingel 63, 9713 EZ Groningen, The Netherlands
[4]Infectious Disease Unit, Veterans Administration Medical Center, West Haven CT 06516, U.S.A.

in vitro, we found the macrophages to be refractory to a second stimulus after the cytotoxic state of a first stimulus has decayed, the observed effect of liposomal MDP on the kinetics of the liver macrophage population may play a decisive role in main taining the cytotoxic state of the macrophage population   required for effective tumor cell killing in vivo.

INTRODUCTION

The successful attempts of Fidler and Poste and their associates to boost the macrophage activating potency of biological response modifiers by encapsulation in liposomes, leading to eradication of established lung metastases in mice after injection of these encapsulated activators (1,2) led us to initiate a study on the activation of liver macrophages by immunomodulators associated with liposomes. A major incentive to start this work was the notion that hepatic metastases from colo-rectal cancers form a major cause of death from cancer in men. No effective therapy of such metastatic liver disease is known to date; yet the clinical practice often involves conditions favorable for an immuno-therapeutic approach, i.e. the existence of a low tumor burden at the time of surgical treatment of the primary tumor. This situation would therefore be ideally suited for an approach with activated macrophages, particularly since the liver, an organ exceptionally rich in macrophages, is the main site of clearance of an injected dose of liposomes from the circulation This, in turn, makes the liposome an ideal carrier for the immuno-activators to be used.

Finally, our previous work on the isolation of liver macrophages and the uptake and processing of liposomes by these cells (3-5), provided a firm experimental background.

METHODS

Isolation of liver macrophages (Kupffer cells).

Liver macrophages were isolated according to established procedures (6) involving brief perfusion of the liver with pronase, digestion of hepatocytes with pronase and purification on a metrizamide gradient followed by counter-flow centrifugation (3,7).

Preparation of liposomes.

Liposomes were prepared as described in detail elsewhere (7), from egg lecithin, cholesterol and dicetylphosphate in a 4 : 5 : 1 molar ratio unless indicated otherwise. The hydrated lipids were extruded through a series of polycarbonate membranes with 0.4 µm as the ultimate pore diameter. Non-encapsulated materials were removed by gelfiltration.

Cytotoxicity assays.

Macrophage-mediated *cytolysis* was assessed by a ^{3}H-deoxythymidine(dThd) release assay (7). Briefly, target cells were labeled with ^{3}H-dThd and added to (activated) macrophages in a 1 : 25 ratio, unless indicated otherwise. Fourty eight hours after the addition of the target cells the culture media were assayed for radioactivity. Specific cytolysis was calculated as

$$\frac{a - b}{c - b} \times 100\ \%, \text{ in which}$$

a = dpm in medium of target cells co-cultured with test macrophages;

b = dpm in medium of target cells co-cultured with control macrophages;

c = total dpm in target cells added.

Macrophage-mediated *cytostasis* was assessed as inhibition of ^{3}H-dThd incorporation into target cells after 24 h incubation with (activated) macrophages.

RESULTS

In vitro activation of Kupffer cells.

Table 1 shows that substantial levels of both cytolysis and cytostasis can be induced in cultured Kupffer cells by incubation with liposome-encapsulated MDP; free MDP at the same dose levels fails to cause either cytolysis or cytostasis (not shown); at all liposome concentrations control liposomes not containing MDP produced the same level of radioactivity release or reduction of label incorporation as medium alone (not shown).

Table 2 demonstrates that also LPS is able to induce a cytolytic effect in cultured cells and that there is a synergism between this activation and either free or liposome-encapsulated MDP. Apparently, the synergistic effect requires the two activators to be present simultaneously.

Of substantial influence is the amount of lipid used for encapsulation. For example, in order to attain a 40 % cytolysis value with a liposome preparation containing 10 ng of MDP per nmol of lipid more than ten times as much MDP was required as of a prepa-

Table 1.   Effect of liposome-encapsulated MDP on macrophage cytolytic and cytostatic activity.

macrophage treatment[a]	liposomal lipid (nmol/well)	dpm released in supernatant[b] (% cytolysis)	dpm incorporated[c] (% cytostasis)
MDP-liposomes (1ng MDP/nmol lipid)	200	1306 ± 3 (56)	121 ± 16 (99)
	100	1082 ± 84 (41)	220 ± 79 (98)
	50	929 ± 64 (31)	962 ± 21 (89)
	25	938 ± 78 (31)	1303 ± 29 (86)
Medium		463 ± 45 (1)	9105 ± 572

a.   *Per well 25×10^4 liver macrophages were incubated with medium,
     control liposomes, or liposomes containing 1 ng of MDP per
     nmol of liposomal lipid.*
b.   *After 4 h, 10^4 [^{3}H]dThd-labeled melanoma cells were added per
     well. After another 48 h, ^{3}H release into the supernatant was
     determined in triplicate experiments. Numbers in parentheses,
     percentage of specific cytolysis; see "Methods".*
c.   *After an incubation of 4 h with the immunomodulators 10^4
     melanoma cells were added per well. After 24 h of cocultivation
     [^{3}H]dThd was added to the wells for another 24 h. At this time
     (48 h of cocultivation) the cultures were washed 3 times with
     PBS, and the cells were lysed with 0.5 M NaOH. Radioactivity of
     the lysate was determined in triplicate experiments. Numbers in
     parentheses, percentage of inhibition; see "Methods".*

ration containing only 1 ng of MDP per nmol of lipid (Table 3).
Although in most of our experiments we applied a macrophage to
target cell ratio of 25 : 1, this is not a prerequisite to obtainmaximal
cytotoxicity ratings, provided that the absolute density of the
macrophages is sufficiently high to allow the formation of a confluent
monolayer (Fig.1). If that condition is fulfilled, a 5 : 1 ratio may
produce the same cytotoxicity as a 30 : 1 ratio. Although not all
tumor cell lines displayed the same sensitivity towards Kupffer cell-
induced cytolysis, the cytolytic action is restricted to tumor cells,
normal cells being virtually fully resistant (Table 4). By contrast, the
inhibitory effect of the activated Kupffer cells on thymidine
incorporation (cytostatic action) was not restricted to tumor cells as
up to 95 % inhibition was found for normal fibroblasts. With respect

Table 2. Synergism of LPS and free or liposome-encapsulated MDP on macrophage cytolytic activity

First macrophage treatment[a]	Second macrophage treatment[b]	dpm released in supernatant[b]
LPS		$464 \pm 36^c(13)^d$
MDP		425 ± 8 (11)
MDP-liposomes		858 ± 54 (36)
LPS + MDP		1264 ± 24 (60)[e]
LPS + MDP-liposomes		1409 ± 6 (68)[f]
LPS	MDP	795 ± 28 (32)[g]
MDP	LPS	799 ± 82 (33)
LPS	MDP-liposomes	871 ± 70 (37)
MDP-liposomes	LPS	799 ± 10 (33)
Medium		237 ± 39
B16 cells alone		220 ± 12

a. *Twenty-five x 10^4 rat liver macrophages were incubated with medium (control) or the indicated immunomodulators. LPS (5 ng/ml), MDP (5 µg/well), and MDP-liposomes (50 ng of MDP per well encapsulated in 50 nmol of liposomal lipid). After 4 h, medium or a second immunomodulator, together with 10^4 [^{3}H]dThd-labeled melanoma cells, was added to the wells without removing the first immunomodulator(s).*
b. *Cytolytic activity was determined after a 48-h coculture of macrophages and [^{3}H]dThd-labeled melanoma cells. ^{3}H release into the supernatant was determined in triplicate experiments.*
c. *Mean $\pm$ SD*
d. *Numbers in parentheses, percentage of specific cytolysis; see "Methods".*
e. *Statistical significance compared to the sum of cytolysis induced by both immunomodulators alone (Student's t test), P<0.005.*
f. *P<0.025.*
g. *P<0.050.*

to the site of action of the various activating substances it is of interest to note the fundamental difference we observed between the effect of liposome encapsulation of MDP on the one hand and LPS

Table 3. **Influence of the amount of encapsulating lipid on liposomal MDP-induced cytolytic activity.**

molar ratio lipid/MDP	amount of liposome-encapsulated MDP per 25 x 10^4 macrophages							
	5	10	25	50	100	250	500	1000
0.1				$14\pm4^*$	18 ± 3	28 ± 5	36 ± 3	47 ± 4
1.0		8 ± 1	19 ± 2	37 ± 3	41 ± 4	39 ± 2		

*) percent specific cytolysis ± standard deviation

25 x 10^4 macrophages were incubated with medium (control) or liposome-encapsulated MDP. MDP was encapsulated in different amounts of lipid: 0.1 or 1.0 nmol of lipid per ng of MDP.
After 4 h, 10^4 [^{3}H]dThd-labeled B16 melanoma cells were added; after another 48 h ^{3}H release into the medium was used to calculate specific cytolysis.

or lipid A on the other hand. Whereas encapsulation of MDP, as outlined above, resulted in a more than 100-fold increase of its activating potency, the liposome entrapment of LPS or lipid A *reduced* the activity of these agents by at least the same factor. This is shown in Fig. 2, which demonstrates that at a concentration at which free, unencapsulated LPS gives rise to a cytotoxicity level of about 40 %, the encapsulated agent still has negligible activating potency. Only at relatively high concentrations (>10^{-1} μg/ml) is the encapsulated LPS equally active as the free LPS; this activity is likely to be accounted for by a small (∼1 %) proportion of non-encapsulated material. For lipid A we found a similar result (not shown), except that for this stimulant no significant level of cytolysis was produced at any of the concentrations tested, when the agent was added in liposome-associated form. Presumably, the lipid A remains more firmly liposome-bound than the more polar LPS.

In view of our observations that LPS and lipid A loose their macrophage-activating potency upon incubation with liposomal fractions at acidic pH (Fig. 3) we presume that the liposome-encapsulated LPS and lipid A are efficiently inactivated in the lysosomal compartment of the Kupffer cells following endocytic uptake. In contrast, MDP is

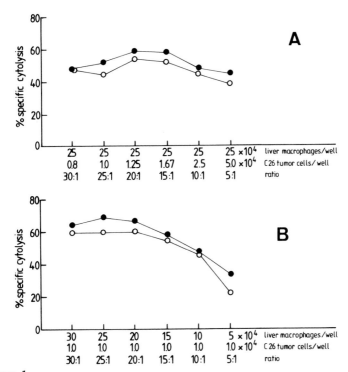

Figure 1.
The effect of the macrophage to tumor cell ratio on macrophage-mediated cytolysis.
Macrophages were incubated with medium (control), with free MDP (50 ug / ml, -O-) or with liposome-encapsulated MDP (500 nmol of lipid containing 500 ng of MDP per ml; -O-). Macrophages and C26 colon adenocarcinoma cells were cultured as described in the Methods section.
A. The ratio was changed by varying the number of tumor cells added to a constant number of macrophages (25×10^4 per well) plated.
B. The ratio was changed by varying the plating density of the macrophages and adding a fixed number of C26 cells (10^4 per well).
The experiment was carried out in triplicate. Plotted are the mean percentages of specific cytolysis (see Methods).

not degraded or modified to an extent that leads to inactivation, but rather becomes available to its intracellular target site(s) upon release from the lysosomal compartment following intralysosomal degradation of the liposomes. Considering the much lower activity of free *vs-*

Table 4. Susceptibility of different tumor cell lines and normal cell lines to macrophage-mediated cytolysis and proliferation inhibition.

Macrophage[a] treatment	dpm released in supernatant (% specific cytolysis)[b]			
(µg MDP/ml)	B16	C26	LLC	Fibroblasts
liposomal-MDP				
(0.5)	929 ± 54 (31)	821 ± 68 (71)	240 ± 20 (4)	2721 ± 97 (4)
free MDP (50.0)	841 ± 99 (26)	761 ± 28 (64)	269 ± 9 (8)	2752 ± 147 (5)
Medium	463 ± 44	195 ± 34	211 ± 19	2597 ± 125
tumor cells alone	440 ± 20	122 ± 27	160 ± 11	2006 ± 90

Macrophage[a] treatment (µg MDP/ml)	dpm incorporated (% proliferation inhibition)[c]			
	B16	C26	LLC	Fibroblasts
liposomal-MDP				
(0.5)	962 ± 21 (89)	109 ± 7 (93)	214 ± 41 (78)	164 ± 21 (96)
free MDP (50.0)	535 ± 23 (94)	134 ± 13 (91)	159 ± 15 (75)	183 ± 18 (95)
medium	9105 ± 572	1441 ± 310	628 ± 65	3940 ± 240
tumor cells alone	8668 ± 556	1790 ± 210	1138 ± 47	9636 ± 649

a. Per well $25x10^4$ liver macrophages were incubated with medium, free MDP or liposome-encapsulated MDP (1 ng of MDP per nmol of liposomal lipid).

b. After 4 h the wells were washed and 10^4 [^{3}H]dThd-labeled target cells were added per well. After another 48 h, ^{3}H release into the supernatant was determined in triplicate experiments. Numbers in parentheses, percentage of specific cytolysis; see "Methods".

c. After an incubation of 4 h with the immunomodulators the wells were washed and 10^4 target cells were added per well. After 24 h of coculture [^{3}H]dThd was added to the wells for another 20 h. At this time, the cultures were washed 3 times with PBS, and the cells were lysed with NaOH. Radioactivity of the lysate was determined in triplicate. Numbers in parentheses, percentage of proliferation inhibition; see "Methods".

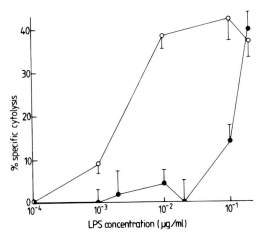

Figure 2
Macrophage-mediated cytolysis with free and liposome-incorporated
LPS. Per well of a 96-well microtiter plate $25x10^4$ liver macrophages
were incubated with medium (control), free LPS (O), or liposomes
containing 0.1 ng of LPS per nmol of liposomal lipid (●). Tumor
cytotoxicity was determined and plotted as described in the legend
of figure 1.

encapsulated MDP, this implies that the (major) target site for the
MDP is located intracellularly, whereas that for LPS or lipid A is
more likely to be at the cell surface. Our results and their
interpretation are compatible with those of Dijkstra et al. (8) who
observed a drastic decrease in LPS-induced interleukin-1 production
by macrophages when the LPS was encapsulated in liposomes. Fogler
et al. (9), on the other hand, reported a stimulatory effect of liposome
encapsulation on LPS-induced macrophage cytotoxicity, similar to
what these authors observed for MDP. On the basis of our experience
with the encapsulation of different types of LPS (8) we think it
likely that this discrepancy relates to the way in which the LPS is
associated with the liposomes, i.e. truly encapsulated vs. bilayer-
associated.

   For a successful immunotherapeutic approach of metastatic growth
in the liver with liposome-encapsulated MDP it is necessary that,
following the intravenous administration of such a preparation, the
liver macrophage population acquires a tumor cytotoxic state. We
found, indeed, that liver macrophages, isolated 18 h after i.v.
injection of liposomal MDP, were cytotoxic to B16 melanoma cells
and C26 colon adenocarcinoma cells in vitro. Moreover, we
demonstrated that five subfractions of macrophages, obtained by a
stepwise increase of the counterflow during centrifugal elutriation,

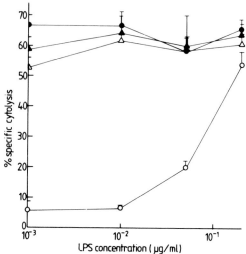

Figure 3

Effect of lysosomal enzymes on LPS induced macrophage cytotoxicity. Per well of a 96-well microtiter plate $25x10^4$ liver macrophages were incubated with medium (control), LPS preincubated without lysosomal fraction at pH 7.4 (▲) or pH 4.8 (●), LPS preincubated with sonicated lysosomal fraction at pH 7.4 (△) or pH 4.8 (O) for 1 h at 37^oC. Tumor cytotoxicity was determined and plotted as described in the legend of figure 1.

were approximately equally active in terms of cytolytic activity. On the other hand, we found that in vivo liposome uptake substantially varies with cell size, larger cells taking up considerably higher amounts of liposomes than the smaller cells, even when corrected for cell size (Fig.4). Thus, it may be that the smaller cells have a higher intrinsic potential to become cytotoxic than the larger cells but that this difference is compensated by higher uptake capacity of the larger cells. In any case, our results show that in vivo induced cytotoxicity is roughly evenly distributed among liver macrophages of different size classes; this suggests that macrophages all through the liver will become activated as a result of an injection with liposomal MDP, a condition favorable for efficient eradication or suppression of liver metastatic growth.

In a liver metastasis model in the mouse, employing C26 colon adenocarcinoma cells injected in the spleen, we showed that treatment with liposome-encapsulated MDP results in a drastic reduction in tumor growth in the liver (Table 5). The effect was more outspoken when treatment was started before tumor cell inoculation, but also when treatment was started 1 or 2 days after injection of the tumor cells, the effect was still highly significant.

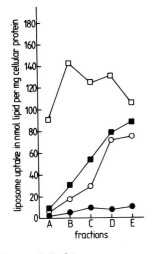

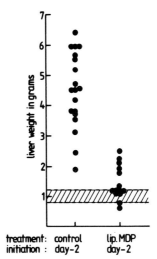

Figure 4 (left)
In vivo uptake of [³H]-cholesteryl hexadecylether(CE)-containing liposomes. Multilamellar vesicles composed of egg-PC:cholesterol:DCP (in a 4:5:1 molar ratio) containing [³H]-CE were injected via the lateral tail vein at the given doses. After 18 h macrophage subfractions were isolated. Aliquots were taken for cell counts and radioactivity measurements.
Given is the mean uptake in nmol of lipid per mg of cellular protein after the injection of 5 μmol (□), 1 μmol (■), 0.5 μmol (O) and 0.1 μmol (●) of lipid. Duplicate experiments agreed within 10%.

Figure 5 (right)
Effect of liposomal MDP therapy on the liver weight of tumor bearing mice on the day of death.
5 x 10⁴ C26 colon adenocarcinoma cells were injected into the spleen of BALB/c mice on day 0; on day 3 the mice were splenectomized. Treatment with liposome-encapsulated MDP (5 ug in 1 umol of lipid daily for 10 consecutive days) was initiated two days prior to tumor cell inoculation. Control mice were injected with buffer. The data represent the results of two experiments. Each point represents the liver weight in grams of an individual mouse on the day the animal died. Shaded area; liver weight of normal mice not bearing a tumor.

In a survival study we also found a significant increase in survival (from 27 days to 36 days, average survival time), but after 45 days still all of 23 mice, except one, were dead (as compared to all of 35 control mice after 33 days). In nearly all cases the cause of death of the treated mice was related to local recurrence of the tumor causing massive tumor growth invading the peritoneal cavity. At the

Table 5.   Reduction of development of liver metastases by
liposome-encapsulated MDP treatment

	% of mice with (number of mice with)[b]:			number of	
Initiation of therapy[a]	more than 10 metastases	1 to 10 metastases	no metastases	mice	experiments
day 2	40% (n= 2)	40% (n= 2)	20% (n= 1)	5	1
day 1	41% (n=12)	38% (n=11)	21% (n= 6)	29	3
day -1	20% (n= 1)	20% (n= 1)	60% (n= 3)	5	1
day -2	4% (n= 1)	52% (n=13)	44% (n=11)	25	3
control[c]	91% (n=53)	8% (n= 5)	0%	58	7

a. *5x10⁴ C26 colon adenocarcinoma cells were injected into the spleen of BALB/c mice on day 0; on day 3 the spleen was resected. Liposome-encapsulated MDP (1 μmol of liposomal lipid containing 5 μg of MDP per treatment per mouse) was injected i.v or i.p.. Treatment was started on the indicated day.*
b. *The mice were killed on day 17 and the number of metastatic foci was counted.*
c. *Control mice were injected with Hepes-NaCl-buffer.*

time of death of the treated animals most livers were free of tumor growth, or tumor growth was limited, as is seen from the liver weights presented in Fig. 5.

During our in vivo studies we noted that the yield of macrophages from rats injected with liposomal MDP was consistently higher than that from control animals. In a detailed study in which we used monoclonal anti-macrophage antibodies to identify the macrophages in liver sections we quantified the dynamics of the macrophage population. Fig. 6 shows how the number of ED_2-positive cells in the liver doubles within about 24 hours after a single injection of MDP-containing liposomes and subsequently declines to control values in the following 48 hours. By using, in addition, fluorescent latex particles to mark the macrophages present before liposomal MDP injection, and by applying another antibody, directed against Br-dUrd, to identify proliferating cells, we were able to conclude that both local proliferation of resident macrophages and recruitment from extrahepatic sources contribute to the population increase.

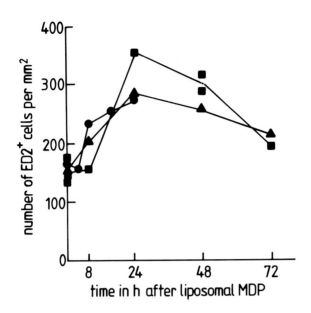

Figure 6
*Effect of injection with liposomal MDP on the population of ED2
antigen expressing liver macrophages.*
*The number of ED2$^+$ cells per mm^2 liver tissue. Each point represents
the mean number of cells counted in minimally 10 microscopic fields
(0.35 mm^2) of an individual rat liver.*
*The results of three different experiments are presented, indicated
by circles, triangles and squares, respectively.*

These preliminary observations may be highly pertinent to the overall
cytotoxic effect of the Kupffer cell population as observed in the
experiments with the metastasizing colon carcinoma cells.

It remains to be seen what the relative contribution of the various
macrophage subpopulations is to the antimetastatic activity observed.
These observations are particularly relevant since we observed before
that, when Kupffer cells have in maintenance culture lost their
cytotoxic activity in the 1-2 days after they were activated, they
are refractory to a second stimulus. Thus, sustained antimetastatic
activity of the liver macrophage population during prolonged
immunotherapeutic treatment may have to rely on the continuous
renewal of the population by influx from the blood (bone marrow)
and/or by local proliferation.

ACKNOWLEDGMENTS

The authors express their gratitude to Aletta Veninga, Sippy Huitema, Bert Dontje and Jan Wijbenga for expert technical assistance and to Lineke Klap for preparing the typescript. Dr. C.D. Dijkstra of the Department of Histology of the Free University of Amsterdam is gratefully acknowledged for providing us with the monoclonal antimacrophage antibodies and Dr. L. de Ley from the Department of Clinical Oncology of the State University at Groningen for a generous gift of the monoclonal anti Br-dUrd antibody.

REFERENCES

1.   Fidler IJ, (1980). Therapy of spontaneous metastases by intravenous injection of liposomes containing lymphokines. Science 208: 1469.

2.   Fidler IJ, Barnes Z, Fogler, WE, Kirsch R, Bugelski P, Poste G (1982). Involvement of macrophages in the eradication of established metastases following intravenous injection of liposomes containing macrophage activators. Cancer Res 42: 496.

3.   Dijkstra J, Van Galen WJM, Hulstaert CE, Kalicharan D, Roerdink FH, Scherphof GL (1984). Interaction of liposomes with Kupffer cells in vitro. Exp Cell Res 150: 161.

4.   Dijkstra J, Van Galen WJM, Scherphof GL (1984). Effects of ammoniumchloride and chloroquine on endocytic uptake of liposomes by Kupffer cells in vitro. Biochim Biophys Acta 804: 58.

5.   Dijkstra J, Van Galen WJM, Regts J, Scherphof GL (1985). Uptake and processing of liposomal phospholipids by Kupffer cells in vitro. Eur J Biochem 148: 391.

6.   Knook DL, Sleijster EC (1976). Separation of Kupffer and endothelial cells of the rat liver by centrifugal elutriation. Exp Cell Res 99: 444.

7.   Daemen T, Veninga A, Roerdink FH, Scherphof GL (1986). In vitro activation of rat liver macrophages to tumoricidal activity by free or liposome-encapsulated muramyldipeptide. Cancer Res 46: 4330.

8.   Dijkstra J, Mellors JW, Ryan JL, Szoka FC (1987). Modulation of the biological activity of bacterial endotoxin by incorporation into liposomes. J Immunol 138: 2663.

9.   Fogler WE, Talmadge JE, Fidler IJ (1983). The activation of tumoricidal properties in macrophages of endotoxin responder and nonresponder mice by liposome-encapsulated immuno-modulators. J Reticuloendothel Soc 33: 165.

Liposomes in the Therapy of Infectious Diseases and Cancer, pages 95–103
© 1989 Alan R. Liss, Inc.

TREATMENT OF ACUTE MYELOGENOUS LEUKAEMIA WITH LIPOSOMES CONTAINING N4-OLEYL-CYTOSINE ARABINOSIDE

R.Schwendener[1],B.Pestalozzi[2],S.Berger[3],
H.Schott[4],H.Hengartner[1], and C.Sauter[2]

Departments of Experimental Pathology[1] and
Medicine[2], University Hospital, Zürich
Institute of Pharmacology[3], University of Zürich, and
Institute of Organic Chemistry[4],University of
Tübingen, FRG.

ABSTRACT

Cytosine-arabinoside (ara-C) is one of the most active
drugs for the treatment of acute myelogenous leukaemia
(AML). Optimal dosage and mode of drug application are,
however, still a matter of debate and new strategies of
therapy are needed.thus, we implemented a phase I/II
study with liposomes containing N4-oleyl-ara-C
(NOAC) in patients resistant to conventional chemo-
therapy.Sterile bilayer liposomes of 80–100nm diameter
were prepared by capillary dialysis.Plasma concentrations of NOAC, ara-C,and ara-U were determined by HPLC.
Among others, one AML patient was treated with NOAC-
liposome infusions of 500 ml containing 420 mg NOAC (=
200 mg ara-C) for 3 cycles on day 1,4,7 and for 3
cycles on day 1–6.
During the day 1–6 cycles NOAC concentration decreased
exponentially, indicating a plasma saturation effect.
The patient achieved a partial remission,thus encouraging further use of the liposomal therapy.

INTRODUCTION

Lipophilic prodrugs of ara-C incorporated into bilayer
liposomes showed significantly   higher therapeutic effects
against L1210 murine leukaemia when compared to the free
drug. Among the prodrugs tested, NOAC had the strongest

cytostatic effect (1). Another lipophilic analogue of ara-C, namely N[4]-behenoyl-ara-C, is presently being tested in clinical trials , but not in a liposomal application form (2). Today the treatment of acute leukaemia with conventional chemotherapy shows not a much better long-term prognosis as in the mid-seventies (3,4). Therefore, new treatment strategies, such as the use of liposomes as drug delivery systems are needed.

Before performing phase I/II trials, we investigated cytotoxic effects and organ distribution of NOAC liposomes in an animal model.

Here, we present the first clinical results of AML patients treated with infusions of NOAC liposomes.

METHODS

Materials

All materials used were the same as described before (1,5).

Preparation of NOAC Liposomes

Sterile and pyrogen free liposomes were prepared as described before (5). Briefly, 28 g soy-phosphatidyl choline (SPC), 2.8 g cholesterol, 5.5 g NOAC and 0.15 g alpha-tocopherol were dissolved together with 34 g Na-cholate in 400 ml methanol/chloroform (1:1 v/v). The organic solvents were removed on a rotatory evaporator. A micellar solution was obtained by addition of 600 ml of PBS to the dry lipid/detergent mixture. After filtration through a 0.2 um sterile filter, the detergent was dialyzed through 3 serially connected cartridges (Travenol[R], ST-12) as described in detail in reference 5. After dialysis, aliquots of the NOAC liposomes were diluted into sterile 0.9% NaCl solutions to give 500 ml infusions containing 420 mg NOAC corresponding to 200 mg of ara-C.

Likewise, reference liposomes (2.5 g SPC, 0.25 g cholesterol and 0.15 g alpha-tocopherol) without prodrug were prepared and diluted into one liter of 0.9% NaCl infusions.

Sterility and absence of pyrogens were tested on CLED agar plates and with the USP rabbit test, respectively.

Liposome size and homogeneity were determined by dynamic laser light scattering (5).

HPLC Assay of the Prodrug and the Metabolite Ara-U

Concentrations of NOAC in the liposome infusions were determined on a C18 reverse phase column (25 x 0.4 cm) with methanol/water (93:7 v/v%) as a solvent phase at a flowrate of 1 ml/min and UV detection at 254 nm. Blood samples from patients were collected in heparinized tubes containing 50 ug tetrahydrouridine as a deaminase inhibitor. NOAC was extracted from plasma aliquots with methanol on Bondelut C18 columns and analyzed as described above. Ara-U (and ara-C) were extracted from plasma by filtration through an Amicon MPS-1 micropartition system. Aliquots of 100 ul plasma filtrate were injected onto a dual column (C18 RP & SCX Partisil) HPLC system as described elsewhere (6).

Whole Body Autoradiography of NOAC Liposomes in Mice.

Ring labelled ^{3}H-NOAC liposomes and ^{3}H-ara-C in PBS, as a reference, were injected i.v. into groups of 3 ICR mice (18-22 g). After 2, 30 min, 6, and 24 hours the animals were killed and whole body sagittal sections of 20 um thickness were prepared (7). The sections were exposed on Hyperfilm [3]H (Amersham) at -20° C for 50 days.

Evaluation of Patients

Patients hospitalized with a malignant haematologic disorder who had normal renal and hepatic functions and gave informal consent were eligible for the phase I study. Each patient received an infusion of 1000 ml drug-free liposomes given over 6 hours. The four patients treated with drug-free liposomal infusions were monitored by various clinical and laboratory parameters before, during, and after the course of infusion.

Patients with an acute leukaemia resistant to standard polychemotherapy or in relapse were eligible for the phase II study if their renal function was normal, their liver enzymes at the most elevated twice above normal, and if thrombocyte substitution was possible. The therapy schedules are given in Table 1.

RESULTS

The NOAC liposomes are highly homogeneous and have a mean diameter of 80-100 nm as determined by laser light scattering. Batches of 10-15 x 500 ml of the NOAC liposomes were prepared and used within 6 months. Shelf stability is greater than 6 months (time of observation) at 4° C.

As shown in Figure 1, the organ distribution of liposomal NOAC in mice is drastically different from free ara-C with a major accumulation of NOAC in the liver. NOAC is preferentially eliminated through the bile, whereas ara-C shows pronounced renal elimination. Six hours after injection both drugs were quantitatively eliminated.

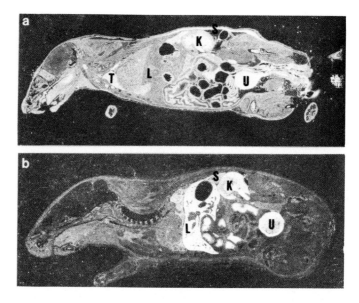

FIGURE 1. Whole-body autoradiography of a) ^{3}H-ara-C and b) ^{3}H-NOAC liposomes, both 30 min after i.v. injection. K,kidney, L,liver, S,spleen, T,thymus and U, urinary bladder.

The patients' plasma levels of NOAC and ara-U, the main metabolite of ara-C, during the day 1-6 cycle are shown in Figure 2. Ara-C could only be detected in nanogram concentrations immediately after infusion. NOAC is eliminated from the circulation at a $t_{1/2}$ of 25 min. Furthermore, plasma saturation occurs during treatment with a decrease from 2 ug/ml on day one to 0.5-1 ug/ml on day 6.

Ara-U maintains a constant level of about 2 ug/ml through
the infusion cycle. Calculated from one single infusion, a
plasma half-time of 8 hours was found for ara-U.

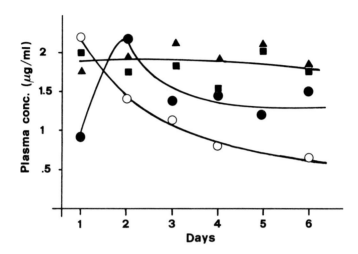

FIGURE 2. Plasma levels of NOAC and ara-U, day 1-6
infusion cycle. Values taken at the end of each single
infusion. o and ● NOAC, ▲ and ■ ara-U from two cycles of
patient No.5 (week 16 and 30, cfr. Table II).

Phase I study
In all four patients who received drug-free liposomes, no
toxic effects could be detected.

Phase II study
In Table 2, treatment and course of the disease of patient
No.5 are summarized. He had a very undifferentiated acute
leukaemia, classified as AML(MO) on the basis of
cytochemical and immunologic typing. His leukaemia was
resistant to two cycles of standard polychemotherapy, and
liposomal therapy with NOAC was initiated (cfr. Table 1).
    Although the effect of the first three therapy cycles
with liposomes on days 1,4, and 7 cannot clearly be
separated from the effect of the initial chemotherapy, it
appears that a partial remission had been achieved after
the first 6 day liposome cycle at week 16 (cfr. Table 2,
bold values).

TABLE 1
PATIENT CHARACTERISTICS AND LIPOSOME THERAPY

Patient	Age/sex	Diagnosis[a]	Liposome therapy
Phase I:			
1 R.A.	72/f	NHL	drug-free x 1[b]
2 R.F.	50/m	NHL	drug-free x 1
3 M.H.	25/f	NHL	drug-free x 1
4 I.B.	37/f	NHL	drug-free x 1
Phase II:			
5 A.C.	50/m	AML(MO)	L3:NOAC,d1,4,7 x 3[c]
			L6:NOAC,d1-6 x 3
6 N.B.	46/m	AML(M2)	L3:NOAC,d1,4,7 x 1
7 P.M.	48/m	AML(M2)	L6:NOAC,d1-6 x 1

[a]NHL, Non Hodgkins lymphoma, AML, acute myelogenous leukaemia; MO..M2, FAB classification.
[b]Infusion of 1000 ml liposomes during 6 hours.
[c]Infusion of 500 ml (420 mg NOAC) during 3 hours.

Blast cells were reduced to zero for the 6 following
weeks and thrombocytes increased to subnormal levels such
that the patient did not require further thrombocyte
substitution for 14 weeks and could thus be managed on an
ambulatory basis. There was no clearcut effect on marrow
morphology. The subsequent 6 day treatment cycles also
showed cytoreductive effects, without much benefit to the
patient who died after 51 weeks with a pararectal abcess.
    Patient No. 6 was in his terminal phase when liposomal
treatment was initiated. He died of thrombocytopenia related subdural haematoma of the spinal chord, unrelated to
liposomal therapy.
    Patient No. 7 developed multiple chloromas, especially
at catheter entry sites when liposome therapy was started
with a day 1-6 infusion cycle. The daily infusions were
administered on an ambulatory basis. He achieved a
reduction of blast cells in the peripheral blood and the
chloromas showed transient regression in size and
consistency. The patient died two months later of
uncontrolled sepsis.

TABLE 2
TREATMENT AND COURSE OF DISEASE OF PATIENT NO.5

Week	Th	BM	Lc	PMN	Bl	Tc	TcS	EcS[a]
1	AD	4/M4	10.0	1.50	8.50	187	–	2
2	O		0.5	0.06	0	93	2	2
3	VM	RL	0.4	0.03	0	9	2	4
4			0.4	0.01	0	14	2	2
5		RL	0.3	0.01	0	21	1	4
6		RL	0.6	0.02	0	6	2	4
7	L3		0.3	0.01	0	14	2	3
8			1.0	0.50	0	13	1	–
9		1/M2	1.8	1.10	0	15	–	–
10	L3		0.7	0.24	0	6	1	4
11			1.5	0.69	0	9	–	–
12		3/M3	2.2	1.20	0.05	23	–	4
13	L3		1.6	0.69	0.02	38	–	2
14			2.9	1.70	–	22	–	–
15		3/M3	4.5	2.80	0.13	58	–	–
16	L6		1.9	1.00	0.09	55	–	4
17			1.6	0.88	0	17	–	2
18		2-3/M4	2.4	1.40	0	18	–	–
20			2.5	0.95	0	58	–	–
22			3.6	1.20	1.20	115	–	–
24			3.8	1.20	1.70	120	–	–
26			3.6	0.88	1.90	84	–	–
28			4.1	0.74	2.50	48	–	–
29		3/M4	5.8	0.83	4.40	48	–	–
30	L6		2.4	0.39	0.12	42	1	2
31			1.9	0.40	0.36	20	1	2
33			1.0	0.03	0.51	24	–	4
36			2.7	0.04	2.10	20	–	3
38			7.2	0.07	6.40	13	–	–
40	L6		9.7	0.10	7.40	12	1	2
41			1.6	0.16	1.20	15	2	4
46			2.1	0.05	1.40	21	1	2
51			2.0	0.07	1.80	13	–	–

Week, indicates the time from diagnosis. Week 1 gives the values before therapy. The given values are from the first day of the week, when the patient was hospitalized (weeks 1-13, 16-17, 29-30, 40, 45, 46-47, 49-51) and are the first values available when the patient was on ambulatory control.

Therapy (Th), consisted initially of free ara-C (A) 100 mg/m^2 daily in continuous infusion over 7 days and of daunorubicin (D) 45 mg/m^2 daily over 3 days. Vincristine (O) 0.8 mg/m^2 was given once on day 10. Starting on day 15, the second course consisted of VP-16 (V) 80 mg/m^2 plus m-Amsacrine (M) 120 mg/m^2 daily for 5 days.

Liposomal therapy(L3,L6),was given as indicated in Table 1. Bone marrow (BM), aspiration cytology was classified according to cellularity (0=aplastic, 1=hypocellular, 2=normocellular, 3=hypercellular, 4=packed) and percentage of blast cells (M1=0-5%, M2=6-25%, M3=26-50%, M4>50%).Residual leukaemia (RL), is the term applied when a hypocellular aspirate (cellularity 0-1) contains malignant cells.

Leukocytes (Lc), Polymorphonuclear neutrophils (PMN), blast cells (Bl), thrombocytes (Th), all in absolute numbers per mm^3 x 1000.

Thrombocyte-substitution (TcS), units of thrombocyte substitutions from random single donors, totalled over each week.

Erythrocyte-substitution (EcS), units of packed red blood cells, totalled over each week.

DISCUSSION

This work describes our pharmacological, experimental, and clinical results with unilamellar liposomes containing N[4]-oleyl-ara-C (NOAC).
The used capillary dialysis method allows fast and reproducible production of large quantities of liposomes containing lipophilic prodrugs.

Due to its prodrug character and the incorporation into lipid vesicles, the biodistribution of NOAC is drastically altered, as compared to free ara-C.

The autoradiography results show that NOAC follows the known pattern of organ distribution of liposomes, namely the preferential accumulation in the reticulo-endothelial system (RES).

The pharmacokinetic parameters of NOAC assessed from patient plasma confirm the data from animal studies. NOAC disappears from circulation at a fast rate, most probably by accumulation in the liver.Thus, the liver functions as a deep tissue deposit for the liposomes from where the prodrug or free ara-C is released. The early detection of ara-U in the plasma indicates that although integrated into liposomes, NOAC is not completely protected from enzymatic cleavage into ara-C and its fatty acid moiety (cfr. Figure 2).

The lipophilic character of these ara-C prodrugs alters their intracellular distribution as demonstrated by Ueda, et al., who found with in vitro studies, marked membrane accumulation of N[4]-behenoyl-ara-C in erythrocytes as well as in L1210 leukaemia cells (8).

Such a cell membrane affinity might also increase the cytostatic effect of liposomal NOAC, especially on tumor cells which are phagocytic.

Several modifications of the drug delivery system may further improve the pharmacological activity of incorporated prodrugs: a) by optimizing the lipid composition of the carrier vesicles, such that RES uptake is minimized, b) by variation of the chemical linkage of the lipophilic sidechain to the active drug moiety and c) by the construction of tumor cell specific liposome-antibody complexes which target the cytotoxic prodrug to the tumor cells.

Our clinical data of the three AML patients treated with NOAC liposomes do not allow us to draw conclusions on the value of liposomal therapy.

Nevertheless, the partial remission achieved in one patient and the effects observed in two others demonstrate the following advantages: a), the cytoreductive effects achieved and, b), the absence of toxic and non-haematological side effects. This encourages us to further use liposomes as carriers for cytostatic drugs or prodrugs.

ACKNOWLEDGEMENTS

The authors wish to thank Profs. R.Zinkernagel and P.Frick for their help. This work is supported by the Krebsliga of the Kanton Zürich and the Deutsche Krebshilfe.

REFERENCES

1. Rubas W,Supersaxo A, Weder, HG, Hartmann HR, Hengartner H, Schott H, Schwendener R (1986). Treatment of murine L1210 leukaemia and melanoma B16 with lipophilic cytosine arabinoside prodrugs incorporated into unilamellar liposomes. Int. J. Cancer 37:149.
2. Kimura K, et al. (1985). Treatment of acute myelogenous leukaemia in adults with N⁴-behenoyl-1-β-D-arabino-furanosylcytosine. Cancer 56:1913.
3. Sauter C,etal.(1984). Acute myelogenous leukaemia: Maintenance chemotherapy after early consolidation treatment does not prolong survival. The Lancet, February 18:379.
4. Sauter C, et al. (1987). Long-term results of two Swiss AML studies. Haematology and Blood Transf. 30:38.
5. Schwendener RA,(1986).The preparation of large volumes of homogeneous, sterile liposomes containing various lipophilic cytostatic drugs by the use of a capillary dialyzer. Cancer Drug Delivery 3:123.
6. Sinkule JA, Evans WE (1983). High-performance liquid chromatographic assay for cytosine arabinoside, uracil arabinoside and some related nucleosides. J.Chromatogr. 274:87.
7. Waser PG, et al.(1987). Localization of colloidal particles (liposomes, hexylcyanoacrylate nanoparticles and albumin nanoparticles) by histology and autoradiography in mice. Int. J. Pharmaceutics 39:213.
8. Ueda T, et al. (1983). Intracellular distribution of N⁴-behenoyl-1-β-D-arabinofuranosylcytosine in blood cells. Gann 74:445.

Liposomes in the Therapy of Infectious Diseases and Cancer, pages 105–116
© 1989 Alan R. Liss, Inc.

STUDIES ON THE MODE OF ACTION OF DOXORUBICIN-LIPOSOMES

G. Storm, U.K. Nässander, F.H. Roerdink[1], P.A. Steerenberg[2], W.H. de Jong[2], D.J.A. Crommelin

Department of Pharmaceutics, University of Utrecht, Croesestraat 79, 3522 AD Utrecht, [1] Laboratory of Physiological Chemistry, University of Groningen, Bloemsingel 10, 9712 KZ Groningen, [2] Department of Pathology, National Institute of Public Health and Environmental Hygiene, P.O. Box 1, 3720 BA Bilthoven, The Netherlands

ABSTRACT   Insights into the mode of action of DXR-liposomes are essential to establish conditions for an optimum therapeutic index by rationale. The results presented in this article point to sustained release as the primary mechanism by which liposome encapsulation of DXR increases the higher therapeutic index of the drug. After i.v. injection of DXR-liposomes two types of drug depots are operational: DXR is released directly from circulating liposomes but also indirectly from the reticuloendothelial system following uptake and processing by macrophages. The relative importance of each depot in the sustained release behavior of DXR-liposomes is dependent on the choice of liposomal lipid composition.

INTRODUCTION

Doxorubicin (DXR) is an established cytostatic drug active in a broad spectrum of human tumors. However, its cardiotoxicity is a major clinical handicap limiting its cumulative dose (1). Reports from several laboratories indicate that encapsulation of DXR into liposomes results in a significantly improved therapeutic index of the drug (2-7). This appears to be due to a reduced toxicity (including its notorious cardiotoxicity) without loss of antitumor activity. These findings prompted several groups to start clinical studies. Until now, no clear insights are available with regard to the mechanism(s) by which liposomes mediate this increase in therapeutic index. Therefore, studies were performed in order to elucidate the mode of action of DXR-liposomes.

METHODS

The experimental details can be found elsewhere (7-12). Here only a brief description is presented.

Liposomes. DXR-liposomes were prepared via the well-known "film method". The resulting multilamellar vesicles were sized by extrusion. Free (non-entrapped) DXR was removed with a cation exchange resin (8). Two types of DXR-liposomes were used: a "fluid" liposome type (egg-phosphatidylcholine (PC)/bovine brain phosphatidylserine (PS)/cholesterol (chol), molar ratio 10/1/4) and a "solid" liposome type (distearoylphosphatidylcholine (DSPC)/dipalmitoylphosphatidylglycerol (DPPG)/chol, molar ratio 10/1/10). The former liposomes are further referred to as PC/PS/chol liposomes and the latter as DSPC/DPPG/chol liposomes. As determined by ^{31}P-NMR measurements, PC/PS/chol liposomes had 1-2 and DSPC/DPPG/chol liposomes 2-3 bilayers.

Evaluation of antitumor activity. Male Lou/M Wsl rats were inoculated s.c. on the left flank with 10^4 IgM immunocytoma cells. Treatment started when the solid tumor had reached a diameter of 20 mm or more. The dose per injection was 2 mg DXR/kg body weight. Injections were performed i.v. on 5 consecutive days (day 0-4) followed by one more injection on day 11.

In vivo studies with radiolabeled DXR-liposomes. In experiments in which the association of liposomes with tumor tissue was studied, tumor-bearing Lou/M rats were given i.v. injections of DXR-liposomes radiolabeled with [^{3}H]inulin. [^{3}H]inulin was used as a marker of the encapsulated aqueous phase since it has proven to be a reliable liposome marker for uptake of intact liposomes (7,9,10,13). It is metabolically inert and has a very long retention time within cells once internalized with the help of liposomes. In free form (e.g. after leakage) it is rapidly cleared from the circulation by the kidneys and not taken up by tissues to any significant amount.

To study the in vivo integrity of DXR-liposomes following i.v. administration both the lipid component and the internal aqueous compartment were radiolabeled. Metabolically inert [^{3}H]inulin was used as radioactive marker of the entrapped aqueous space. Cholesteryl-1-[^{14}C]oleate was employed as marker of the lipid phase. In contrast to cholesterol, cholesteryl-1-[^{14}C]oleate does not interact with lipoproteins (14). Furthermore, this compound is susceptible to lysosomal esterase-activity resulting in the liberation of the labeled oleate from the cholesterol moiety (10,11). Consequently, as [^{3}H]inulin remains metabolically inert in the cells, intracellular degradation of the liposomes will result in an increase in the ^{3}H/^{14}C ratio of the injected liposome preparation.

In a next set of experiments, DXR-liposomes were double-radiolabeled with [^{3}H]inulin and [^{14}C]DXR in order to follow the fate of the encapsulated drug. Plasma pharmacokinetic studies have shown that i.v.

administered DXR disappears from the plasma very fast (15). Therefore, if [³H]inulin remains in circulating liposomes (9), release of DXR from circulating liposomes will be detected as an increase in the ³H/¹⁴C ratio of the injected liposome preparation.

In vitro studies on the processing of DXR-liposomes by liver macrophages. Kupffer cells were isolated from female Wistar rats by pronase digestion of the liver and purified by centrifugal elutriation, basically according to Knook and Sleyster (16) with some modifications as described by Dijkstra et al. (17). Release of DXR from the Kupffer cells into the supernatant following internalization of DXR-liposomes was monitored with the use of a HPLC method capable to detect not only intact DXR but also major metabolites (18).

RESULTS

Antitumor Activity

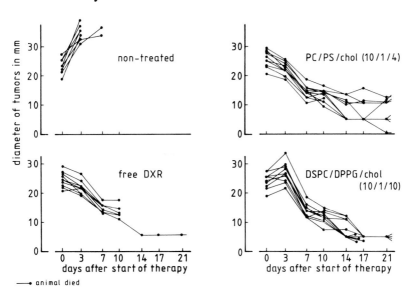

FIGURE 1. Antitumor activity of free DXR and DXR entrapped in different liposome types in solid IgM immunocytoma bearing Lou/M Wsl rats. 2 mg DXR/kg body weight was injected i.v. daily for 5 days (0-4) followed by one additional injection at day 11 after start of therapy. Results obtained during the first 21 days after start of treatment are shown. Treatment groups consisted of 10 animals.

Free DXR and DXR entrapped in the fluid PC/PS/chol liposomes induced a similar pattern of tumor regression (Fig.1). However, during the first three days after start of therapy, the solid DSPC/DPPG/chol liposomes did not induce tumor regression but only tumor growth retardation. After that initial period, the tumor showed regression similarly to the regression induced by PC/PS/chol liposomes and free DXR. Apparently, the antitumor activity of the DSPC/DPPG/chol liposomes was delayed significantly.

Detection of Radiolabeled Liposomes in Tumor Tissue

[^{3}H]Inulin-labeled DXR-liposomes were injected i.v. into tumor-bearing rats. Results are presented in Table 1. As it was found (results not shown) that 4 h after injection all PC/PS/chol liposomes were cleared from the circulation but that DSPC/DPPG/chol liposomes were still present in the blood in a considerable amount (about 20% of injected ^{3}H-dose), the association of the latter liposomes with tumor tissue was also studied 24 h after injection.

TABLE 1
DETECTION OF RADIOLABELED DXR-LIPOSOMES IN TUMOR
TISSUE

Liposome type	Time after injection (h)	Tumor-associated radioactivity (% of injected ^{3}H-dose)
Free [^{3}H]inulin	4	0.4 ± 0.1
PC/PS/chol	4	0.8 ± 0.2
DSPC/DPPG/chol	4	0.9 ± 0.2
	24	0.6 ± 0.1

DXR-liposomes radiolabeled with [^{3}H]inulin were administered i.v. to rats bearing a solid IgM immunocytoma (2 mg DXR/kg body weight). As a control, also free [^{3}H]inulin was injected at a label dose similar to that used for injection of liposomes. Results are expressed as mean ± SD of 3 animals.

Based on [^{3}H]inulin recovery, only a very low percentage of the injected amount of liposomes was found to be present in tumor tissue. No substantial difference in tumor-associated amounts of label between PC/PS/chol liposomes and DSPC/DPPG/chol liposomes was observed.

In Vivo Integrity with respect to the Liposomal Carrier:
Double-radiolabeling with [^{3}H]Inulin and Cholesteryl-1-[^{14}C]oleate

As pointed out in Methods, changes in the ^{3}H/^{14}C ratio associated with

DXR-liposomes double-radiolabeled with [^{3}H]inulin and cholesteryl-1-[^{14}C]oleate indicate that the structural integrity of the injected liposomes is affected. Leakage of [^{3}H]inulin from circulating liposomes will lead to a decrease and intracellular degradation of liposomes to an increase in ^{3}H/^{14}C ratio.

TABLE 2
IN VIVO RETENTION OF STRUCTURAL INTEGRITY OF
DXR-LIPOSOMES

Liposome type	Tissue	Ratio ^{3}H/^{14}C		Initial ratio ^{3}H/^{14}C of the liposome preparation
		1 h	4 h	
PC/PS/chol	Blood	5.0 ± 0.1	-[a]	5.1 ± 0.1 (n = 3)
	Liver	ND[b]	7.9 ± 0.6	
	Spleen	ND	53.3 ± 14.2	
DSPC/DPPG/chol	Blood	5.4 ± 0.1	5.7 ± 0.1	5.3 ± 0.1 (n = 3)
	Liver	ND	4.8 ± 0.4	
	Spleen	ND	6.9 ± 0.4	

DXR-liposomes, double-labeled with [^{3}H]inulin as a marker of the aqueous phase and cholesteryl-[^{14}C]oleate as a marker of the lipid phase were administered i.v. to rats (2 mg DXR/kg body weight). The results are expressed as the mean ± SD of 4 animals.
[a] Amounts of radioactivity too low for accurate determination
[b] ND, not determined

Following i.v. injection, most injected double-radiolabeled liposomes were taken up by liver and spleen (results not shown). Table 2 shows that both markers were cleared at similar rates from the circulation as the observed ^{3}H/^{14}C ratios equal those of the liposome preparations before injection up to at least one hour indicating that the vesicles remained intact during their stay in the bloodstream. The ^{3}H/^{14}C ratios measured in liver and spleen homogenates 4 h after injection denote that once within liver and spleen PC/PS/chol liposomes were degraded much faster than DSPC/DPPG/chol liposomes. In the spleen the ^{3}H/^{14}C ratio increased to a much higher extent for PC/PS/chol liposomes than for DSPC/DPPG/chol liposomes. In the liver the ^{3}H/^{14}C ratio also increased in case of the fluid liposome type, whereas for the solid liposome type the ratio did not increase at all. These observations indicate that the fluid PC/PS/chol liposomes are much more susceptible to intracellular degradation than the solid DSPC/DPPG/chol liposomes.

Processing of DXR-Liposomes by Liver Macrophages *In Vitro*

The difference in susceptibility to intracellular degradation of the two liposome types could also be demonstrated by incubating the vesicles, labeled with cholesteryl-1-[^{14}C]oleate, with cultured rat Kupffer cells (liver macrophages): PC/PS/chol liposomes were degraded considerably faster than DSPC/DPPG/chol liposomes. Similar results were found by incubating the two liposome types at pH 4.8 with lysosomal fractions isolated from rat liver homogenates: PC/PS/chol liposomes were much more sensitive to lysosomal esterase activity than DSPC/DPPG/chol liposomes (results not shown).

In order to investigate whether DXR and/or degradation products are released by macrophages after phagocytosis of DXR-containing liposomes and whether the observed differences in intracellular degradation rate between both liposome types are reflected in different release profiles of the drug, DXR-liposomes were incubated with Kupffer cell monolayers. After removal of unbound liposomes from the medium the cells were incubated for another 30 min in the presence of ammonium chloride to allow endosomes (containing liposomes) to fuse with primary lysosomes. An HPLC method was applied to monitor the release of not only intact DXR but also possible metabolites. From Table 3 it is clear that DXR was released from liposome-loaden Kupffer cells into the medium in a chemically intact form. However, the release of DXR from cells loaden with DSPC/DPPG/chol liposomes was significantly delayed as compared to the release from cells loaden with PC/PS/chol liposomes. Only minimal amounts of degradation products were detected in supernatants after prolonged incubation.

TABLE 3
RELEASE OF DXR FROM LIPOSOME-LOADEN KUPFFER CELLS

Liposome type	Percent DXR release				
	0 min	60 min	120 min	240 min	24 h
PC/PS/chol	n.d.[a]	11.9	5.8	6.1	84.9
DSPC/DPPG/chol	n.d.	n.d.	n.d.	n.d.	17.1

Kupffer cells in maintenance culture were incubated with DXR-liposomes at 37 °C for 60 min in the presence of 10 mM ammonium chloride. 2.5 µmol liposomal lipid was added to 5.7 x 10^6 cells. Unbound liposomes were washed away and the liposome-loaden cells were incubated for another 30 min in the presence of ammonium chloride. Thereafter (indicated as zero time) the medium was replaced by ammoniumchloride-free medium. At times indicated the medium was pipetted off, centrifuged and analysed for the amount of DXR released by the cells using HPLC. Data are expressed as percent of total cell-associated DXR at t = o.
[a] n.d., not detectable

In Vivo Integrity with respect to the <u>Encapsulated Drug</u>:
Double-radiolabeling with [^{3}H]Inulin and [^{14}C]DXR

DXR-liposomes were double-labeled with [^{3}H]inulin and [^{14}C]DXR. If DXR-liposome integrity is preserved on injection in the blood compartment, then the ratio between ^{3}H and ^{14}C should remain constant.

TABLE 4
DXR-LIPOSOME INTEGRITY IN BLOOD AFTER I.V. INJECTION

Time (min)	Ratio ^{3}H/^{14}C PC/PS/chol	DSPC/DPPG/chol
0[a]	2.4 ± 0.1	5.1 ± 0.1
10	3.6 ± 0.1	5.5 ± 0.1
30	6.1 ± 0.1	5.6 ± 0.1
60	11.2 ± 0.3	6.1 ± 0.1
120	25.0 ± 0.1	ND[b]

DXR-liposomes, double-radiolabeled with [^{3}H]inulin and [^{14}C]DXR were administered i.v. to rats at equal DXR (2 mg DXR/kg body weight) and lipid doses (170 μmol lipid/kg body weight). Results are expressed as mean ± SD of 3 animals.
[a] Initial ratio ^{3}H/^{14}C of the liposome preparation before injection (n=6)
[b] ND, not determined

As indicated by the increase in ^{3}H/^{14}C ratio upon i.v. injection (Table 4), DXR is released from circulating liposomes. The extent of DXR-release appeared to be liposome-type dependent. A much greater part of the liposomal DXR content is lost from PC/PS/chol liposomes than from DSPC/DPPG/chol liposomes. It can be estimated that PC/PS/chol liposomes lost about 65% and DSPC/DPPG/chol about 20% of the initially injected amount liposome-bound [^{14}C]DXR. The major part of the leaked amount of DXR was released within 30 min after injection: during this initial time period PC/PS/chol liposomes lost about 50% and DSPC/DPPG/chol liposomes about 10% of the injected liposomal DXR dose.

DISCUSSION

For a realistic assessment of the potential of DXR-liposomes in the clinical setting as well as for optimizing the results of chemotherapy with this novel treatment modality, a better understanding of the specific variables responsible for the superior therapeutic index induced by liposome encapsulation is needed.

Several hypotheses can be formulated for the mode of action of DXR-liposomes. There is experimental data suggesting that intact liposomes are capable of penetrating solid tumors *in vivo* (19). Therefore, a *site specific delivery* to the tumor can be proposed. However, to date most evidence available indicates that tumors do not take up substantial amounts of i.v. administered liposomes. The results concerning the association of DXR-liposomes with tumor tissue (Table 1) are in agreement with that view. As during DXR induced regression of the solid IgM immunocytoma a massive accumulation of macrophages at the tumor site occurs, we recently investigated the intriguing possibility that cells of the mononuclear phagocyte system are involved in transport of DXR-liposomes into the tumor (10). However, the results obtained suggest that DXR-liposomes do not enter the solid tumor, even when during therapy macrophages accumulate. In general, considering the inability of especially larger liposomes to pass through the vascular endothelium (20), the uptake of liposomal DXR may depend strongly on the structure and physiological condition of the tumor blood vessels (21).

The findings presented in this article and described more extensively in ref. 7 point to *sustained release* as the primary mechanism by which liposome encapsulation of DXR achieves a higher therapeutic index. This proposal for the mode of action is based on observations which are discussed in the following. Treatment of tumor-bearing rats with DXR-liposomes composed of solid-phase lipids in combination with relatively high amounts of cholesterol ("solid" liposomes, herein represented by DSPC/DPPG/chol (10:1:10)) resulted in a delayed tumor regression as compared to treatment with DXR-liposomes composed of fluid-phase lipids in combination with relatively low amounts of cholesterol ("fluid" liposomes, represented by PC/PS/chol (10:1:4)). During the first three days after start of therapy the solid liposomes did not induce tumor regression whereas the fluid liposomes were already as effective as free DXR. This delayed antitumor effect observed during treatment with DSPC/DPPG/chol liposomes (Fig. 1) was regarded as a useful phenomenon for the study of the path along which DXR-liposomes exert antitumor activity.

Because of the very low and similar recoveries of [^{3}H]inulin for PC/PS/chol and DSPC/DPPG/chol liposomes in tumor tissue (Table 1), the delayed antitumor effect can not be ascribed to differences in liposome uptake by the tumor. Instead, we hypothesized that during the first three days after start of treatment less DXR was released *in vivo* from the solid liposome type than from the fluid liposome type. To collect experimental evidence for this hypothesis, experiments on the *in vivo* integrity of both liposome types under investigation were performed. The double label method using [^{3}H]inulin and cholesteryl-1-[^{14}C]oleate provided data suggesting that the bilayer structure of both PC/PS/chol liposomes and

DSPC/DPPG/chol liposomes remained intact in the circulation (Table 2). The majority of injected liposomes accumulated in liver and spleen. Liposome uptake by liver and spleen occurs predominantly by way of endocytosis, although especially in the case of the DSPC/DPPG/chol liposomes adsorption to the cell surface without internalization can not be totally excluded (22). After internalization the liposomes end up in the lysosomal system (23). Intralysosomal degradation of liposome structures is reflected by an increase in $^3H/^{14}C$ ratio. The degradation rate appeared to be dependent on the lipid composition of the liposomal membranes: PC/PS/chol liposomes were degraded much faster than DSPC/DPPG/chol liposomes (Table 2). After injection of PC/PS/chol liposomes, the increase of the $^3H/^{14}C$ ratio with time was much more pronounced in the spleen than in the liver suggesting a higher rate of liposomal degradation in the spleen as compared to the liver. However, this observation may be misleading as we showed earlier (9) that in the liver efficient reutilization of [^{14}C]oleate, liberated from the liposomal bilayers during intralysosomal degradation, for lipid synthetic pathways in hepatocytes can easily lead to an underestimation of the actual rate of intrahepatic degradation. On the basis of ^{14}C-label release from spleen cells it can be estimated that 4 h after i.v. injection the fluid liposomes were degraded for more than 90% whereas the solid liposomes were degraded for only 20-25%. Recent results show that this large difference in "state of degradation" persisted over an observation period of 48 h (results not shown).

Correlation of the relatively slow degradation of the DSPC/DPPG/chol liposomes (Table 2) with the delayed antitumor activity exhibited by these liposomes *in vivo* (Fig. 1) suggests that the antitumor activity exerted by DXR-liposomes *in vivo* is dependent on the rate of degradation of the liposome structures within mononuclear phagocytes of the reticuloendothelial system (RES). Liposome degradation within mononuclear phagocytes seems to be the rate-limiting step in the expression of antitumor activity. We proposed that macrophages residing in liver and spleen and other sites of the body might act as reservoirs for DXR, slowly releasing the drug as a result of intracellular processing of the liposome components.

Crucial for the performance of such a drug delivery system is, of course, that DXR is released from these phagocytic cells after uptake of DXR-liposomes. Indeed previous results indicate that it is possible that DXR is released from peritoneal macrophages which have phagocytosed DXR-liposomes (11). In view of the delayed antitumor effect, differences in the degradation rate of DXR-liposomes in macrophages are expected to cause different DXR-release profiles. This topic was investigated with *in vitro* cultured rat liver macrophages (Kupffer cells). The results provide further evidence in favour of the proposed concept of drug depot formation in macrophages. PC/PS/chol liposomes are more susceptible to intracellular degradation as well as *in vitro* degradation by lysosomal enzymes than DSPC/DPPG/chol liposomes (results not shown). Importantly, after uptake of DXR-liposomes by the cells, DXR was released from the cells into the medium in a chemically intact form (Table 3). In addition, the release of DXR from cells which internalized DSPC/DPPG/chol liposomes was significantly delayed as compared to the release of DXR from cells which internalized PC/PS/chol liposomes (Table 3). Thus, these *in vitro* data obtained at a cellular as well as subcellular level are consistent with the proposal that the antitumor activity displayed by DXR-liposomes is dependent on the rate of intralysosomal degradation of the liposome structures within RES macrophages.

In order to obtain *in vivo* evidence for the role of macrophages in the mode of action of DXR-liposomes, the *in vivo* integrity of DXR-liposomes with respect to the encapsulated drug was followed (Table 4). Rather unexpectedly, the experiments using double-labeling with [^{3}H]inulin and [^{14}C]DXR show that DXR is lost in the circulation from intact liposome structures in a liposome-type dependent rate. It is estimated that about 65% of the injected amount of liposome-bound DXR was released from PC/PS/chol liposomes and about 20% from DSPC/DPPG/chol liposomes. These data point to differences in the extent of DXR-leakage between circulating PC/PS/chol and DSPC/DPPG/chol liposomes as the underlying mechanism of the delayed antitumor effect associated with treatment of tumor-bearing rats with the latter liposomes. However, drug depot formation in macrophages still can be an important aspect of the mode of action of DXR-liposomes. After the delay in antitumor activity, DSPC/DPPG/chol liposomes induced complete tumor regression (Fig. 1). Therefore, in view of the relatively small fraction of bound DXR leaking into the blood compartment, RES-mediated release of drug might contribute significantly to the mechanism of antitumor activity of DSPC/DPPG/chol liposomes.

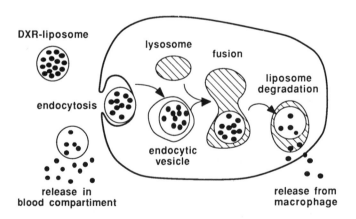

FIGURE 2.   Mode of action of DXR-containing liposomes.

In conclusion, the results indicate that after i.v. injection of DXR-liposomes two different pathways for sustained release of DXR exist: DXR is released directly from liposomes still being present in the blood but also indirectly from the RES following uptake and processing by macrophages (Fig. 2). The relative importance of each pathway in the mode of action of DXR-liposomes is dependent on the lipid composition of the liposomes. Peak concentrations of "free" DXR in organs which are particularly sensitive to the toxic action of the drug, like the heart, are avoided, while apparently the prolonged presence of relatively low "free" (i.e. non-liposomal) DXR levels in the blood can result in sufficient exposure levels for tumor cells. That avoidance of peak plasma levels is an important component of the mode of action of DXR-liposomes was recently confirmed by the observation that in the IgM immunocytoma system administration of DXR as a continuous infusion is as effective as PC/PS/chol liposomes in reducing cardiotoxicity with preservation of the antitumor effect.

The sustained release effects may be profitable in the treatment of a variety of neoplasms with their metastases, if any. The observed effect of liposomal lipid composition on the sustained release processes suggests that the *in vivo* rate of DXR-release from i.v. injected DXR-liposomes is a controllable and predictable variable. Therefore, proper selection of the liposomal lipid composition may lead to an optimal therapeutic availability of liposomal DXR.

REFERENCES

1. Lefrak EA, Pitha J, Rosenheim S, Gottlieb JA (1973). A clinicopathologic analysis of adriamycin cardiotoxicity. Cancer (Phila.) 32: 302.
2. Forssen EA, Tökes ZA (1983). Improved therapeutic benefits of doxorubicin by entrapment in anionic liposomes. Cancer Res 43: 546.
3. Van Hoesel QGCM, Steerenberg PA, Crommelin DJA, Van Dijk A, Van Oort W, Klein S, Douze JMC, De Wildt DJ, Hillen FC. Reduced cardiotoxicity and nephrotoxicity with preservation of antitumor activity of doxorubicin entrapped in stable liposomes in the LOU/M Wsi rat (1984). Cancer Res 44: 3698.
4. Rahman A, White G, More N, Schein PS. Pharmacological, toxicological, and therapeutic evaluation in mice of doxorubicin entrapped in cardiolipin liposomes (1985). Cancer Res 45: 796.
5. Gabizon A, Goren D, Fuks Z, Meshorer A, Barenholz Y (1985). Superior therapeutic activity of liposome-associated adriamycin in a murine metastatic tumour model. Br J Cancer 51: 681.
6. Gabizon A, Meshorer A, Barenholz Y (1986). Comparative long-term study of the toxicities of free and liposome-associated doxorubicin in mice after intravenous administration. JNCI 77: 459.

7. Storm G (1987). Liposomes as delivery system for doxorubicin in cancer chemotherapy. Thesis, University of Utrecht, The Netherlands, September 1987 (available upon request).

8. Storm G, Van Bloois L, Brouwer M, Crommelin DJA (1985). The interaction of cytostatic drugs with adsorbents in aqueous media. The potential implications for liposome preparation. Biochim Biophys Acta 818: 343.

9. Storm G, Roerdink FH, Steerenberg PA, De Jong WH, Crommelin DJA (1987). Influence of lipid composition on the antitumor activity exerted by doxorubicin-containing liposomes in a rat solid tumor model. Cancer Res 47: 3366.

10. Storm G, Van Gessel HJGM, Steerenberg PA, Speth P, Roerdink FH, Regts J, Van Veen M, De Jong WH (1987). Investigation of the role of mononuclear phagocytes in the transportation of doxorubicin containing-liposomes into a solid tumor. Cancer Drug Delivery 4: 89.

11. Storm G, Steerenberg PA, Emmen F, Van Borssum-Waalkes M, Crommelin DJA (1988). Release of doxorubicin from peritoneal macrophages exposed in vivo to doxorubicin-containing liposomes. Biochim Biophys Acta, in press.

12. Storm G, Steerenberg PA, Van Borssum-Waalkes M, Emmen F, Crommelin DJA (1988). Potential pitfalls in in vitro antitumor activity testing of free and liposome-encapsulated doxorubicin. J Pharm Sci, in press.

13. Abra RM, Hunt CA (1981). Liposome disposition in vivo. III. Dose and vesicle-size effects. Biochim Biophys Acta 666: 493.

14. Barter PJ, Lally JI (1978). The activity of an esterified cholesterol transferring factor in human and rat serum. Biochim Biophys Acta 531: 233.

15. Parker RJ, Priester ER, Sieber SM (1982). Effect of route of administration and liposome entrapment on the metabolism and disposition of adriamycin in the rat. Metabol Disp 5: 499.

16. Knook DL, Sleyster E Ch (1976). Separation of Kupffer and endothelial cells of the rat liver by centrifugal elutriation. Exp Cell Res 99: 444.

17. Dijkstra J, Van Galen WJM, Hulstaert CE, Kalicharan D, Roerdink FH, Scherphof GL (1984). Interactions of liposomes with Kupffer cells in vitro. Exp Cell Res 150: 161.

18. Cummings J (1985). Method for the determination of 4'-deoxydoxorubicin, 4'-deoxydoxorubicinol and their 7-deoxyaglycones in human serum by high-performance liquid chromatography. J Chromatography 341: 401.

19. Poste G, Kirsch R, Bugelski P (1984). Liposomes as drug delivery system in cancer therapy. In Sunkara PS (ed): "Novel Approaches to Cancer Chemotherapy", New York: Academic Press, p 165.

20. Crommelin DJA, Storm G (1988). Review of progress in drug targeting. In Taylor JD (ed): "Medicinal Chemistry", Oxford UK: Pergamon Books, in press.

21. Shubik P (1982). Vascularization of tumors: a review. J Cancer Res Clin Oncol 103: 211.

22. Pagano RE, Schroit AJ, Struck DK (1981). Interactions of phospholipid vesicles with mammalian cells in vitro: Studies of mechanism. In Knight CG (ed): "Liposomes: from physical structure to therapeutic applications", New York, Elsevier/North-Holland Biomedical Press, p 323.

Liposomes in the Therapy of Infectious Diseases and Cancer, pages 117–124
© 1989 Alan R. Liss, Inc.

THERAPY OF METASTASIS IN CANINE OSTEOSARCOMA[1]

E. Gregory MacEwen, Ilene D. Kurzman,
Bernard W. Smith, and Robert C. Rosenthal

Department of Medical Sciences
School of Veterinary Medicine
University of Wisconsin
Madison, Wisconsin 53706

ABSTRACT Canine osteosarcoma is a spontaneous
malignancy in dogs which is characterized by
micrometastases to pulmonary and extrapulmonary
tissues at the time of diagnosis. The standard
treatment involves amputation of the affected leg, but
the median survival time is 3–4 months with death due
to pulmonary and extrapulmonary metastases. We have
been conducting a randomized double-blind trial to
evaluate liposome-encapsulated muramyl tripeptide-
phosphatidylethanolamine (liposome/MTP-PE) as a
treatment for metastases in dogs undergoing amputation
for osteosarcoma. To date we have entered 27 dogs
into the study. Dogs were treated with MTP-PE at a
dose of 2 mg/m^2 I.V. starting 24 hours after
amputation. Treatments were given twice weekly for 8
weeks. The liposomes were a mixture of
phosphatidylserine and phosphatidylcholine at a 3:7
molar ratio. Thirteen dogs were treated with empty
liposomes and 14 were treated with liposome/MTP-PE.
The median survival time for the dogs treated with
empty liposomes was 77 days (range: 31–438 days) as
compared to dogs treated with liposome/MTP-PE for
which the median survival was 222 days (range:
81–820+); $p < 0.004$. In the liposome/MTP-PE group
there are 5 dogs alive and free of metastases at one
year post surgery.

[1]This work was supported by CIBA-GEIGY Limited,
Basel, Switzerland and The Morris Animal Foundation,
Englewood, Colorado.

INTRODUCTION

One of the most devastating aspects of neoplasia is its ability to spread from the primary site to distant metastatic sites, such as the liver and lungs. Although many neoplasms can be controlled locally through the use of conventional methods of treatment, such as surgery, radiation and chemotherapy, failure results when heterogenous clones of tumor cells emerge from the primary tumor forming metastases that are resistant to standard treatment (1). These resistant cells must, therefore, be eradicated by some other therapeutic regimen. One way in which metastases might be controlled is through the body's own natural defenses, such as the reticuloendothelial system.

Macrophages, when functionally activated, can destroy drug-resistant cancer cells in vitro (2). There are a variety of cytokines and bacterial agents that can activate macrophages to become cytotoxic. One of these agents is muramyl dipeptide (MDP), a synthetic molecule that resembles a fragment of the peptidoglycan cell wall of Mycobacterium and other bacteria. MDP has been shown to activate rat alveolar macrophages (3) and mouse peritoneal macrophages (4) to a tumoricidal state. In recent studies in our laboratory, we found that MDP will activate canine adherent mononuclear cells to become cytostatic against canine osteosarcoma cells (5). A lipophilic derivative of MDP, known as muramyl tripeptide-phosphatidylethanolamine (MTP-PE) has been shown to activate human monocytes to become cytotoxic to cancer cells (6,7). Both of these macrophage-activating agents can be easily encapsulated in liposomes.

Liposomes are microscopic membrane structures composed of phospholipids. When injected intravenously, liposomes are endocytosed or phagocytosed by cells of the reticuloendothelial system. Once taken into the cell, the liposomes are degraded through the effect of cytoplasmic enzymes and the encapsulated drug is slowly released into the cell. Liposome-encapsulated MDP and MTP-PE have been shown to have antitumor activity in rodent tumor models. In studies utilizing the B-16 melanoma cell line in mice, it was found that administration of liposome/MDP resulted in regression of spontaneous lung metastases when compared to mice treated with empty liposomes, saline, and free muramyl peptides (8). Similar studies in other murine metastatic tumors of systemic administration of liposomes containing different immunomodulators have shown similar antitumor activity (9-13). Liposome-encapsulated MTP-PE has been shown to activate peripheral blood monocytes when injected into humans (7). Recent, yet unpublished studies in our laboratory show that when liposome-encapsulated MTP-PE is injected into normal dogs, it will induce adherent mononuclear cells to become cytostatic.

The phospholipid composition of liposomes will influence the success of the their being phagocytosed or endocytosed by the macrophage. Liposomes containing negatively charged phospholipids have enhanced uptake by blood monocytes and tissue macrophages. In addition, the presence of phosphatidylserine in the liposome has been shown to result in enhanced binding and phagocytosis to all cells of the reticuloendothelial system. Negatively charged liposomes containing phosphatidylserine are phagocytosed up to 10-fold faster than are positively charged liposomes of the same size and configuration (14). The liposomes we used in this study consisted of phosphatidylserine and phosphatidylcholine at a 3:7 molar ratio.

The purpose of this study was to evaluate the effectiveness of liposome-encapsulated MTP-PE in controlling or preventing distant metastasis in dogs with spontaneous osteosarcoma. Canine osteosarcoma is a rapidly metastasizing tumor and probably all dogs have micrometastases at the time of diagnosis (15). The most commonly reported metastatic site in the dog is the lung (15,16). Despite various therapeutic regimens, mostly involving amputation, survival times remain short; median survival times range from 3 to 6 months, only about 10% of the dogs survive a year or longer (15-21). Since most dogs die of metastatic disease in a short period of time, we chose this malignancy as a model to evaluate the effectiveness of liposome-encapsulated MTP-PE.

MATERIALS AND METHODS

Animals. Dogs with primary osteosarcoma of the extremity, without evidence of distant metastases, were eligible for entry into this study. All dogs were evaluated with a complete blood count, serum chemistry profile, and radiographs of the primary tumor and thorax. Only dogs with histologically proven osteosarcoma were entered.

Treatment. Surgery consisted of complete amputation of the affected limb. Immediately following surgery, dogs were randomized to receive either liposome-encapsulated MTP-PE (liposome/MTP-PE) or empty liposomes. All treatment assignments were double-blind. The liposome preparation was given twice weekly for eight weeks by a slow intraveous infusion over a 5 to 8 minute period. The dose of liposome/MTP-PE was 2 mg/m^2.

Liposome Preparation. Lyophilized liposomes with or without MTP-PE were supplied by CIBA-GEIGY Limited, Basel, Switzerland. Liposomes were prepared from the freeze-dried preparations by adding 2.5 ml of phosphate buffered saline, without calcium or magnesium, to the vials containing dioleoyl-phophatidylserine and 1-palmitoyl-2-oleoyl-phosphatidylcholine at a 3 to 7 molar ratio (250 mg of total lipid per vial), with or without MTP-PE. After 15 seconds, the vial contents were mechanically agitated on a vortex mixer at high speed for one minute and then each vial was diluted to a total of 10 ml with PBS. The preparation was then ready for intravenous administration.

Follow-Up Studies. A complete physical examination and a complete blood count were performed each time the dog received the liposome treatment. Thoracic radiographs were taken at 2 month intervals following amputation. Follow-up continued for as long as necessary to determine metastasis-free interval and survival time for each dog.

Statistical Considerations. The metastasis-free intervals and survival times were compared between the liposome/MTP-PE treatment group and the empty liposome group. The differences between the groups were analyzed using the Kaplan-Meier method and the Breslow and Mantel-Cox tests of significance between survival curves. A p value of less than 0.05 was considered significant.

RESULTS

Twenty-seven dogs with osteosarcoma were admitted into this study. Of these, 14 received liposome/MTP-PE and 13 received empty liposomes. There was no apparent toxicity associated with the administration of the MTP-PE or empty liposomes. All dogs tolerated the treatment very well. There were no consistent changes in the complete blood count or serum chemistry profile for dogs in either treatment group. The only side effect noted was an elevation in body temperature by 1 to 2°C which occurred

from 1 to 3 hours after the liposome injection. Body
temperature returned to normal by 6 hours post injection.
The temperature elevations usually occurred during the
first 3 to 4 treatments, and less often towards the end of
therapy. Temperature elevations were more frequent in dogs
receiving liposome/MTP-PE than in those receiving empty
liposomes, however, this difference was not significant.

The median survival time for the dogs receiving
liposome/MTP-PE was 222 days (range: 81-820+ days) as
compared to 77 days (range: 31-438 days) for the group
receiving empty liposomes; $p < 0.004$ (Figure 1). In the
liposome/MTP-PE group, there are five dogs alive of which
four are free of metastases at one year post surgery and
one is free of metastases at two years post surgery. In
the placebo group, all 13 dogs have died as a result of
metastatic disease.

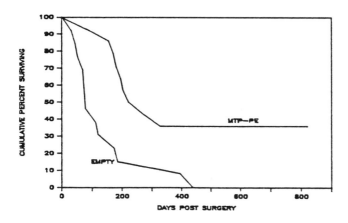

FIGURE 1. Survival of osteosarcoma dogs receiving
liposme/MTP-PE versus those receiving empty liposomes.

The median time from surgery to metastasis was significantly longer in the liposome/MTP-PE group compared to the empty liposome group; 168 days (range: 54-820+ days) and 58 days (range: 31-227 days), respectively; p = 0.002 (Figure 2).

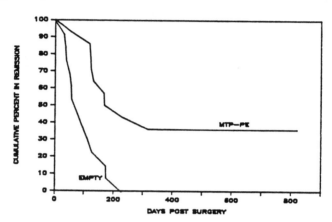

FIGURE 2. Metastasis-free intervals of osteosarcoma dogs receiving liposme/MTP-PE versus those receiving empty liposomes.

DISCUSSION

Based on these results, it would appear that MTP-PE, when encapsulated in liposomes, has similar antitumor activity in dogs with spontaneously occurring osteosarcoma as that found in the rodent tumor models. Liposome/MTP-PE therapy significantly delayed the time to metastasis and prolonged survival when compared to dogs receiving empty liposomes. Five of 14 dogs (36%) receiving liposome/MTP-PE have survival times in excess of one year with one dog alive at two years. Although these results are quite encouraging and show that liposome/MTP-PE treatment is more effective than surgery alone, even with this treatment over 50% of the dogs are dead by 9 months post surgery. Since most dogs are presumed to have micrometastases at the time of amputation, it may be that the tumor burden post surgery is too great for liposome/MTP-PE therapy alone. Further studies are warranted to evaluate liposome/MTP-PE therapy in combination with other treatment modalities.

ACKNOWLEDGEMENTS

The authors thank Ms. Cynthia Broderick and Dr. Lisa Lindesmith for their assistance throughout this study.

REFERENCES

1. Fidler IJ, Poste G (1985). The cellular heterogeneity of malignant neoplasms: Implications for adjuvant chemotherapy. Semin in Oncol 12:207.
2. Fidler IJ (1985). Macrophages and metastasis—a biological approach to cancer therapy. Cancer Res 45:4714.
3. Sone S, Fidler IJ (1981). In vitro activation of tumoricidal properties in rat alveolar macrophages by synthetic muramyl dipeptide encapsulated in liposomes. Cell Immunol 57:42.
4. Phillips NC, Moras ML, Chedid L, et al (1985). Activation of macrophage cytostatic and cytotoxic activity in vitro by liposomes containing a new lipophilic muramyl peptide derivative, MDP-L-alanyl-cholesterol (MTP-CHOL). J Biol Resp Modif 4:464.
5. Smith BW, Kurzman ID, Schultz KT, et al (1988). Muramyl dipeptide augments in vitro cytostatic activity of canine plastic-adherent mononuclear cells for canine osteosarcoma cells. Veterin Immunol Immunopathol (submitted).
6. Kleinerman ES, Erickson KL, Schroit AJ, et al (1983). Activation of tumoricidal properties in human blood monocytes by liposomes containing lipophilic muramyl tripeptide. Cancer Res 43:2010.
7. Fidler IJ, Jessup JM, Fogler WE, et al (1986). Activation of tumoricidal properties in peripheral blood monocytes of patients with colorectal carcinoma. Cancer Res 46:994.
8. Fidler IJ, Poste G (1982). Macrophage-mediated destruction of malignant cells and new strategies for the therapy of metastatic disease. Springer Semin Immunopathol 5:161.
9. Poste G, Kirsch R, Fogler W, Fidler IJ (1979). Activation of tumoricidal properties in mouse macrophages by lymphokines encapsulated in liposomes. Cancer Res 39:881.

10. Deodhar SD, Borna BP, Edinger M, et al (1982). Inhibition of lung metastases by liposomal immunotherapy in a murine fibrosarcoma model. J Biol Resp Modif 1:27.

11. Key ME, Talmadge JE, Fogler WE, et al (1982). Isolation of tumoricidal macrophages from lung melanoma metastases of mice treated systemically with liposomes containing a lipophilic derivative of muramyl dipeptide. JNCI 69:1189.

12. Philips NC, Moras ML, Chedid L, et al (1985). Activation of alveolar macrophage tumoricidal activity and eradication of experimental metastases by freeze-dried liposomes containing a new lipophilic muramyl dipeptide derivative. Cancer Res 45:128.

13. Talmadge JE, Lenz BF, Klabansky, et al (1986). Therapy of autochthonous skin cancers in mice with intravenously injected liposomes containing muramyltripeptide. Cancer Res 46:1160.

14. Schroit AJ, Fidler IJ (1982). Effects of liposome structure and lipid composition on the activation of the tumoricidal properties of macrophages by liposomes containing muramyl dipeptide. Cancer Res 42:161.

15. Brodey RS, Abt DA (1976). Results of surgical treatment in 65 dogs with osteosarcoma. JAVMA 168:1032.

16. Weiden PL, Storb R, et al (1978). Canine osteosarcoma: Results of amputation with and without adjuvant immunotherapy. Cancer Immunol Immunother 5:181.

17. Henness AM, Theilen GH, et al (1977). Combination therapy for canine osteosarcoma. JAVMA 170:1076.

18. Cotter SM, Parker IM (1978). High-dose methotrexate and leucovorin rescue in dogs with osteogenic sarcoma. AJVR 39:1943.

19. Madewell BR, Leighton RL, et al (1978). Amputation and doxorubicin for treatment of canine and feline osteosarcoma. Europ J Cancer 14:287.

20. Weiden PL, Deeg HJ, Graham TC, et al (1981). Canine osteosarcoma: Failure of intravenous or intradermal BCG as adjuvant immunotherapy. Cancer Immunol Immunother 11:69.

21. Meyer JA, Dueland RT, et al (1982). Canine osteogenic sarcoma treated by amputation and MER: Adverse effect of splenectomy on survival. Cancer 49:1613.

Liposomes in the Therapy of Infectious Diseases and Cancer, pages 125–134
© 1989 Alan R. Liss, Inc.

HUMAN MONOCYTE ACTIVATION TO THE TUMORICIDAL STATE
BY LIPOSOME-ENCAPSULATED MURAMYL TRIPEPTIDE
AND ITS THERAPEUTIC IMPLICATION[1]

Saburo Sone

Third Department of Internal Medicine,
The University of Tokushima School of Medicine
Kuramoto-cho 3, Tokushima 770, Japan

ABSTRACT Human alveolar macrophages and blood
monocytes can be activated to the tumoricidal state by
incubation in vitro with liposomes containing muramyl
dipeptide (MDP) or its lipophilic muramyl tripeptide
phosphatidylethanolamine (MTP-PE). Macrophages activated
by this procedure are cytotoxic to allogeneic tumor cells,
but not to non-tumorigenic cells. MDP or its lipophilic
MTP-PE encapsulated in multilamellar vesicle (MLV)
liposomes activated human monocyte-macrophages at lower
concentrations than free MDP and also maintained the
activated state for a longer period than free MDP. Blood
monocytes obtained from lung cancer patients were less
responsive to MDP analog and lipopolysaccharide (LPS) than
those of healthy donors, but there was no difference in
antitumor potential of monocytes activated with liposome-
MTP-PE between these two groups. Interferon (IFN) α, β and
γ also rendered human monocytes tumoricidal, but IFN γ had
a much higher synergistic effect than IFN α or IFN β with
soluble MDP analog for monocyte activation. Similarly, a
combination of IFN γ and liposome-entrapped MTP-PE at
suboptimal concentrations also induced synergistic
activation of monocytes to the tumoricidal state. Thus,
encapsulation of macrophage activators in liposomes may be
a valuable approach in in situ activation of monocyte-
macrophages for treatment of cancer metastases in humans.

---

[1]This work was supported by a Grant-in-Aid for Cancer
Research from the Ministry of Education, Science and
Culture of Japan, and by the Ministry of Health and
Welfare of Japan

INTRODUCTION

Increasing evidence in murine systems that activated macrophages are important in host defense against primary and/or metastatic neoplasias has resulted in the development of new biological response modifiers (BRMs) that can enhance macrophage-mediated tumor cell killing (reviewed in ref. 1, 2). Structurally-defined BRMs such as synthetic chemical immunoadjuvants or recombinant cytokines obtained by DNA technology are now available for clinical trials. Recently, much attention has been paid to the use of liposomes as carriers to deliver BRMs to monocyte-macrophages in vivo (1, 2). There is encouraging evidence for the efficacy of liposomal BRM (MDP and MTP-PE) in treatment of cancer metastases in murine systems (1, 3). Similar therapeutic approaches with liposomal BRMs are expected to be effective clinically in treating patients with disseminated malignant diseases. Nevertheless, little is known about the mechanism by which liposomes containing BRMs render human monocyte-macrophages tumoricidal. In this review, we address the values of MDP or its analogs encapsulated in liposomes in human monocyte-macrophage activation and the activation mechanism.

LIPOSOMES AS CARRIERS TO DELIVER
BRM TO MACROPHAGES

Activation of human macrophages to the tumoricidal state by BRM has been achieved in two main ways: 1) by direct interaction of the macrophages with bacterial preparations such as LPS and MDP (4-6), and 2) by indirect mechanisms involving lymphokines, such as macrophage-activating factor (MAF) and interferon γ (IFN γ) or cytokines (IFN α and β) (7-9). Recent studies have shown that the minimal principle unit of Mycobacterium in Freund's adjuvant is N-acetyl-muramyl-L-alanyl-D-isoglutamine (MDP) (10, 11), which can be synthesized, and has potent effects on a varieity of host defense cells, including causing macrophage activation (12). These chemically defined compounds allowed us to elucidate the mechanism by which macrophages can be rendered tumoricidal. In attempts to potentiate the macrophage-activating effect of diffusible BRM in vivo, we used liposomes as carriers to deliver BRM to macrophages. In vitro kinetic studies showed that liposomes containing BRM

(IFN γ or MDP) rendere human monocyte-macrophages tumoricidal at far lower concentration and for a longer period than their free counterparts (5, 7, 13). The ability of liposome-BRM to activate macrophages in vitro and in vivo is influenced by the characters of the liposomes, such as their size, structure and lipid composition. Negatively charged MLV liposomes prepared from PS and PC were found to provide a suitable carrier vehicle for delivery of BRMs (MAF, IFN γ, MDP or MTP-PE) to macrophages in vitro and in vivo, leading to their activation to the tumoricidal state (2, 14). These findings raise the possibility that these activated macrophages could enhance host defense against tumor meatstasis. Indeed, intravenous injection of MLV liposomes containing BRMs (MAF, MDP, IFN γ, C-reactive protein or poly(I).poly(C)) have been demonstrated to be effective in the destruction of established pulmonary metastases in murine tumor sytems (1, 2).

The mechanism responsible for the regression of tumor metastases after systemic administration of MLV liposome-BRM probably involves the activation of circulating monocytes to the tumoricidal state (2). Thus, the interaction of monocytes as precursors of tumor-infiltrating macrophages with liposome-entrapped activation stimuli seem to be important for eradication of tumor metastases. Recently, the tumoricidal activity of blood monocytes from patients with colorectal carcinoma was observed even after multiple treatments by

TABLE 1
ANTITUMOR POTENTIAL OF BLOOD MONOCYTES
FROM LUNG CANCER PATIENTS

	% Cytotoxicity against A375 melanoma cells		
Subject	LPS	norMDP	Liposome-MTP-PE
Heatlhy donors	34.8 + 4.5 (20)[a]	47.8 + 6.0 (8)	27.6 + 3.6 (17)
Lung cancer patients	23.4 + 3.4 (23)	26.0 + 4.4 (11)	30.0 + 3.2 (23)

[a]Values in parentheses indicate number of subjects tested.

radiotherapy or chemotherapy (15). We also examined whether blood monocytes of lung cancer patients can respond to activation stimuli to become tumoricidal (Table 1). We observed that blood monocytes obtained from lung caner patients were rendered tumoricidal following interaction in vitro with MTP-PE in liposomes, but these monocytes responded to LPS or MDP analog at lesser extent than those of healthy donors. These findings suggest that in vivo activation of macrophages by liposome–MTP-PE may be feasible.

PRIMING EFFECT OF IFN γ ON HUMAN MONOCYTE ACTIVATION FOR TUMOR CELL KILLING

The exact mechanism by which IFN γ activates macrophages is unknown, but studies in human and rodent systems suggest that it involves at least two main steps (Fig. 1). Recently, we observed synergism between IFN γ and MDP or its analog (norMDP) in activation of human monocytes to the tumoricidal state (6, 16). In contrast, IFN α and IFN β with monocyte-activating potential, unlike IFN γ, had additive effects with norMDP in human monocyte activation (6). For synergistic activation of the tumoricidal properties of monocytes, the cells had to be treated first with IFN γ and then with a second stimulus, such as LPS or MDP (6). The activation of monocyte-

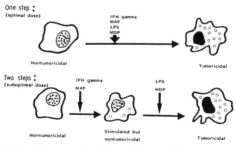

FIGURE 1. Proposed kinetics of human monocyte activation to the tumoricidal state by two BRMs.

macrophages to the tumoricidal state by a lymphokine, such as IFN γ has been shown to involve two main steps. For example, once IFN γ is bound to the specific receptors on the surface, it is internalized to act on intracellular sites and cause macrophage activation (17). If the IFN γ molecule does not bind to the cell surface, it cannot be

internalized into macrophages, as shown by the fact that
the proteolytic enzyme pronase can alter the macrophage
surface so much that their activation by free INF γ no
longer takes place (18). This is not the case with MDP,
since MDP enters macrophages by pinocytosis. Moreover,
studies with (^{3}H)norMDP revealed that the activation of
monocytes by norMDP was not attributable to its
interaction with a specific cell surface receptor and did
not result merely from internalization of glycopeptide by
monocytes (19). The intracellular interaction of (^{3}H)-
norMDP with IFN γ-primed monocytes was specific, in that
the intracellular radiolabeled material could be displaced
by unlabeled norMDP and recovered as intact molecules, but
not by a biologically inactive MDP stereoisomer (19),
suggesting that activation of the tumoricidal properties
of human blood monocytes by MDP occurs subsequent to its
intracellular interaction with specific MDP receptors.

SYNERGISM OF IFN γ WITH LIPOSOME-MTP-PE
IN ACTIVATION OF HUMAN MONOCYTES

We reported that IFN γ and MDP showed synergism in
monocyte activation when they were encapsulated in the
aqueous space of MLV liposomes, and that when these two
agents were incorporated into liposomes, they were
effective at far lower cocentrations than when they were
added directly to the medium (16). Nevertheless, since
the use of liposomes poses some problems, such as leakage
of encapsulated soluble agents from the liposomes and
instability of the preparations, we examined the effect of
liposomes containing lipophilic MTP-PE inserted into the
membrane bilayers of the liposomes. We found that a dried
preparation of liposomes contained a lipophilic analog of
MDP (MTP-PE), which can be standardized and has a
reproducible effect in human monocyte activation (20).

FIGURE 2.
Synergism between
IFN γ and liposome-
MTP-PE for human
monocyte activation

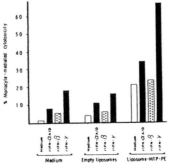

Furthermore, we found that IFN γ acted synergistically
with liposome-MTP-PE as a second stimulus for induction of
tumoricidal monocytes (21). We also examined whether
other types of human IFN, such as IFN α and IFN β could
act synergistically with liposome-MTP-PE to render
monocytes tumoricidal. As shown in Fig. 2, recombinant
IFN α A/D and IFN β acted additively rather than
synergistically with liposome-MTP-PE in activation of
human monocytes to the tumoricidal state.

We previously found that phagocytosis by monocyte-
macrophages is a prerequisite for induction of tumoricidal
activity by liposomes containing MDP and its lipophilic
derivative, MTP-PE (21). IFN γ was found to cause
significant increase in the uptake of liposomes by
monocytes. Although the mechanism of the synergistic
actions of IFN γ and MTP-PE in liposomes may be very
complex, a major factor contributing to development of the
observed synergism in monocyte activation is a significant
increase in phagocytosis of liposomes by IFN γ-treated
monocytes. Possibly cytoplasmic receptors for a second
activator (liposome-MTP-PE) may increase the interaction
of cells with IFN γ. This may be involved in the synergism
between IFN γ and liposome-MTP-PE, judging from the
following findings: i) expression of the tumoricidal
activity of monocytes treated with liposome-entrapped
macrophage activators required intracellular interaction
between macrophage activators and cytoplasmic receptor
sites ; ii) in murine systems IFN γ was found to increase
binding of the MDP analog to macrophages and so to have a
synergistic effect with a suboptimal dose of the MDP
analog in activation of macrophages to the tumoricidal
state. Further studies are required to elucidate the
events occurring in monocytes after phagocytosis of
liposomal MTP-PE.

EFFECTOR MECHANISM OF TUMOR-CELL KILLING BY BLOOD
MONOCYTES ACTIVATED BY LIPOSOMAL ACTIVATORS

Human AM and monocytes were found to secrete a tumor
cytotoxic factor (TCF) into the supernatant when they were
rendered tumoricidal by incubation with lipopolysaccharide
(LPS) or MDP (22-24). These molecules have been referred
to as TCF. The synergistic activation of the tumoricidal
properties of human monocytes by IFN γ and norMDP was also
found to be correlated with the release of TCF into the

culture supernatant by monocytes (24). On the other hand, interleukin 1 (IL-1) and tumor necrosis factor (TNF) are known to be one of the antitumor monokines responsible for monocyte-mediated cytotoxicity against tumor targets such as human A375 melanoma cells (25, 26). The problem of whether human monocyte-macrophages require cell-to-cell contact for expression of their tumoricidal activity still seems controversial. We recently showed that monocytes activated to the tumoricidal state by liposome-MTP-PE did not produce intra- or extracellular IL-1 (27). Moreover, supernatants obtained from cultures of these activated monocytes did not kill A375 melanoma cells (Fig. 3), suggesting that monocytes activated by liposomal MTP-PE do not secrete any monokines responsible for tumor cell killing.

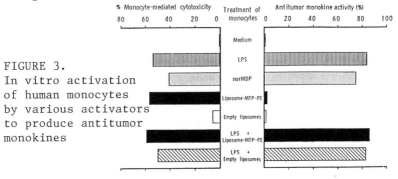

FIGURE 3.
In vitro activation of human monocytes by various activators to produce antitumor monokines

These findings, together with our previous findings that MLV liposomes are preferentially phagocytized by monocytes, suggest that triggering of monokine synthesis by soluble macrophage activators involves membrane-associated events, whereas liposome-encapsulated activators interact with intracellular sites rendering the cells tumoricidal but not stimulating production of monokines (TCF and IL-1). There are two ways in which activated monocytes may kill tumor cells: 1) tumor cytotoxicity mediated by antitumor monokines secreted by activated monocytes and 2) killing by direct cell-to-cell contact of activated monocytes and tumor target cells. These findings suggest that human monocytes activated by liposomal stimuli may require cell-to-cell contact for expression of antitumor activity. It is noteworthy that systemic administration of MLV liposomes is safe and results in no adverse side effect. These observations, together with the previous findings (1, 2) that liposome-entrapped MDP or MTP-P can activate human monocyte-macrophages to the tumoricidal state, and results on the therapeutic effect of these liposomes on murine cancer metastasis, indicate that administration of MLV liposomes should be useful for the treatment of disseminated metastatic diseases in humans.

ACKNOWLEDGEMENTS

I am grateful to many colleagues for collaboration in the work mentioned in this review. I wish to thank Drs. I. J. Fidler and T. Ogura for their encouragement.

REFERENCES

1. Fidler IJ (1985). Macrophages and metastasis-A biological approach to cancer therapy: Presidential address. Cancer Res 45:4714.
2. Sone S (1986). Role of alveolar macrophages in pulmonary neoplasias. Biochim Biophys Acta 823:227.
3. Fidler IJ, Sone S, Fogler WE, Barnes ZL (1981). Eradication of spontaneous metastases and activation of alveolar macrophages by intravenous injection of liposomes containing muramyl dipeptide. Proc Natl Acad Sci USA 78:1680.
4. Sone S, Moriguchi S, Shimizu E, Ogushi F, Tsubura E (1982). In vitro generation of tumoricidal properties in human alveolar macrophages following interaction with endotoxin. Cancer Res 42:2227.
5. Sone S, Tsubura E (1982). Human alveolar mcrophages: potentiation of their tumoricidal activity by liposome-encapsulated muramyl dipeptide. J Immunol 129: 1313.
6. Utsugi T, Sone S (1986). Comparative analysis of the priming effect of human interferon α, β and γ on synergism with muramyl dipeptide analog for antitumor expression of human blood monocytes. J Immunol 136:1117.
7. Kleinerman ES, Schroit AJ, Folger WE, Fidler IJ (1983). Tumoricidal activity of human monocytes activated in vitro by free and liposome-encapsulated human lymphokines. J Clin Invest 72:304.
8. Fidler IJ, Kleinerman ES (1984). Lymphokine-

activated human blood monocytes destroy tumor cells but not normal cells under cocultivation condition. J Clin Oncol 2:937.

9. Sone S, Utsugi T, Shirahama T, Ishii K, Mutsuura S, Ogawara M (1985). Induction by interferon-α of tumoricidal activity of adherent mononuclear cells from human blood: Monocytes as responder and effector cells. J Biol Resp Modif 4:134.

10. Ellouz F, Adam A, Ciobaru R, Lederer E (1974). Minimal structural requirements for adjuvant activity of bacterial peptidoglycan derivative. Biochem Biophys Res Commun 59:1317.

11. Kotani S, Watanabe Y, Shimono T, Narita T, Koto K, Stewart-Tull DES, Kinoshita F, Yokogawa K, Kawata S, Shiba T, Kusumoto S, Tarumi Y. Immunoadjuvant activities of cell walls, their water-soluble fractions and peptidoglycan subunits, prepared from various gram-positive bacteria, and of synthetic N-acetyl-muramyl peptide. Z Immun Forsch Exp Ther 149:302.

12. Chedid L, Carelli L, Adudibert F (1979). Recent development concerning muramyl dipeptide, a synthetic immunoregulating molecule. J Reticuloendothel Soc 26: 631.

13. Sone S, Mutsuura S, Ogawara M, Tsubura E (1984). Potentiating effect of muramyl dipeptide and its lipophilic analog encapsulated in liposomes on tumor cell killing by human monocytes. J Immunol 132:2105.

14. Fidler IJ, Sone S, Fogler WE, Smith D, Braun DG, Tarcsay L, Gisler RJ, Schroit A (1982). Efficacy of liposomes containing a lipophilic muramyl dipeptide derivative for activating the tumoricidal properties of alveolar macrophages in vivo. J Biol Resp Modif 1:43.

15. Fidler IJ, Jessup SM, Fogler WE, Staerkel R, Mazumder A (1986). Activation of tumoricial properties in peripheral blood monocytes of patients with colorectal carcinoma. Cancer Res 44:994.

16. Saiki I, Sone S, Fogler WE, Kleinerman E, Lopez-Berestein G, Fidler IJ (1985). Synergism between human recombinant γ-interferon and muramyl dipeptide encapsulated in liposomes for activation of antitumor properties in human blood monocytes. Cancer Res 45:6188.

17. Celada A, Gray PW, Rinderknecht E, Schreiber RD (1984). Evidence for a gamma interferon receptor

that ragulated macrophage tumoricidal activity.
J Exp Med   160:55.

18. Fidler IJ, Fogler WE, Kleinerman ES, Saiki I (1985).
Abrogation of species specificity for activation of
tumoricidal properties in macrophages by recombinant
mouse or human interferon-γ encapsulated in
liposomes.   J Immunol 135:4289.

19. Fogler WE, Fidler IJ (1986). The activation of
tumoricidal properties in human blood monocytes by
muramyl dipeptide requires specific intracellular
interaction.   J Immunol 136:2311.

20. Sone S, Utsugi T, Tandon P, Ogawara M (1986).   A
dried preparation of liposomes containing muramyl
tripeptide phosphatidylethanolamine as a potent
activator of human blood monocytes to the tumoricidal
state.   Cancer Immunol Immunother   22:191.

21. Sone S, Tandon P, utsugi T, Ogawara M, Shimizu E,
Ogura T (1986). Synergism of recombinant human
interferon gamma with liposome-encapsulated muramyl
tripeptide in activation of the tumoricidal
properties of human monocytes.   Int J Cancer 38:495.

22. Sone S, Tachibana K, Ishii K, Ogawara M, Tsubur E
(1984). Production of a tumor cytolytic factor(s) by
activated human alveolar macrophages and its action.
Cancer Res   44:646.

23. Sone S, Lopez-Berestein G, Fidler IJ (1985).
Kinetics and function of tumor cytotoxic factor(s)
produced by human blood monocytes activated to the
tumoricidal state.   J Natl Cancer Inst 74:583.

24. Sone S, Lopez-Berestein, G, Fidler IJ (1986).
Potentiation of direct antitumor cytotoxicity and
production of tumor cytolytic factors in human blood
monocytes by huamn recombinant interferon-gamma and
muramyl dipeptide. Cancer Immunol Immunother 21:93.

25. Lachman LB, Dinarello CA, Llansa ND, Fidler IJ
(1986). Natural and recombinant human interleukin 1
is cytotoxic for human melanoma cells.
J Immunol 136: 3098.

26. Feinman R, Henriksen-DeStefano H, Tsujimoto M, Vilcek
J (1987). Tumor necrosis factor is an important
mediator of tumor cell killing by human monocytes.
J Immunol   138:635.

27. Tandon P, Utsugi T, Sone S (1986). Lack of
production of interleukin 1 by human blood monocytes
to the antitumor state by liposome-encapsulated
muramyl tripeptide.   Cancer Res   46:5039.

Liposomes in the Therapy of Infectious Diseases and Cancer, pages 135–154
© 1989 Alan R. Liss, Inc.

LIPOSOMES IN DRUG DELIVERY:
FROM SERENDIPITY TO TUMOR TARGETING

D. Papahadjopoulos,† N. Lopez‡ and A. Gabizon†*

†Cancer Research Institute and ‡Department of Pharmacology,
University of California, San Francisco, California 94143.
*Liposome Technology Inc., Menlo Park, California 94025

ABSTRACT
Liposomes have several important characteristics that define their potential as drug
carriers in four distinct areas:
Localized slow release: Liposomes can be
used as a slow-release system, following local
application either directly on the skin, by
inhalation or by injection into an anatomi-
cally protected area.
Site avoidance: Since uptake of liposomes by some sensitive tissues such as
heart, kidneys and gut is very limited, encapsulation of certain drugs produces a lowering
of their toxicity to these critical tissues.
Clearance by the reticuloendothelial
system (RES): Natural affinity of microorganisms.
Site-directed targeting: A relatively
high uptake of liposomes by specific "target"
cells in some tissues is theoretically
possible as indicated by extensive *in vitro*
studies. However, the applicability of this
approach to clinically relevant situations has
been limited by the following two aspects: the
short residence time of he liposomes in blood,
and the variable accessibility to the target
cells, which is determined by the location of

the target cells and the relative permeability
of the endothelial barrier within each tissue.
    Recent work in this area has revealed
some new and important characteristics of
liposomes: Inclusion of certain glycolipids
within liposomes composed of phosphatidylcholine and cholesterol or sphingomyelin
drastically prolongs the circulation time and
reduces their uptake by liver and spleen.
Concomitantly, their accumulation in several
implanted tumors is substantially increased.
These studies suggest that controlling the
circulation time of liposomes and limiting
their non-specific uptake by the RES opens up
new opportunities for achieving specific
targeting to tumors *in vivo*, with both diag-
nostic and therapeutic possibilities.

INTRODUCTION

    An impressive evolution has occurred in the
field of liposomes since the first publication by
Bangham in 1965 on the properties of swollen phospholipid lamellae (1). Those initial experiments
set the stage for a whole series of studies in membrane biophysics, examining the role of lipid
structure and permeability in membrane function (2). In addition, liposomes have become the
preferred system for studying the reconstitution of
membrane transport proteins and enzymes, ionophoric
peptides and a variety of anesthetics and other
drugs (4). Thus, liposomes have played an essential role in developing our current understanding
of the structure and function of biological membranes in such subjects as membrane fusion (5)
antigen-antibody interactions (6,7), the complement system (8) blood coagulation (9,10) and
atherosclerosis (11,12).
    During the early seventies, work on liposomes
went beyond membrane biophysics and into the area
of therapeutic applications, as a vector system for

altering the tissue disposition of various macro-molecules *in vivo* and also for enhancing the cyto-plasmic delivery of foreign macromolecules into cells *in vitro* (13). Since then liposomes evolved as a field at the interface between Biophysics, Cell Biology and Medicine. The synergy between these three essentially different areas of research activity is responsible for the current vitality of the field (14,15).

The first major example of the ability of liposomes to increase the therapeutic index of drugs was the use of antimonials against parasitic diseases such as leishmaniasis (16-18). Although, this has not reached the stage of clinical trials as yet, several other applications of liposomes are currently being tested in human patients with encouraging results. These include the use of anthracyclines in cancer patients (19-20), ampho-tericin B to combat fungal infections (21), and muramyl-dipeptide derivatives for immunomodulation (22). In addition liposomes are being tested in humans as carriers of bronchodilators (23) and of tumor imaging agents (24).

This conference is a testimony to the progress that has been achieved so far with liposomes in various medical applications. So far, however, liposome therapy has been based on three main properties of liposomes as a delivery system.

a) Solubilization of water-insoluble and amphipathic drugs within the bilayer, with primary examples, amphotericin B and Adriamycin. Such solu-bilization provides a thermodynamically stable com-plex, which facilitates intravenous administration and may allow the drugs to stay longer in circula-tion (25,26,27).

b) Avoidance of certain sensitive tissues where liposomes do not normally accumulate, such as heart, kidneys and gastrointestinal tract. Examples of this are the lowering of cardiotoxicity of Adriamycin (28,29) and of nephrotoxicity of amphotericin B (30) resulting from drug's encapsu-lation in liposomes.

c) Uptake of drug-loaded liposomes by the reticuloendothelial (RES) cells of the liver and spleen (31,32). In this case liposomes can concentrate drugs within the RES cells of these tissues, where many parasitic and microbial infections are often localized. Such concentration can drastically increase the therapeutic index of these drugs (16).

In order to enhance the ability of liposomes to deliver drugs to cells or tissues other than the RES, considerable effort has been mounted both in our own and other laboratories. This effort resulted in the advent of methods for conjugation of antibodies on the liposome surface (33-35), temperature sensitive liposomes (36,37) which can be used in conjunction with hyperthermia (38) and pH sensitive liposomes either for localization of drugs in low pH areas (39) or for release of the liposome-encapsulated drugs following endocytosis (40-42).

Until recently such systems could not be developed further into practical applications because of the characteristic tendency of liposomes to be taken up rapidly by the RES (31) and by the limited permeability of the endothelial barrier in most tissues to particles of the size usually encountered in liposome preparations (43). Recent work, however, has shown that specific changes in the liposome composition can drastically reduce their uptake by the RES of liver and spleen (44-46). Such liposomes can circulate in the blood for much longer periods of time, compared to the usual compositions presently tested in clinical trials. Eventually, intact liposomes can be found in relatively high amounts in many tissues. Most fortunately, however, we have found them to accumulate in the areas of implanted tumors at concentrations higher than any other organ or tissue of the body outside the RES. Furthermore, when liposomes are conjugated to monoclonal antibodies that recognize antigens on the tumor cell surface, there is a further increase in liposome uptake by the tumor, as opposed to other parts of the body. Such targeting effect to diseased parts of the body, could revolutionize drug delivery for such life threatening diseases as cancer and AIDS. However, much more work is needed before the preliminary results reported here can be considered of potential application to human patients.

RESULTS & DISCUSSION

Our strategy in formulation design was based on the following information regarding stability and blood half-life of liposomes and other particulate carriers. First, the inclusion of cholesterol (Ch) and high-temperature phase transition phospholipids such as sphingomyelin (SM) and distearoylphosphatidylcholine (DSPC) has been shown to increase liposome stability in plasma as determined by the degree of retention of various liposome-encapsulated markers *in vitro* (47–49). Second, formulations containing SM or DSPC are cleared more slowly after intravenous injection than those made with low phase transition temperature lipids such as phosphatidylcholine (PC) from egg yolk (50–52). Third, the inclusion of certain gangliosides, conferring to the vesicle surface a negative charge and increased hydrophilicity, synergizes with cholesterol to enhance liposome stability in plasma (53) and prolongs liposome half-life in blood with a concomitant decrease in liver and spleen uptake (44,45). Hydrophilic coating of polystyrene particles with polymeric glycols also results in significantly enhanced blood half-lives (54). Finally, it has been generally observed that reduction of vesicle size, contributes to slower clearance rate from the circulation (55).

Effect of Lipid Composition on the Tissue Distribution of Liposomes in Normal Mice.

In order to study the effect of lipid composition on tissue distribution *in vivo* we have screened a variety of liposome formulations for their localization in various tissues after i.v. injection in mice. All liposomes were made by thin lipid film hydration, followed by extrusion through polycarbonate membranes of 0.08 or 0.05 μm-pore as previously described (46). The vesicles were radiolabeled with [67]-Gallium deferoxamine according

to a method previously reported (56). To facilitate the analysis of the tissue distribution data,
we have divided the body into 4 arbitrary anatomic
compartments (blood, liver-spleen, carcass-skin,
other organs) and calculated the percentage of
recovered and injected dose for each of them.
Blood represents the pool of circulating liposomes
available for homing to tissues. Liver-spleen is
taken as an approximation to the uptake by the RES.
Carcass-skin includes all bones, muscles, and skin.
Other organs include gut and appendages, kidneys,
heart, and lungs.

To illustrate the various factors that play a
role in prolonging circulation time and improve
biodistribution of liposomes, we have presented in
Figure 1, the percentage of recovered dose in the
various body compartments at 4 hours and 24 hours
after injection using PG and GM1-containing liposomes. The effect of liposome configuration and
size can be clearly recognized when comparing the
unextruded MLV preparation of PG-PC-Ch (size
distribution range 0,5 - 5.0 μm) to the extruded
liposomes (mean size range 70 - 120 nm) of the same
composition at 4 hours after injection (Figure 1A).
A 14-fold increase in the amount remaining in blood
is noticed. However, in both cases the majority of
the label is recovered in liver-spleen. When the
negatively-charged PG is replaced at the same molar
fraction by a negatively-charged glycolipid, GM1,
there is a drastic reduction in the amount accumulated in the liver-spleen compartment, and, as a
result, the circulating liposome pool is significantly larger (~6-fold) than with PG liposomes.

Figure 1B shows the distribution of the GM1-
PC-Ch liposomes 24 hours after injection and
compares them to two more preparations where PC
(derived from egg yolk and forming a fluid bilayer
at body temperature) is replaced by DSPC which
forms a more rigid bilayer at body temperature.
The relative distribution of the liposome
radiolabel was found to be similar when GM1-
containing fluid vesicles (GM1-PC-Ch) are compared
to DPPG-containing solid vesicles (DPPG-DSPC-Ch).
However, with GM1-containing solid vesicles (GM1-

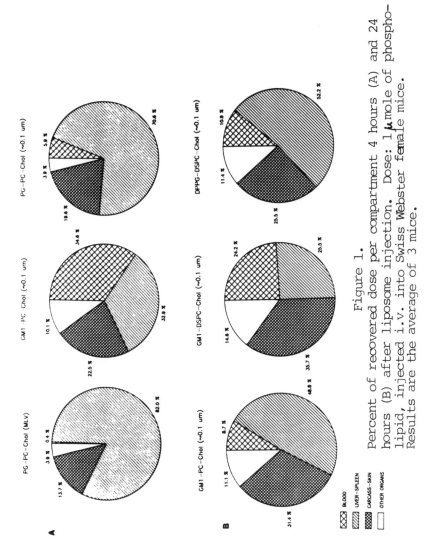

Figure 1.

Percent of recovered dose per compartment 4 hours (A) and 24 hours (B) after liposome injection. Dose: 1 μmole of phospholipid, injected i.v. into Swiss Webster female mice. Results are the average of 3 mice.

DSPC-Ch) the distribution was favorably changed toward higher concentration in blood, and decreased accumulation in liver-spleen. In this case, more than 50% of the recovered dose is found in carcass-skin and other organs, suggesting that liposomes can localize in significant amounts in tissues other than liver and spleen, provided that a long circulation time is achieved. Thus it appears from the comparison shown in Figures 1A and 1B that liposome size, type of surface charge and bilayer fluidity all play a role in determining the optimal characteristics associated with prolonged circulation time of liposomes.

Figure 2 shows the percentage of recovered dose in blood, liver-spleen, and carcass-skin at 24 hours after injection for 20 different liposome compositions, all of which were sized down by extrusion to a mean vesicle diameter of approximately 100 nm (range 70-120 nm). Clearly, as the amount recovered in liver-spleen decreases, the amount remaining in circulation increases. With formulations 1 and 2 (GT1-PC-Ch and PS-PC-Ch), the liposome content of liver-spleen is about 200-fold that of the blood. With formulation 20 (GM1-DSPC-Ch), the liposome contents of blood and liver-spleen are approximately equal. Another observation from Figure 2 is that the liposome uptake of the carcass-skin compartment appears to increase gradually in parallel with the increase in the fraction of circulating liposomes.

To examine whether the trends observed in Figure 2 follow a statistically significant correlation, we performed linear regression analysis of the percentage of recovered dose in blood on the one hand, and the percentages of recovered dose in liver-spleen and carcass-skin on the other hand for each formulation tested in Figure 2. This is displayed graphically in Figure 3. Statistical analysis indicates a correlation coefficient of -0.88 ($p < 10^{-6}$) for RES versus blood, and -0.95 ($p < 10^{-3}$) for RES versus carcass-skin. Multiple regression analysis, using blood and RES as independent variables and carcass-skin as a dependent variable, gives a correlation coefficient of 0.96

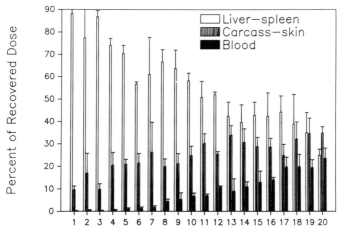

FORMULATION TESTED

Figure 2

Distribution of liposomes in blood, liver-spleen and carcass-skin, at 24 hours post-injection. The numbers correspond to different liposome compositions as follows: (numbers in parenthesis indicate molar ratios).
1, GT1-PC-Ch (1-10-5). 2, PS-PC-Ch (1-10-5). 3, GL4-PC-Ch (1-10-5). 4, PG-PC-Ch (1-10-5). 5, DSPC-Ch (10-5). 6, Sulf-PC-Ch (1-10-5). 7, SM-PC-Ch (8-2-5). 8, HPI-DOPC-Ch (1-10-5). 9, CS-DSPC-Ch (1-10-5). 10, PC-Ch (10-5). 11, GM1-SM-PC-Ch (1-8-2-5). 12, DPPG-DSPC-Ch(1-10-5). 13, PG-DSPC-Ch (1-10-5). 14, PI-PC-Ch (1-10-5). 15, Sulf-DSPC-Ch (1-10-5). 16, GM1-DSPC-Ch (1-10-5). 17, HPI-DSPC-Ch (1-10-5). 18, GM1-SM-DSPC-Ch (1-8-2-5). 19, HPI-HPC-Ch (1-10-5). 20, GM1-DSPC-Ch (1-10-5).

ABBREVIATIONS:
Ch, cholesterol; CS, cholesterol-sulfate; PG, phosphatidylglycerol; DPPG, dipalmitoylphosphatidylglycerol; DSPC, distearoylphosphatidylcholine; GMI, monosialoganglioside; HPI, hydrogenated soybean PI, phosphatidylinositol; Sulf, bovine brain sulfatides; GT1, trisialoganglioside; PS, phosphatidylserine; GL4, globoside;SM, sphingomyelin

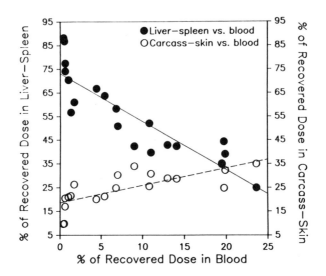

Figure 3

Linear regression analysis of the percent of
recovered dose in blood, versus the percent of
recovered dose in either liver-spleen or carcass-
skin, 24 hours after i.v. injection of various
liposome compositions. Each point represents one
of the liposome compositions presented in Figure 2.

$(p<10^{-3})$. These results strengthen the conclusion
that prolonged circulation of liposomes in blood is
dependent on a reduced and/or retarded uptake by
RES, and that their accumulation in carcass-skin is
determined in turn by the fraction of liposomes
remaining in circulation.

To assess the pharmacological impact of the
observed differences in liposome distribution, we
calculated the area under the curve (AUC) values in
blood and liver for several formulations (Table 1).
When PG-PC-Ch liposomes are compared to GM1-DSPC-Ch
liposomes, the most favorable formulation studied

so far, a 3.8-fold increase in the blood AUC and a 11.2-fold decrease in the liver AUC can be noticed. These results are encouraging inasmuch as the liver AUC can be significantly reduced by manipulating lipid composition. This diminishes the likelihood of toxicity to the RES and enhances the liposome blood pool available for homing to other tissues.

Effect of Lipid Composition on the Tissue Distribution of Liposomes in Tumor-bearing Mice.
Some of the liposome compositions tested in normal mice were also injected in tumor bearing mice to examine their localization in tumors and compare them with that of other tissues. The J6456 tumor, a T-cell-derived lymphoma (57) was inoculated IM in the hind limb of syngeneic BALB/c mice. Liposomes were injected intravenously into mice with tumor implants weighing between 0.5 to 2 g. The results obtained 24 hours after injection are presented in Table 2. A highly significant increase in tumor uptake (up to 25-fold) was observed with liposome formulations selected for longer circulation times in normal mice. The highest tumor uptake (5.3% of injected dose/g) was obtained with GM1-DSPC-Ch liposomes. Another interesting finding is that liposome concentration in tumors is higher than that seen in all other tissues except for liver and spleen (data not shown for spleen). These values were obtained after correcting for the blood content of tumors of similar size as determined by [111]Indium-oxine-labeled red blood cells (58). Therefore, indicated that the increased liposome concentration in tumors was not due to the tumor vascular blood pool. When free [67]Gallium-deferoxamine was injected, the uptake by tumor at 24h was <0.1% of injected dose per gram. Preliminary results from our laboratory indicate that liposomes with long circulation times show a similarly enhanced accumulation in two other tumor models, mouse B16 melanoma, and human LS174 colon carcinoma. These data support the hypothesis that accumulation of liposomes in tumors depends on a prolonged circulation time. If localization in other important tissues is not enhanced to the same

degree, as suggested in this study, the new liposome formulations would provide an opportunity for
selective delivery of drugs to tumors.

TABLE 1
AUC (1-24 HRS) IN BLOOD AND LIVER[1]

Composition (Molar Ratio)	$\dfrac{\mu\text{moles Phospholipid} \times \text{hr}}{\text{g tissue}}$		
	Liver	Blood	Ratio: Liver/ Blood
PG-PC-Ch (1:10:5)	7.34	0.52	14.1
DPPG-DSPCh-Ch (1:10:5)	4.27	3.52	1.2
HPI-DSPC-Ch (1:10:5)	3.31	3.82	0.9
GM1-SM-DSPC-Ch (1:8:2:5)	1.76	2.21	0.8
GM1-PC-Ch (1:10:5)	1.68	2.66	0.6
GM1-DSPC-Ch (1:10:5)	1.95	5.84	0.3

[1] Data obtained from 3 time points (3 hr, 24 hr)
and from 3 mice for each time point and each
formulation tested. Dose 1μmol phospholipid per
mouse, iv. in Swiss Webster female mice.

CONCLUDING REMARKS

The significance of the studies reported here
is related to the possibility of increasing concentrations of anti-cancer agents in tumors   Our
recent studies indicate that this can be achieved
by using liposomes with   reduced rate of RES-
mediated clearance, thereby diminishing the likeli-

TABLE 2
TISSUE DISTRIBUTION OF LIPOSOMES IN TUMOR-BEARING MICE
% Injected Dose/G (SD)

Liposome Composition (Molar Ratio)	Tumor	Blood	Liver	Kidney	Lung	Skin
PG-PC-C(1-9-5)	0.2(0.0)	0.5(0.2)	36.4(6.3)	1.9(0.8)	0.8(0.2)	0.7(0.2)
SULF-DSPC-C(1-10-5)	2.1(0.3)	0.5(0.1)	32.1(4.5)	2.1(0.4)	1.5(0.4)	0.6(0.2)
DSPC-C(10-5)	2.1(0.3)	0.2(0.0)	36.5(7.6)	1.3(0.2)	0.9(0.0)	0.6(0.0)
CS-DSPC-C(1-10-5)	2.5(0.2)	0.2(0.0)	29.7(1.4)	1.5(0.3)	1.4(0.1)	0.6(0.1)
DPPG-DSPC-C(1-10-5)	4.1(1.7)	0.3(0.0)	38.3(0.5)	1.9(0.1)	1.7(0.4)	0.7(0.1)
HPI-DSPC-C(1-10-5)	4.1(1.2)	1.4(0.3)	37.8(0.4)	2.3(0.6)	2.1(0.3)	0.9(0.3)
GM1-PC-C(1-9-5)	3.5(0.6)	2.6(0.2)	20.7(1.0)	2.8(0.9)	2.9(0.9)	0.8(0.1)
GM1-DSPC-C(1-10-5)	5.3 (1.0)	3.1 (0.5)	31.7 (1.5)	4.7 (1.1)	1.7 (0.4)	1.3 (0.1)

- BALB/c female mice were inoculated IM with 10^6 J6456 tumor cells in the hind leg. Two to three weeks later, mice received each of the indicated formulations at a dose of 1 μmol phospholipid per mouse and were sacrificed 24 hours later. Average tumor weight ranged from 0.5 to 2.0 g. Total body recovery of radiolabeled material ranged from 50-70% of injected dose.

hood of RES toxicity. RES blockade has been used for increasing the tumor uptake of subsequently administered sonicated neutral DSPC-Ch liposomes (52). However, RES blockade may result in toxicity (59,60), and adds complexity to the pharmacokinetic and pharmacodynamic analysis. The data reported here are also of significance in the context of the broadest use of liposomes as drug carriers. Manipulations in formulation can have profound effects on the *in vivo* clearance and disposition of liposomes, reflecting the extreme versatility of this carrier, and the possibility of tailoring its design to various applications.

The accumulation of liposomes into the implanted tumors reported here, could be due to convective transport through leaky endothelia, as has been noted before for various tumors (61). Such accumulation should be differentiated from the serendipitous targeting of most liposomes (62) to liver and spleen which involves their recognition by the RES cells. Accumulation in tumors is apparently related to the ability of liposomes to stay in the circulation for longer periods of time, which in turn is controlled by the surface chemical characteristics that determine the extent of their recognition by the RES. Since we have no information that the observed accumulation in tumors depends on specific recognition, we define the phenomenon as non-specific targeting. This definition helps to differentiate it from ligand-specific targeting (33-35) which has also been demonstrated with tumor cells *in vivo* (45). Such non-specific tumor targeting with liposomes may have the advantage of general applicability and simplicity compared with other approaches relying on recognition of specific antigens expressed by tumor cells, such as antibody conjugation to toxins, liposomes, drugs or radionuclides (45,61,62)

ACKNOWLEDGEMENTS

We thank Renee Shiota for technical assistance.
This work was supported until November 1987 by a grant from the National Cancer Institute (CA 35340)

and subsequently by Liposome Technology, Inc., (Menlo Park, CA).

REFERENCES

1. Bangham AD, Standish MM, Watkins JC (1965). Diffusion of univalent ions across the lamelae of swollen phospholipids J Mol Biol 13:238.
2. Bangham AD, Hill MW, Miller NGA (1974). Preparation and use of liposomes as models of biological membranes. In Korn ED, (ed): "Methods in Membrane Biology," New York: Plenum Press, p 1.
3. Papahadjopoulos D, Kimelberg HK (1973).A recent review on reconstitution of membrane proteins etc on liposomes. In Davidson SG, (ed): "Progress in Surface Science," Pergamon Press, p 141.
4. Jost PC, Thompson TE, Weinstein JN, Parsegian VA (1982). Protein-lipid interactions in membranes. Biophys J 37:1.
5. Düzgünes N, Papahadjopoulos D (1983). Ionotropic effects on phospholipid membranes: Calcium/magnesium specificity in binding, fluidity and fusion. In Aloia RC (ed): "Membrane Fluidity in Biology," Vol. 2, New York: Academic Press, p 187.
6. Honegger JL, Isakson PC, Kinsky SC (1980). Murine immunogenicity of N-substituted PE derivatives in liposomes: Response to the hapten P.C. J Immunol 124:669.
7. Hafeman D, Lewis J, McConnel H (1980). Triggering of the macrophage and neutrophil respiratory burst by antibody bound to a spin-label phospholipid hapten in model lipid bilayer membranes. Biochemistry 19:23.
8. Müller-Eberhard HJ (1988) Molecular Organization and Function of the Complement System. Ann Rev Biochem 57:321.
9 . Bangham AD, (1961) A correlation between surface charge and coagulant action of phospholipids. Nature 192:1197.
10. Papahadjopoulos D, Hougie D, Hanachan D (1962). Influence of surface charge of

phospholipids on their clot-promoting activity. Proc Soc Exper Biol 111:412.

11. Papahadjopoulos D, (1974). Cholesterol and cell membrane functions: A hypothesis concerning the etiology of atherosclerosis. J Theoret Biol 43:329.

12. Small DM, Shipley GG (1974) Physical-chemical basis of lipid deposition in atheroschrosis. Science 185:222.

13. Papahadjopoulos D (1978). Liposomes and their uses in biology and medicine. Ann NY Acad Sci Vol: 308.

14. Gregoriadis G (1988). Liposomes as drug carriers: Trends and Progress, London, John Wiley Ltd.

15. Ostro MJ (1987). "Liposomes From Biophysics to Therapeutics." New York: Marcel Dekker, Inc.

16 Black ED, Watson GJ, Ward RJ (1977). The use of pentostam liposomes in the chemotherapy of experimental leishmaniasis. Trans R Soc Trop Med Hyg 71:550.

17. New RR, Chance ML, Thomas SC, Peters W (1978). Antileishmanial activity of antimonials entrapped in liposomes. Nature 272:55.

18. Alving CR, Steck EA, Chapman WL Jr, Waits VW, Hendricks LD, Swartz GM, Hanson WL (1978). Therapy of leishmaniasis: Superior efficacies of liposome-encapsulated drugs. Proc Natl Acad Sci (USA) 75:2959.

19. Gabizon A, Peretz T, Ben-Yosef R, Catane R, Biran S, Barenholz Y (1986). Phase I study with liposome-assoc. Adriamycin: preliminary report. Proc Am Soc Clin Oncol 5:43

20. Treat J, Roh JK, Woolley PV, Neefe J, Schein PS Rahman A, (1987). A phase I study: Liposome-encapsulated doxorubicin. Proc Am Soc Clin Oncol 6:31.

21. Lopez-Berestein, Fainstein GV, Hopfer R, Mehta K, Sullivan MP, Keating M, Rosenblum MG, Mehta R, Luna M, Hersh EM, Reuben J, Juliano RJ, Bodey GP (1985). J Inf Dis 151:704.

22. Koff WC, Showalter SD, Hounpar D, Fidler IJ (1985). Science 228:495.

23. Mihalco PJ, Schreier H, Abra RM (1988). Liposomes: a pulmonary perspetive. In

Gregoriadis G (ed): "In Liposomes as drug arrives: Trends and progress," John Wiley Ltd.

24. Turner AF, Presant CA, Proffitt RJ, Williams LE, Windsor DW,Werner JL (1988). In-111-labeled Liposomes: Dosimetry and Tumor Depiction. Radiology 166:761.

25. Sculier JP, Coune A, Meunier F, Brassinne C, Laduron C, Hollaert C, Collette N, Heymans C, Klastersky J (1988). Pilot Study of Amphotericin B Entrapped in Sonicated Liposomes in Cancer Patients with Fungal Infections. Eur. J. Cancer Clin. Oncol. 24:527.

26. Rahman A, Carmichael D, Harris M, Roh JK (1986). Comparative Pharmacokinetics of Free Doxorubian and Doxorubian Entrapped in Cardiolipin Liposomes. Cancer Res. 46:2295.

27. Forssen EA, Tokes ZA (1981). Use of anionic liposomes for the reduction of chronic doxorubicin-induced cardiotoxicity. Proc Natl Acad Sci USA, 78:1873.

28. Olson F, Mayhew E, Maslow D, Rustum Y, Szoka F (1982). Characterization toxicity and therapeutic efficacy of adriamycin encapsulated in liposomes. Eur J Cancer Clin Oncol 18:167.

29. Gabizon A, Meshorer A, Barenholz Y (1986a). Comparative long-term study of the toxicities of free and liposome-associated doxorubicin in mice after intravenous administration. J Natl Cancer Inst 77:459.

30. Lopez-Berestein G, Mehta R, Hopfer R,Mills K, Kasi L, Mehta K, Fainstein V, Hersh E, Juliano R, (1983). J Inf Dis 147:939.

31. Gregoriadis G, Senior J. In: Targeting of drugs with synthetic systems. Gregoriadis G, Senior J, Poste G, (eds):"Plenum Press," New York, p. 183.

32. Scherphof G, Roerdink F, Dikstra J, Ellens H, DeZanger R, Wisse E (1983) Biol. Cell. 47: 47.

33. Heath TD, Fraley R, Papahadjopoulos D, (1980). Conjugation of Ab on Liposomes. Science, 210: 539.

34. Leserman LD, Barbet J, Kourilsky FM, Weinstein JN, (1980). Nature, (London) 288:602.
35. Huang A, Huang L, Kennel SJ (1980). J. Biol. Chem. 255:8015.
36. Papahadjopoulos D, Jacobson K, Nir S, Isac, T (1973). Phase transitions in phospholipid vesicles: Fluorescence polarization and permeability properties concerning the effect of temperature and cholesterol. Biochim Biophys Acta 311:330.
37. Yatvin MB, Weinstein JN, Dennis WH Blumenthal R (1978). Design of liposomes for enhanced local release of drugs by hyperthermia. Science 202:1290.
38. Weinstein JN, Magin RL, Yatvin MB, and Zaharko DS (1979). Liposomes and local hyperthermia: selective delivery of methotrexate to heated tumors. Science 204:188.
39. Yatvin MB, Kreutz W, Horwitz BA Shinitzky M (1980). pH-sensitive liposomes: possible clinical implications. Science 210:1253.
40. Duzgunes N Straubinger RM, Baldwin PA Friend DS, Papahadjopoulos D (1985). Proton-induced fusio of oleic acid/phosphatidylethanolamine liposomes. Biochemistry 24:3091.
41. Ellens H, Bentz J, Szoka F (1984). H^+ and Ca^{2+} Induced fusion and destabilization of liposomes. Biochemistry 23:1532.
42. Connor J, Yatvin MB, Huang L (1984). pH-sensitive liposomes: Acid-induced liposome fusion. Proc. Natl Acad. Sci USA 81:1715.
43. Poste G (1983). Liposome targeting in vivo: problems and opportunities. Biol. Cell, 47:19.
44. Allen TM, Chonn A (1987). Large unilamellar liposomes with low uptake into the reticuloendothelial system. FEBS Lett. 223:42-46.
45. Papahadjopoulos D, Gabizon A. (1987). Targeting of liposomes to tumor cells in vivo. Ann NY Acad Sci 504:64.
46. Gabizon A, Papahadjopoulos D (1988).Liposome formulations with prolonged circulation time

in blood and enhanced uptake by tumors. Proc Natl Acad Sci (in press).

47.   Senior J, Gregoriadis G (1982).Stability of small unilamellar liposomes in serum and clearance from the circulation: effect of phospholipid and cholesterol components. Life Sci 30:2123.

48.   Mayhew E, Rustum Y, Szoka F, Papahadjopoulos D (1979). Role of cholesterol in enhancing the antitumor activity of cytosine arabinoside entrapped in liposomes. Cancer Treat Rep 63:1923.

49.   Allen TM, (1981).A study of phospholipid interactions between high density lipoproteins and small unilamellar vesicles. Biochim Biophys Acta 640:385.

50.   Gregoriadis G, Senior J (1986). Liposomes in vivo: A relationship between stability and clearance. In Gregoriadis G, Senior J Poste G (eds.) "Targeting of drugs with synthetic Systems," New York: Plenum Press, p 183.

51.   Hwang KJ, Luk KK, Beaumier PL (1980). Hepatic uptake and degradation of unilamellar sphingomyelin/cholesterol liposomes: A kinetic study. Proc Natl Acad. Sci 77:4030.

52.   Proffitt RT, Williams LE, Presant CA, Tin GW, Uliana JA, Gamble RC, Baldeschwieler JD (1983). Liposomal blockage of the reticuloendothelial system: improved tumor imaging with small unilamellar vesicles. Science 220:502.

53.   Allen TM, Ryan JL, Papahadjopoulos D (1985). Gangliosides reduce leakage of acqueous-space markers from liposomes in the presence of plasma. Biochim Biophys Acta 818:205.

54.   Illum L, Davis SS (1983). J Pharm Sci 72:1086.

55.   Senior, J.H.. (1987) Crit. Rev. Ther. Drug Carrier Systems. 3:123-193.

56.   Gabizon A, Huberty J, Straubinger RM, Price DC Papahadjopoulos D (1988). An improved method for in vivo tracing and imaging of liposomes using a gallium[67]-deferoxamine complex. J Liposome Res 1:124.

57. Gabizon A, Trainin N (1980). Enhancement of growth of a radiation-induced lymphoma by T cells from normal mice. Br J Cancer 42:551.

58. Heaton WA, Davis HH, Welch MJ, Mathias, CJ, Joist, HH, Sherman LA, Siegel BA (1979). Br. J. Haematol. 42:613.

59. Zimmerman HJ (1986). Progress in Liver Disease. 8:621.

60. Allen TM, Murray L, MacKeigan S, Shah M (1984). Chronic liposome administration in mice: Effects on reticuloendothelial function and tissue distribution. J Pharmacol Exp Ther 229:267.

61. Jain RK, Gerlowski LE (1986). Extravascular transport in normal and tumor tissues. Crit Rev Oncol Hematol 5:115.

62. Mayhew E, Papahadjopoulos D (1983). Therapeutic applications of liposomes. In Ostro, MJ (ed): "Liposomes," New York: Marcel Dekker, Inc p 289.

63. Davies AJS, Crumpton MJ, Eds. (1982). In "Experimental Approaches to Drug Targeting." Cancer Surveys 1(3):347.

64. Order S, Ed. (1987). In "Labeled and Unlabeled Antibody in cancer Diagnosis and Therapy." NCI Monger 3.

Liposomes in the Therapy of Infectious Diseases and Cancer, pages 155–163
© 1989 Alan R. Liss, Inc.

LIPOSOMES - FROM THE BENCH TO THE MARKETPLACE:
DOXORUBICIN LIPOSOMES AS AN EXAMPLE

Marc J. Ostro, Ph.D.

The Liposome Company, Inc., One Research Way
Princeton, New Jersey 08540

The motivation for encapsulating doxorubicin in
liposomes stems from the desire to develop a
commercializable form of the drug which has diminished
acute and chronic toxicity while exhibiting efficacy at
least equivalent to unencapsulated drug at a comparable
dose. It is presumed that if the drug in the liposome is
less toxic, higher doses can be administered which would
result in enhanced efficacy.

Liposome encapsulated doxorubicin has a long
history. In fact, there have been well over thirty
publications in the field using a wide variety of
liposome types and compositions. In spite of the study
to study variations in vesicle structure, most of the
work has demonstrated (in mice) reduced acute toxicity
without compromising activity against several ascitic and
solid experimental tumors. In addition, it has been
demonstrated by several laboratories in rodents, and dogs
(1-3) that liposomal encapsulation of doxorubicin results
in a significant reduction in cardiotoxicity compared to
unencapsulated drug. This has been primarily attributed
to the fact that encapsulated drug does not accumulate in
the heart tissue. Work in this area has progressed to
the point where preparations made by Rahman, et al. (4)
and Gabizon, et al. (5) and The Liposome Company are
currently undergoing clinical testing in Israel, England,
Canada and the U.S.

However, in spite of all the work that has been done
on liposomal doxorubicin, a product has not yet been
commercialized. The reasons for this are many, but

certainly the fact that much of the early work was done
in academic settings where the rigors of the
pharmaceutical industry as monitored by the Food and Drug
Administration (FDA) have not been routinely addressed is
a contributing factor. Now that liposome-encapsulated
drugs are being tested in humans, these pharmaceutical
demands must be met. Problems such as scale-up to
thousands of liters, sterility, reproducibility of the
preparations, pyrogen content, integrity of the raw
materials, acute, subacute and chronic toxicity, quality
control methods, regulatory issues, patentability and
cost must be resolved. In this chapter, I will attempt
to briefly discuss all of these issues.

When one considers embarking on the development of a
new pharmaceutical product, several criteria must be
satisfied. Clearly, there must be a reason to believe
that the proposed product will satisfy a clinical need.
If this requirement is not fulfilled, then the
continuation of the project would be precluded. The drug
must be efficacious, it must have an acceptable toxicity
profile, it must be stable, manufacturable, economical
and patentable. The process for sorting out all of these
issues is complex. The research and development sequence
begins in the exploratory mode which then leads into the
development of a prototype product which undergoes
preclinical testing and finally clinical evaluation. Of
course, towards the end of this sequence, the FDA plays a
major role in determining how fast one can progress.
Each one of the steps in this sequence will be discussed
briefly.

While this sequence could be applicable to the
development of any new drug, there are specific steps
which are unique to the development of a liposome-
encapsulated drug. For example, the first task that must
be accomplished is the efficient encapsulation of the
drug in a liposome. In the case of doxorubicin, this has
represented a significant impediment to commercial
development of a product. Doxorubicin is amphipathic
and, as such, represents a class of molecules which
cannot be efficiently and stably encapsulated in a lipid
vesicle. The drug does not recognize the lipid bilayer
as a permeability barrier. Therefore, once encapsulated,
the drug rapidly leaks out of the liposome. For example,
the half-life of leak in saline at 37°C of doxorubicin

from liposomes composed of egg phosphatidylcholine is
approximately one hour. Given that one needs to develop
a product with at least 18 months of stability, the
classical approach to encapsulation must be changed. One
method of overcoming this problem was developed by Mayer,
et al. (6) and shall be referred to as "remote
loading". The mechanism for remote loading involves the
generation of an electric potential across a liposome
membrane. This is accomplished by creating a pH
differential between the inside of the liposome and the
extra liposomal buffer. It has been found that a $\triangle$
pH of 3.0 to 3.5 units will create approximately 150
millivolts of electric potential. For example, if one
entraps buffer at pH 4 and suspends the liposome at pH
7.5, a 3.5 log differential in the hydrogen ion
concentration will be created. Since protons will
permeate lipid bilayers in the direction of the
concentration gradient, an electric potential is
generated. If one mixes these liposomes with a molecule
that has some degree of lipid solubility and is cationic,
the molecule will get pulled through the liposome
membrane and accumulate on the inside of the vesicle.
When one uses this technique to encapsulate doxorubicin,
up to a 500 millimolar concentration of the drug within
the liposome can be achieved.

From a commercialization standpoint, this approach
for encapsulating doxorubicin has several advantages.

1. Since the drug and the liposomes are not mixed
    together until just prior to use, the issue of drug
    leakage over time is condensed from years to hours.

2. In the past, unsuccessful attempts to stably
    encapsulate doxorubicin by classical means have
    involved the use of anionic phospholipids such as
    phosphatidyglycerol and cardiolipin in an attempt to
    develop a charge/charge interaction between the
    positively charged drug and the vesicle membrane.
    These phospholipids are extremely expensive and add
    possibly unacceptable cost to the doxorubicin
    product. When remote loading is used, there is no
    constraint on the choice of vesicle composition,
    thereby permitting the use of inexpensive
    phosphatidylcholine as a major component of the
    liposome membrane.

3. The best encapsulation of doxorubicin that has been
    reported in the literature is approximately 50% (1).
    Remote loading allows for the encapsulation of close
    to 100% of the drug. This, once again, impacts on
    the overall cost of the product since elaborate drug
    recovery systems do not need to be established.
    Disposal of unencapsulated doxorubicin is not
    practical since its wholesale cost is $177 per 50 mg
    vial.

4. To date, the best lipid:drug ratio that has been
    achieved is 12:1 (1). The remote loading process
    routinely generates 3:1 lipid to drug ratios.

5. One must consider when thinking about commercializing
    a doxorubicin liposome product the process for
    eventual large scale manufacturing. Classical
    liposome encapsulation involves the physical handling
    of the doxorubicin itself. This drug is highly
    caustic and must be handled only under specialized
    conditions. This requires the construction of a
    facility capable of handling this compound, once
    again adding to the overall cost of the product.
    With the remote loading system, the unencapsulated
    doxorubicin is never removed from its vial. No
    contact is made during the manufacture of the
    liposome.

Once the doxorubicin is encapsulated, preliminary
toxicity and efficacy studies must be performed.
Liposome encapsulation of doxorubicin increases the
LD_{50} from 20mg/kg for unencapsulated drug to 57 mg/kg,
thereby enabling one to give more than twice the amount
of drug before acute toxicity is encountered. This
concept is important when one tries to improve the drug's
efficacy. Table 1 is a compilation of the data generated
from six different animal tumor models where the efficacy
of free and encapsulated doxorubicin were compared. In
five out of six instances, (L1210 leukemia, P388
leukemia, Shinogi breast carcinoma, P815 mastocytoma and
B16 melanoma) comparable doses of free and liposome
encapsulated drug resulted in the same therapeutic
benefit. In the case of M5076, liposomal doxorubicin was
more potent than free drug. In all cases, higher doses
of liposome encapsulated doxorubicin could be
administered resulting in increases in efficacy. In the

case of the Shinogi breast carcinoma, when 13 mg/kg of
encapsulated drug was administered, the mass of the tumor
was reduced to the point where it could no longer be
palpated.

Once the optimal encapsulation of doxorubicin has
been achieved and its preliminary efficacy and toxicity
determined, the exploratory phase of the research program
is concluded and product development begins. One of the
most crucial aspects of product development is the
establishment of validated analytical methods which can
be used to guarantee that the drug which is produced is
the same from lot to lot and is stable over time.
Developing the methods to measure the "intactness" of a
"conventional" drug is often difficult since one must
prove that the assays used can detect any changes in the
structure of the molecule. This difficulty is compounded
when one considers the liposomal form of a drug since one
now must consider the integrity of a three dimensional
structure in addition to the identity of the active
ingredient. To accomplish this, validated assays for the
lipid raw materials, the particle itself and the drug
must be established. Once all relevant variables are
identified, a specification sheet can be written which
defines the limits within which each parameter may vary.
For example, egg phosphatidylcholine (EPC) is used as one
of the membrane constituents of liposomal doxorubicin.

TABLE 1
TREATMENT OF MURINE TUMORS WITH THE OPTIMAL DOSE OF
UNENCAPSULATED AND ENCAPSULATED DOXORUBICIN

TUMOR	Dosing Schedule (Days Post Tumor Innoculation)	Long Term Survivors (Number/Total) ([Days]) FREE	LIPO	Maximum % T/C[+] FREE	LIPO	% Tumor Reduction FREE	LIPO
*L1210 Leukemia	1	0/10 [60]	2/10 [60]	189	222	—	—
*P388 Leukemia	1	0/10 [48]	2/10 [48]	181	224	—	—
*B16 Melanoma	1,5,9	6/6 [48]	6/6 [48]	119	119	—	—
*M5076 Reticulosarcoma	1,5,9	9/10 [30]	10/10 [30]	148	204	—	—
Shinogi Breast Carcinoma	7,14,21	—	—	—	—	50	100
P815 Mastocytoma	1	6/10 [90]	8/10 [90]	—	—	—	—

*All experiments done under GLP.
[+]Median day of survival in treated groups/median day of survival in untreated group X 100

Table 2 shows the parameters measured and the techniques used to establish its specifications. If a lot of EPC does not meet the narrow range of values chosen to be be acceptable for each assay, then the EPC is not used. Each raw material must comply with its own list of specifications. Once the liposomes are produced, the final product (both pre- and post- reconstitution) must also meet the appropriate specifications.

TABLE 2
METHODS USED TO ANALYZE EGG PHOSPHATIDYLCHOLINE

Test	Method
Total Phospholipid Content	Bartlett Phoshpate Assay
EPC Purity	(TLC)Thin Layer Chromatography
Lyso PC Content	TLC
Sphingomyelin Content	TLC
Neutral Lipid Content	TLC
PE Content	TLC
H_2O Content	Karl Fischer Titration
Peroxide Value	Iodometric Spectrophotometry
Acid Value	Sodium Hydroxide Titration
Heavy Metal	Sodium Sulfide Precipitation

Once validated, stability indicating assays have been established, the formulations must be assessed for stability at several temperatures. For liposomal doxorubicin, GLP (Good Laboratory Practice) tests have been run at 5°, 20°, 35° and $60^\circ C$. After 90 days, the buffer-filled pH 4 liposomes have shown no sign of change at either 5° or $20^\circ C$. These studies are continuing. Non-GLP studies have demonstrated an excess of 14 months of stability at $5^\circ C$.

The last part of the product development phase involves the creation of processes (Process Development) which can be used to produce pilot scale quantities of liposomes. To put this in perspective, at the exploratory stage of development, liposomes are typically made in volumes of 10-100 ml. At the pilot scale, liposomes would be produced in 10-100 liter lots. For liposomal doxorubicin, buffer filled liposomes have been

produced in 10-20 liter batch sizes. Commercial scale
would probably entail a 10-50 fold scale up from pilot
production.

The next step in the product development cascade is
to initiate preclinical efficacy and toxicity studies.
Formal preclinical studies are preferrably done using
material manufactured by good manufacturing practices
(GMP) and carried out under GLP. The specific purpose of
these studies is to support the filing of an
investigational new drug application (IND) with the FDA.
Remote-loaded liposomal doxorubicin has been tested
against 4 tumor models (see Table 1) and found to be at
least as efficacious as free drug at comparable doses
and, in most cases, more efficacious at higher doses.

One and five day toxicology studies have also been
completed in mice and dogs. In both species, following
the 1 and 5-day dosing schedule, liposomal drug proved to
be better tolerated than free doxorubicin. In the single
dose study, approximately two times as much drug could be
given in the liposomes as in the free form before dose
limiting toxicity was encountered.

In addition to efficacy and toxicity studies, one
must evaluate the distribution, metabolism and excretion
(DME) of the drug in experimental animals. It is
important to note that this aspect of preclinical
development does not have to be completed for IND
approval. However, completed DME studies must be
available prior to the submission of a new drug
application (NDA) to the FDA.

The data generated thus far plus a detailed
description of the manufacturing process and the clinical
protocols (approved by the relevant institutional review
board) can now be codified in an IND submission
eventually leading to the initiation of the Phase I, II
and III clinical assessment of the drug. At present,
remote-loaded doxorubicin liposomes are entering Phase I
studies in the United States. The purpose of this study
is to determine the maximum tolerated dose of the drug in
cancer patients with advanced disease. Once this goal
has been achieved, Phase II studies designed to assess
efficacy of liposomal doxorubicin against specific
indications and eventually Phase III studies designed to

gather statistically significant efficacy data in large numbers of patients compared to the best known existing therapy can be initiated. Of course, the ultimate goal is to collect enough meaningful clinical data to convince the FDA to allow the drug to be sold for general use.

While much has been accomplished to reach this goal with liposomal doxorubicin, there are still several hurdles to overcome. A sobering thought is that after many years of progress in the liposome field, it is still not reasonable to expect the first liposome-based therapeutic products to reach the market until 1991 or 1992.

ACKNOWLEDGEMENTS

This work was actually done by numerous scientists at The Liposome Company, The Canadian Liposome Company and Roswell Park Memorial Institute.

Specifically at The Liposome Company: Richard Ginsberg, Jacqueline Coelln, George Mitilenes, Frank Pilkiewicz and Joel Portnoff.

The Canadian Liposome Company: Pieter Cullis and Lawrence Mayer.

Roswell Park Memorial Institute: Peter Kanter.

REFERENCES

1. Herman EH, Rahman A, Ferrans VJ, Vick JA, Schein, PS (1983). Prevention of chronic doxorubicin cardiotoxicity in beagles by liposomal encapsulation. Cancer Res. 43:5427.

2. Forssen EA, Tokes ZA (1981). Use of anionic liposomes for the reduction of chronic doxorubicin-induced cardiotoxicity. Proc. Nat'l Acad Sci 78:1873.

3. Van Hoesel QGCM, Steerenberg PA, Crommelin DJA, vanDijk A, vanOrt W, Klein S, Douze JMC, deWildt DJ, Hillen, FC (1984). Reduced Cardiotoxicity and nephrotoxicity with preservation of antitumor activity of doxorubicin entrapped in stable liposomes in the LOU/M Wsl. rat. Cancer Res. 44:3698.

4. Treat J. This volume.

5. Gabizon A. This volume.

6. Mayer LD, Bally MD, Hope MJ, Cullis PR (1985). Uptake of antineoplastic agents into large unilamellar vesicles in response to a membrane potential. Biochim. Biophys. Acta 816:294.

III. LIPOSOMES IN INFECTIOUS DISEASES-I

Liposomes in the Therapy of Infectious Diseases and Cancer, pages 167–176

LIPOSOME COMPOSITION AND ACTIVATION OF MACROPHAGES FOR ANTIMICROBIAL ACTIVITIES AGAINST LEISHMANIA PARASITES

Carol A. Nacy, Micheal J. Gilbreath, Glenn M. Swartz Monte S. Meltzer, and Carl R. Alving

Departments of Immunology and Membrane Biochemistry Walter Reed Army Institute of Research Washington, DC 20307-5100

ABSTRACT   In vitro activation of macrophages by lymphokines induces the intracellular destruction of **Leishmania major**, a parasite that replicates in macrophages of infected individuals. Lymphokines encapsulated in liposomes that had as a constituent phosphatidylserine (PS) did not activate macrophages for eradication of the intracellular parasite. The addition of PS liposomes by themselves abrogated macrophage intracellular killing induced by free lymphokines. Liposome-induced suppression occurred during the priming phase of macrophage activation, and was specific for macrophage killing of intracellular parasites: PS liposomes did not affect macrophage killing of tumor targets or performance of several other effector functions of activated macrophages. This dissociation of liposome effects on macrophage functions resulted from a breakdown product of one of the constituent lipids. Liposome composition will be a critical element in designing therapies for immunomodulation of these parasitic diseases.

INTRODUCTION

Liposome-encapsulated drugs are successful therapeutic modalities for treatment of certain systemic parasitic infections in experimental animals (1-3). The administration of encapsulated antimony or amphotericin B prevents lethal visceral disease in hamsters and monkeys infected with the obligate intracellular parasite, **Leishmania donovani** (3). Concentrations of the drugs required for effective therapy are substantially less (100-fold) than that required for cure without encapsulation (3). The targets for drug delivery by liposomes are phagocytic macrophages of liver and spleen, cells that also serve as host cells for replication of this parasite (4). In 1984, Reed and coworkers reported that mice treated with liposome-encapsulated lymphokines (soluble products of stimulated lymphocytes) had fewer hepatic parasites than control groups infected with the New World agent of visceral leishmaniasis, **L. chagasi** (5). Injection of lymphokines by itself (no liposomes) had little effect on the intrahepatic replication of the parasite. The differences in parasite burden in liposome-treated animals, although small, suggested that liposomes might also be useful for immunotherapy of parasitic diseases. Indeed, the same theory behind the successful delivery of chemotherapeutic agents to macrophages of infected animals could be postulated for delivery of macrophage activating lymphokines to infected cells. We initiated a series of studies to examine the **in vitro** activation of macrophages by liposome-encapsulated lymphokines for intracellular destruction of **L. major,** a parasite that causes cutaneous ulcers with systemic complications in humans and certain mouse strains. Rather than an augmentation of killing, however, we found that lymphokines encapsulated in liposomes composed of phosphatidylserine (PS) were totally ineffective for activating macrophages to eradicate the intracellular parasite (6-9).

RESULTS

Resident peritoneal macrophages from C3H/HeN mice develop potent antimicrobial activities against intracellular amastigotes of the protozoan parasite **L. major** following treatment with lymphokines. Table-1 shows a dose response curve of macrophages treated with lymphokines, with or without encapsulation in liposomes. Cells treated with unencapsulated lymphokines develop the ability to kill almost all the intracellular parasites (80-100% decrease in infected cells). In contrast, cells treated with lymphokines encapsulated in phosphatidylcholine/phosphatidylserine liposomes (PC/PS, 7:3 molar ratio) had markedly diminished antimicrobial activity (7).

TABLE 1
LYMPHOKINE ACTIVATION OF MACROPHAGES FOR
ANTIMICROBIAL ACTIVITY AGAINST LEISHMANIA

Treatment	Conc.	Percent infected macrophages	Microbicidal activity (%)
Medium		68 ± 3	0
Medium + PC/PS liposomes		68 ± 5	0
Lymphokines	1/6	3 ± 2	93
	1/18	8 ± 4	88
	1/54	16 ± 3	76
PC/PS liposome-encapsulated lymphokines	1/6	58 ± 4	15
	1/18	67 ± 2	2
	1/54	69 ± 4	0

That the failure of liposome-encapsulated lymphokines to activate macrophages was an intrinsic property of the liposome itself was demonstrated by adding empty PC/PS liposomes to unencapsulated lymphokines (Figure 1). To provide a control for the effects of macrophage phagocytosis of non-specific particles, we exposed certain of the cultures to lymphokines plus latex beads. As you can see from Figure 1, cells treated with lymphokines alone or in the presence of latex beads develop potent antimicrobial activity, while cells treated with lymphokines in the presence of empty PC/PS liposomes are essentially inactive for intracellular destruction of the parasite. The degree of suppression of lymphokine-induced effector activities is directly related to the concentration of PC/PS liposomes in the lymphokine preparation: 100 nmol/ml PC/PS liposomes is sufficient to completely block the induction of intracellular killing by lymphokines (7). Despite the potent effect of liposomes on the induction of activated microbicidal macrophages, we could not document any toxic effect of the liposomes on the macrophages themselves: macrophage viability, phagocytosis by several receptors, and performance of a number of other effector reactions remain the same as medium control cells.

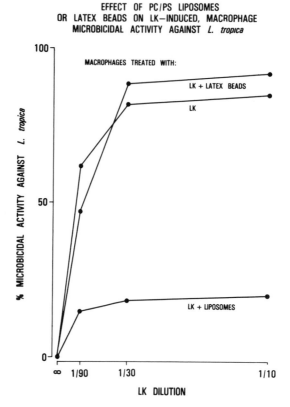

EFFECT OF PC/PS LIPOSOMES
OR LATEX BEADS ON LK—INDUCED, MACROPHAGE
MICROBICIDAL ACTIVITY AGAINST *L. tropica*

FIGURE 1.   ACTIVATION OF MACROPHAGES BY LYMPHOKINES

The effect of PC/PS liposomes on macrophage effector functions was specific for intracellular killing of **Leishmania**. Treatment of macrophages with lymphokines before exposure to parasites profoundly alters the capacity of these cells to phagocytose amastigotes, and fewer cells become infected in lymphokine-pretreated macrophage cultures than medium-treated controls (10). This macrophage antimicrobial effector function is called "resistance to infection", since it is not yet clear whether the parasites are killed extracellularly, or only prevented from entry by lymphokine-induced modulation of macrophage receptors for parasite entry. Macrophages treated with lymphokines also develop the capacity to kill the fibrosarcoma TU-5 (11). Figure 2 shows a lymphokine dose response for induction of intracellular killing, resistance to infection, and tumor cytotoxicity. In each case, lymphokines alone induced potent killing of the intracellular and extracellular targets; addition of PC/PS liposomes affected the induction of intracellular killing by lymphokines, but expression of resistance to infection and tumoricidal activity was indistinguishable in cultures treated with lymphokines with or without the addition of PC/PS liposomes (6).

FIGURE 2. INDUCTION OF MACROPHAGE EFFECTOR ACTIVITIES

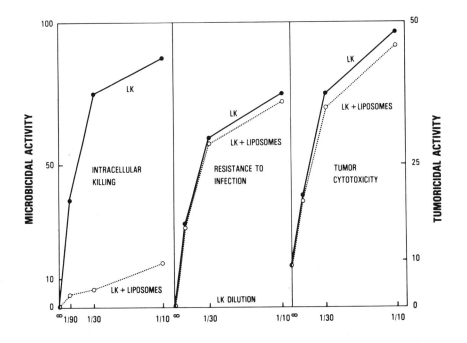

To examine whether the PC/PS liposomes interfered with the effector mechanism of activated macrophages for intracellular destruction of the parasite, we injected mice intraperitoneally with several macrophage activation agents: **Mycobacterium bovis**, strain BCG and **Corynebacterium parvum (Propionibacterium acnes)**. Macrophages obtained from in vivo-treated animals are activated at the time of explantation, and spontaneously kill a variety of obligate and facultatively intracellular microorganisms (11). The high spontaneous intracellular killing activity of these in vivo activated cells (90-100%) was not diminished in the presence of PC/PS liposomes (Table 2). The effect of liposomes, then must not be on the effector mechanism of activated macrophages, but on the early events that occur during lymphokine induction of intracellular killing (7).

TABLE 2
EFFECT OF PC/PS LIPOSOMES ON IN VIVO
ACTIVATED MACROPHAGE ANTIMICROBIAL ACTIVITIES

Macrophages from:	Cells treated with:	Microbicidal activity (%):
Control mice	Medium	0
	Medium + liposomes	2
	Lymphokines	78
	Lymphokines + liposomes	9
BCG-infected mice	Medium	90
	Medium + liposomes	96
C. parvum treated mice	Medium	97
	Medium + liposomes	100

The induction of a number of activated macrophage effector activities, including intracellular killing, occurs by sequential interaction of endogenous lymphokines and accessory factors (11). Factors generated during an immune response "prime" the cell for killing activities, but the actual microbicidal effector function occurs after a "trigger" signal is received by the primed macrophage. Certain aspects of this priming phenomenon can be recapitulated by experiments with brief pulses of lymphokine in vitro. Treatment of macrophages with lymphokines for 4-8 hr elicits microbicidal activity at 72 hr equivalent to that induced by treatment with lymphokine throughout the entire culture period (11). Macrophages pulsed with lymphokine for less than 4 hr fail to develop microbicidal activity. During this 4 hr time period, the physiology of the resting macrophage is changed. Analysis of the time course for suppression of macrophage activation suggests that PC/PS liposomes interfere with one (or more) of the intracellular signals that are required for the priming stage of macrophage activation: liposomes added before, but not after 6 hr exposure of macrophages to lymphokines are suppressive (8).

The constituent lipid responsible for the rapid and profound suppression of macrophage antimicrobial activities induced by PC/PS liposomes was PS (6). Figure 3 demonstrates that macrophages treated with lymphokines in the presence of liposomes composed of only PC were equally active for the intracellular destruction of L. major as cells treated with lymphokines alone.

FIGURE 3.   LIPID COMPOSITION AND ACTIVATION OF MACROPHAGES

INHIBITION OF LK-INDUCED, MACROPHAGE MICROBICIDAL ACTIVITY BY PC/PS LIPOSOMES : DOSE RESPONSE

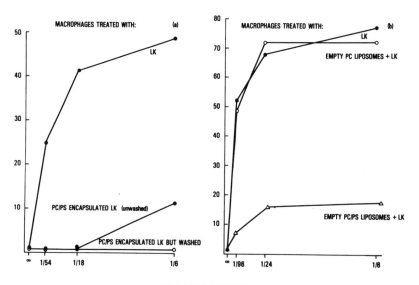

LYMPHOKINE DILUTION

Altering the lipid composition to include increasing concentrations of cholesterol did not affect the ability of PC/PS liposomes to inhibit microbicidal activity. Further, replacement of PS with any number of other lipids , such as phosphatidylinositol or dicetylphosphate totally abolished the ability of liposomes to inhibit the development of activated macrophage antimicrobial activities (8).

A possible insight into the mechanism of inhibition by PS liposomes came from experiments with the synthetic phospholipid DMPS: cells treated with lymphokines in the presence of PC/DMPS developed full capacity to kill the intracellular parasite (8). By replacing PS in liposomes with DMPS, at least two simultaneous changes occur. First, the normal unsaturated fatty acids of PS are replaced by a saturated fatty acid. Second, this saturated PS is now much less susceptible than highly unsaturated PS to digestion by phospholipase A_2 into lysophosphatidylserine (lysoPS). Indeed, liposomes composed of PC/lysoPS were strongly inhibitory for the development of macrophage intracellular killing activities. That the lysoPS was a breakdown product induced by **macrophage** lysosomal phospholipase A_2 activity (12) on PC/PS liposomes was demonstrated by analysis of the PC/PS liposomes for the presence of lysoPS: quantities were less than detectable levels (0.4%) by thin layer chromatography, and were, if present, substantially less than the minimal amount of lysoPS required for induction of the liposome suppressive effects (2%) by PC/lysoPS liposomes.

More recently, we examined the efficacy of different synthetic phospholipids for inhibition of macrophage activation for intracellular destruction of L. major (9). These studies showed that both the number of saturated bonds and the composition of the headgroups of the fatty acid influenced the ability of the phospholipid to inhibit intracellular killing. In all cases, however, the inhibitory activity could be attributed to the conversion of the fatty acid to lysoPS by by metabolic conversion to PS and cleavage by phospholipase A_2.

DISCUSSION

There is increasing interest in the use of liposomes as drug delivery agents or as adjuvants in vaccine preparations. Obviously, selection of a particular liposome for these uses will depend upon the balance between efficacy and toxic side effects. Quite apart from the discussion above on the possible mechanisms of action, the data we present clearly demonstrates that changes in liposome phospholipid composition dramatically affect cell function and, in turn, the pharmacology of any given agent. The liposome activities we describe are not generalized toxic effects (PC/PS liposome inhibition of intracellular killing was reversible) but rather selective alterations in cell biology. Careful definition of these liposome-macrophage interactions **in vitro** may provide a physiologic basis for selection of liposomes for therapeutic use.

REFERENCES

1.   Heath S, Chance ML, New RR (1984) Quantitative and ultrastructural studies on the uptake of drug loaded liposomes by mononuclear phagocytes infected with **Leishmania donovani.** Mol Biochem Parasitol 12:49.
2.   Panosian CB, Barza M, Szoka F, and Wyler DJ (1984) Treatment of cutaneous leishmaniasis with liposome-intercalate amphotericin B. Antimicrob Agents Chemother 25:655.
3.   Berman JD, Hansen WL, Chapman WL, Alving CR, Lopez-Berestein G (1986) Antileishmanial activity of liposome-encapsulated amphotericin B in hamsters and monkeys. Antimicrob Agents Chemother 30:847.
4.   Alving CR, Weldon JS, Munnell JF, and Hansen WL (1985) Liposomes in leishmaniasis: the lysosome connection. In Gregoriadis G, Poste G, Senior J, and Trouet A (eds): "Receptor-mediated Targeting of Drugs," New York: Plenum Press, p 317.
5.   Reed SG, Barral-Netto M, Inverso JA (1984) Treatment of experimental visceral leishmaniasis with lymphokine encapsulated in liposomes. J Immunol 132:3116.
6.   Gilbreath MJ, Swartz GM Jr, Alving CR, Nacy CA, Hoover DL, and Meltzer MS (1985) Differential inhibition of macrophage microbicidal activity by liposomes. Infect Immun 47:567.
7.   Gilbreath MJ, Nacy CA, Hoover DL, Alving CR, Swartz GM Jr, and Meltzer MS (1985) Macrophage activation for microbicidal activity against **Leishmania major:** inhibition of lymphokine activation by phosphatidylcholine-phosphatidylserine liposomes. J Immunol 134:3420.
8.   Gilbreath MJ, Hoover DL, Alving CR, Swartz GM Jr, and Meltzer MS (1986) Inhibition of lymphokine-induced macrophage microbicidal activity against **Leishmania major** by liposomes: characterization of the physicochemical require-

ments for liposome inhibition. J Immunol 137:1681.
9. Gilbreath MJ, Fogler WF, Swartz GM Jr., Alving CR, and Meltzer MS Inhibition of Intergeron gamma-induced macrophage microbicidal activity against Leishmania major by liposomes: inhibition is dependent upon composition of phospholipid headgroups and fatty acids. (submitted).
10. Nacy CA, Meltzer MS, Leonard EJ, and Wyler DJ (1981) Intracellular replication and lymphokine-induced destruction of Leishmania tropica in C3H/HeN mouse macrophages.   J Immunol 127:2381.
11. Nacy CA, Oster CN, James Sl, and Meltzer MS (1984) Activation of macrophages for destruction of intracellular and extracellular parasites. Cont Topics Immunobiol 13:147.
12. Snyder DS and Unanue ER (1982) Corticocosteroids inhibit murine macrophage Ia expression and interleukin 1 production. J Immunol 129:1803.

Liposomes in the Therapy of Infectious Diseases and Cancer, pages 177–190
© 1989 Alan R. Liss, Inc.

COMPARATIVE ACTIVITIES OF FREE AND LIPOSOME ENCAPSULATED AMIKACIN AGAINST MYCOBACTERIUM AVIUM COMPLEX (MAC)[1]

Pattisapu R.J. Gangadharam[2], Veluchamy K. Perumal[2],
L. Kesavalu[2] Robert J. Debs, Jayne Goldstein[3]
and Nejat Duzgunes[3]

Mycobacteriology Research Laboratories, National Jewish Center
for Immunology and Respiratory Medicine, Denver, Colorado 80206
and Cancer Research Institute, University of California,
San Francisco, San Francisco, California

ABSTRACT   Mycobacterium avium complex (MAC) causes
serious disseminated disease in normal and immune deficient
individuals, more so in AIDS victims. In a multifaceted
approach to identify new drugs active against MAC, we
discovered   that   amikacin   at   50   mg/kg   dose   given
intramuscularly (IM) daily exhibited high activity against
experimental MAC infections in the beige mouse model. In
order to reduce the dose and duration of treatment, we
investigated   the   liposome-encapsulated   amikacin   in
comparative studies with the standard IM dose in the same
model. The drug was encapsulated in phosphatidyl–glycerol
(PG)/phosphatidyl-Choline (PC) liposomes, at a dose of 5 mg/kg
(1/10 the IM dose), given intravenously in four injections at 1
day, and weekly intervals up to 3 weeks; this regimen was
compared with the 50 mg/kg dose given 6 injections a week for
8 weeks. Liposome-amikacin inhibited the growth of MAC in
the liver over an 8 week period retaining the colony forming
unit (CFU) counts 3 orders of magnitude below that in untreated
animals whereas free amikacin or buffer loaded liposomes were
ineffective.   Amikacin encapsulated in liposomes was also
effective against MAC in the spleen and kidneys reducing the
CFU counts by 1,000 fold compared to untreated controls and
free drug. A reduction in the counts was observed in the lungs
only at 8 weeks in mice given the liposome formulation and in
lymph nodes the counts were not effected by either free or
encapsulated amikacin. In confirmation with earlier findings,
IM dose showed remarkable reduction of the counts in the
organs.   Liposome encapsulated amikacin showed marked
inhibition of intracellular multiplication of MAC inside resident

---

[1]This investigation is supported by NIH Contract No. AI 76236,
NIH grant AI 21897 and grant from AIDS Task Force University
Systems of California.

and activated macrophages from beige, C57Bl/6 or S/W mice; in these situations, free amikacin was not active. In contrast, both free and liposome encapsulated forms were equally active against MAC growth in J-774 A.1 cell lines.

INTRODUCTION

Mycobacterium avium intracellulare complex (MAC) group of organisms cause serious pulmonary and disseminated disease in normal and immune compromised individuals, more so in acquired immune deficiency syndrome (AIDS) patients (1). More than 50% of AIDS victims have this opportunistic infection and many succumb to it within one year after diagnosis (2). Chemotherapeutic management of this disease with available drugs is poor because most of the available drugs are ineffective against this organism (3). Discovery of potential drugs active against this disease, more so in AIDS patients has become an urgent necessity. With our beige mouse model for MAC disease (4), we tested several compounds which were found to be active in vitro by conventional and radiometric (BACTEC) procedures (5). Among these, amikacin proved to be the most effective in dynamic in vitro and in vivo studies (6,7). When MAC infected beige mice were treated intramuscularly (IM) daily (6 days a week) for 8 weeks with amikacin, (50 mg/kg), a remarkable in vivo chemotherapeutic activity was evident, with a highly significant reduction in the colony forming unit (CFU) counts of the recoverable organisms from the spleen, liver, lungs, kidneys and lymph nodes in the drug treated group as compared to the controls. However, the dose of 50 mg/kg given daily for 8 weeks, necessitated in the mouse model as equivalent to 15 mg/kg given to humans, as demonstrated by serum levels is high, and involves multiple injections over a prolonged period. Attempts were therefore made to reduce the dosage and number of injections, with parallel lowering of toxicity and cost. One approach deals with the liposome encapsulation of this drug, whose comparative chemotherapeutic activity with free drug is assessed and discussed in this communication.

Amikacin sulphate was obtained from Sigma Chemical Company (St. Louis, MO). The infecting organism, MAC strain 101 (serotype 1) was isolated from the blood of an AIDS patient (8). A single cell suspension of a predominantly (> 95%) of transparent colony suspension of this strain was obtained using the procedures previously described (9,10). Each animal received 10^6 to 10^7 viable units of the organism through a caudal vein. Treatment, either with free amikacin given IM 50 mg/kg, 6 days a week for 8 weeks or 5 mg/kg given in 4 IV injections or with liposome encapsulated form at the same dose (5 mg/kg) with 4 injections (1 day and 1, 2, and 3, weeks) was started after challenge. The animals were followed for mortality and CFU counts.   At each time point at 1 day and weekly intervals after challenge, 3 randomly selected animals were sacrificed and the number of organisms of MAC from spleen, liver, lungs, kidney and pooled lymph nodes (superficial inguinal, mesenteric, superficial deep cervical and renal) were obtained by plating aliquots of the dilutions of the ground suspension of the tissues on to 7H11 agar medium.   The inoculated plates were incubated at 37° C for three weeks after which the CFU counts were enumerated.

Standard randomization procedures were employed in selecting the animals to be killed at scheduled intervals.   To avoid bias, the identity of the group of animals was concealed from the observer until the CFU counts were enumerated. Student's t test and analysis of variance were used in individual experiments to analyze the data.

Amikacin was encapsulated in liposomes composed of phosphatidyl-glycerol/phosphatidyl-choline/cholesterol (1:1:1 molar ratio), by reverse phase evaporation followed by extrusion through polycarbonate membranes (11).   A sterile solution of amikacin (50 mg/ml) in 10 mM KCl 5 mM glycine, pH 9.6, adjusted to an osmolarity of 300 mM with NaCl, was added to a solution of lipids in diethyl ether (5.0 mu mole lipid in 2 ml) at a 1:3 ratio, and the mixture was sonicated under argon for 5 minutes.   The resulting emulsion was evaporated under controlled vacuum in a rotary evaporator as described previously (13). To eliminate residual ether, the suspension was supplemented with a 1.32 ml of amikacin solution and placed in the evaporator for an additional 20 minutes.   The liposomes were extruded through polycarbonate membranes of 0.2 mu M pore diameter (Nuclepore, Pleasanton, California) under Argon pressure.   Unencapsulated amikacin was eliminated by chromatographing the liposome suspension on sterilized Sephadex G-75 using 140 mM NaCl, 10 mM KCl, 10 mM glycine, pH 9.6 as the elusion buffer.   Liposome suspension was filtered through 0.22 mM filter (Schleicher and Schuell, Keene, New Hampshire) to insure sterility.   The size distribution of the liposomes was ascertained in a Coulter NP-4 Dynamic Light scattering instrument.   The mean diameter of the vesicles was in the range of 400 nm with standard deviation of 140 nm.

The amount of unencapsulated amikacin was determined by an ELISA assay after lysing the liposomes with 0.5% Triton X-100 using DuPont ACA discrete clinical analyzer. The assay is based on the activity of glucose-6 phosphate dehydrogenase conjugated to amikacin.   The enzyme is inhibited when the conjugate is bound to anti-amikacin antibody.   The amount of bound conjugate is determined by the concentration of free amikacin which competes for the antibody.   Phospholipid concentrations were determined by phosphate analysis (13).   Control liposomes containing buffer only without amikacin were prepared with 140 mM NaCl, 10 mM KCl, 5 mM glycine, pH 9.6 as the aqueous medium.

The effect of treatment with the free and liposome encapsulated forms of amikacin on the progress of MAC disease in the beige mouse model over a period of 8 weeks is discussed separately for each tissue.

Spleen

Figure 1

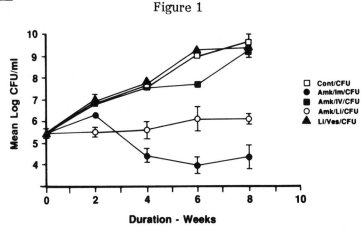

Intravenous administration of 4 weekly low doses of amikacin (5 mg/kg) encapsulated in liposomes prevented the in vivo multiplication of MAC in spleen even though the overall reduction during the period of 8 weeks was greater with the intramuscular dose (Figure 1). The results with intramuscular dose are similar to those obtained by us in other studies. By two weeks, the CFU counts in animals with liposomal amikacin treatment were 1.5 log units lower than the CFU counts in untreated animals and those receiving the free drug. At 8 weeks i.e., 5 weeks after the end of treatment, the CFU counts were approximately 3 log units lower in liposome amikacin treated animals than in controls or those receiving free IV amikacin at 5 mg/kg. The CFU in the spleen of free amikacin treated mice increased by five orders of magnitude in 8 weeks, whereas in liposome-amikacin treated animals, the increase was only two orders of magnitude. It is of interest, that liposome-amikacin treated animals showed a considerable reduction in CFU counts compared to controls at a 2 week point at which time the daily IM treatment, with a high dose, did not show any effect (P < 0.0005). In four weeks the CFU counts in the two groups were similar despite the 60-fold higher dose of IM amikacin.

Liver

Essentially similar results were obtained with liver as with the spleen (Figure 2). Intramuscular treatment caused significant reduction in CFU counts and the control animals as well as those receiving empty vesicles or the intravenous dose of amikacin showed no effect. The liposome amikacin treated group with four intravenous injections of the low dose (5 mg/kg) prevented the in vivo multiplication of MAC over the 8 week period. At 8 weeks, the CFU counts in the liposome group were more than three orders of magnitude below the buffer or empty liposome controls or the free amikacin group. The effect of the liposome amikacin persisted at least 5 weeks after cessation of treatment.

Figure 2

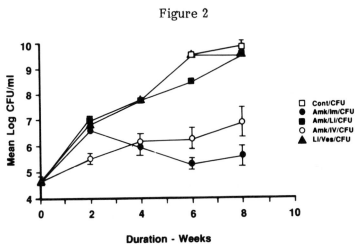

Kidneys

Figure 3.

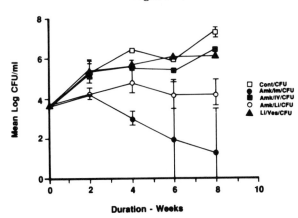

In the kidneys, liposome encapsulated amikacin prevented the increase of CFU counts as in the spleen and liver; however, unlike those tissues, no difference in CFU counts between the liposome group and the IM group was observed at 2 weeks in the tissue (Figure 3). At the end of 8 weeks, the CFU counts in mice treated with lipsome amikacin were a 1000-fold lower than the untreated animals

(P < 0.025), whereas in mice given free intravenous amikacin at a low dose the reduction in CFU counts was less than 10-fold.

Lungs

Lung CFU levels were not effected by the intravenous administration of free or liposome encapsulated amikacin over a 6 week period (Figure 4).

Figure 4

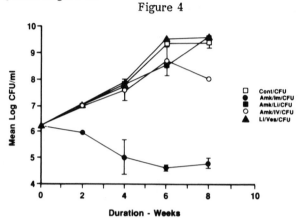

At 8 weeks the liposome amikacin groups exhibited a slight reduction in CFU counts compared to the untreated control groups (P < 0.025). Intramuscular administration of amikacin at high doses reduced the CFU counts below the baseline day 1 level starting at the 2 week point, reaching 1.6 log units below this level by the 6th week. It is suggested that the vesicle size may be instrumental in limiting the availability of the drug in this tissue; this aspect is considered in the design of the next batch of experiments discussed later.

Lymph Nodes

Essentially similar results as with lungs were obtained with lymph nodes (Figure 5).

Figure 5

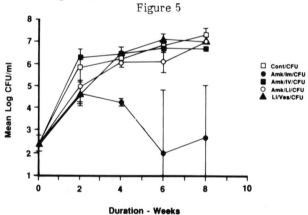

Neither the free nor encapsulated amikacin was effective over an 8 week period while the control intramuscular group was effective in reducing the counts over the 8 week period. The reduction of the CFU counts in the IM group was significant from 4 weeks onwards.

Overall Comparison of IV and IM Doses

In order to facilitate a direct and easy comparison of the liposome encapsulated and free amikacin forms of amikacin against MAC disease in the beige mouse model, the results obtained in various tissues are summarized in Table 1.

Table 1. Comparison of the reduction in CFU counts in Beige mice treated with free or liposome-encapsulated amikacin administered intravenuously, or amikacin given intramuscularly. The reduction is given log CFU relative to the control animals.

			REDUCTION OF MEAN LOG CFU RELATIVE TO CONTROL				
TIME	TREATMENT	TOTAL DOSE (µg)	LIVER	SPLEEN	LUNGS	KIDNEYS	LYMPH NODES
2 WEEKS	EMPTY LIPOSOMES	0	-0.07	0.11	0.03	-0.10	1.18
	AMIKACIN LIPOSOMES	200	1.37	1.46	0.08	1.11	0.85
	FREE AMIKACIN	200	-0.10	0.00	0.03	-0.11	-0.44
	IM AMIKACIN	12000	0.62	0.32	1.10	1.15	1.16
4 WEEKS	EMPTY LIPOSOMES	0	-0.04	-0.02	0.05	0.71	-0.29
	AMIKACIN LIPOSOMES	400	2.12	1.56	0.21	1.57	0.13
	FREE AMIKACIN	400	0.10	-0.06	-0.10	0.73	-0.24
	IM AMIKACIN	24000	3.34	1.77	2.76	3.43	1.95
6 WEEKS	EMPTY LIPOSOMES	0	-0.20	-0.03	-0.15	-0.10	-0.32
	AMIKACIN LIPOSOMES	400	2.97	3.17	0.66	1.98	0.71
	FREE AMIKACIN	400	1.36	0.99	0.80	0.78	0.08
	IM AMIKACIN	36000	5.12	4.14	4.71	4.18	4.78
8 WEEKS	EMPTY LIPOSOMES	0	0.10	0.25	-0.21	1.16	0.24
	AMIKACIN LIPOSOMES	400	3.45	2.95	0.57	3.14	0.24
	FREE AMIKACIN	400	0.26	0.28	-0.22	0.86	0.54
	IM AMIKACIN	.48000	5.23	4.23	4.59	6.01	4.54

Considerable reduction in CFU counts compared to controls were observed in IM and liposome and amikacin groups. At two weeks, the liposome group showed greater reduction than the IM group in the liver and spleen. If the reduction in CFU count is expressed with respect to the unit dose of drug administered, the liposome amikacin group showed a remarkable efficiency of therapeutic response. For example, at two weeks, the reduction of the CFU in the spleen per unit dose of liposome encapsulated amikacin was 1,280-fold greater than the IM amikacin group and 394-fold greater in the liver. At 4 weeks, these values were 3.6-fold in the liver and 38-fold in the spleen. Although the CFU counts in the IM group were reduced below the baseline (day 1 levels) over the 8 week period the reduction of CFU in the liver and spleen per unit drug dose was greater in the liposome amikacin group than the IM group (2 and 6.34-fold) respectively.

Summarizing the results discussed so far, it can be said that liposome encapsulation facilitated reduction of the CFU counts in the spleen, liver and kidneys although not in the lungs and lymph nodes. In the next series of experiments, we extended these investigations in three directions: (i) by increasing the dose of liposome encapsulated form from 5 mg/kg to 10 mg/kg, (ii) increasing the number of injections from 4 to 5 i.e., at 1 day, and weekly intervals up to 4 weeks instead of 3 weeks and (iii) increasing the vesicle size of the liposomes, with the hope that more drug would be delivered to the lungs. The choice of animals, challenge with MAC strain and follow-up of the animals were essentially the same as in the earlier studies. As before, the results were discussed separately for the spleen, liver and lungs.

Spleen

The CFU counts in tissues of animals receiving various regimens (liposome amikacin with 5 and 10 mg/kg in small and large vesicles, free amikacin given intravenously, empty liposome vesicles and buffer control) are given in Figure 6.

Figure 6

SMALL & LARGE LIPOSOME AMIKACIN ON MAC IN BEIGE MICE.

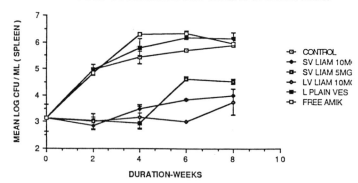

The liposome amikacin at 5 mg/kg in small vesicles gave comparable results with previous experiments (Figure 6). Increasing the dose to 10 mg/kg body weight, which is 1/5th the intramuscular dose, showed better response than the 5 mg/kg dose. The vesicle size adds more to the killing effect in that the 10 mg/kg in the large vesicles showed higher results than the small vesicles. As in previous experiments, both controls (buffer alone or empty liposome vesicles) as well as free intravenous amikacin showed negligible effect on the growth rate of the organisms.

Liver

Figure 7.

SMALL & LARGE LIPOSOME AMIKACIN ON MAC IN BEIGE MICE.

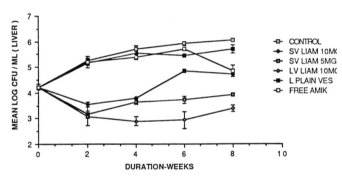

Essentially similar results were obtained as with the spleen and the effect of the vesicle size and dosage is more pronounced in the liver than the spleen (Figure 7).

Lungs

One of the main purposes of using the larger vesicles in the second series of experiments was to find out whether the effect would be seen to a greater extent in the lungs than the small vesicles. Only slight effect was seen in the 8th week as seen in earlier studies with larger vesicles containing 10 mg dose (Figure 8)

Figure 8

SMALL & LARGE LIPOSOME AMIKACIN ON MAC IN BEIGE MICE.

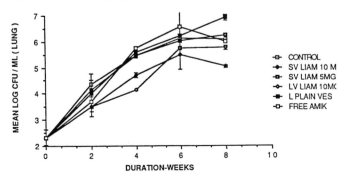

The animal experiments discussed above gives the indication that it is possible to reduce the amount of amikacin with added advantage of the reduction of trauma of multiple injections and savings in cost, yet getting beneficial results with respect to the control of MAC infections. The results are all the more valuable since we the immune deficient beige mouse model. Increasing the dose to 10 mg from 5 mg showed better effect, but increasing the vesicle size does not seem to offer the expected advantage in the lungs. Even with 10 mg/kg dose given for 5 injections as done in the second series, the amount and number of doses was significantly lower than the standard intramuscular injections of 50 mg/kg dose given 6 days a week for 8 weeks These results warrant explorations to develop a feasible and acceptable form of chemotherapy of MAC infections in humans.

In other studies, we have compared the effects of free and liposome amikacin against phagocytosis and intracellular multiplication of MAC in resident and activated macrophages and J-774 A.1 macrophage cell lines. These studies were done with the belief that any chemotherapeutic agent for mycobacterial diseases should be able to to kill all persisting bacilli inside the macrophages.

Earlier studies by us with free amikacin on MAC inside resident and activated macrophages in beige mice showed negligible effect (14). Extension of these studies to C57Bl/6 and S/W mice gave the same results. Following the encouragement from animal data discussed above, we explored whether the liposome encapsulated amikacin will be more effective against intracellularly multiplying MAC inside macrophages and cell lines.

In these studies macrophages to the bacteria and drug were exposed either in vitro or in vivo either simultaneously or one before the other, separated by an interval of 48 hours. Macrophages were harvested by lavaging the peritoneal cavity with Hanks Balanced Salt Solution containing heparin and after allowing the suspension to adhere for 2 hours, the nonadherent cells were washed out. The medium was replaced with fresh RPMI 1640 medium and the macrophages allowed to incubate at 37° C in 5% CO_2 for 24 hours. In all these studies, one day old adherent macrophages are used. The number of AFB inside the macrophages were counted after lysing the macrophages at various time periods with 0.25% sodium dodecyl sulphate (SDS) and plating aliquots of lysates on 7H11 agar medium.   The inoculated plates were read after three weeks incubation at 37° C. In in vivo studies with macrophages, healthy animals were given free or liposome amikacin for an arbitrary period of 2 weeks, at which time the macrophages were harvested and allowed to adhere and after 1 day were exposed either to MAC or to MAC and free or liposome amikacin as the case may be.

Considering the situation where peritoneal macrophages were exposed in vitro simultaneously to MAC, only liposome encapsulated amikacin shows marked inhibitory activity (Figure 9).

Figure 9

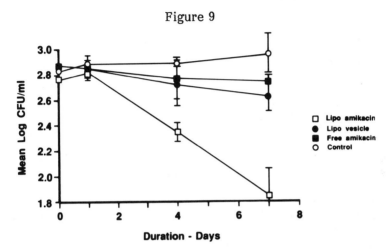

Similar results were obtained when the bacteria were exposed to the macrophages 48 hours prior to the effect of the drugs (Figure 10).

Figure 10

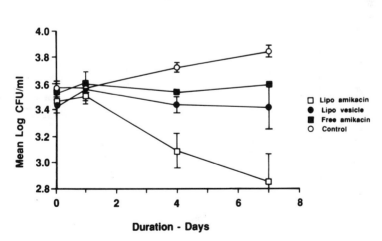

Figure 11

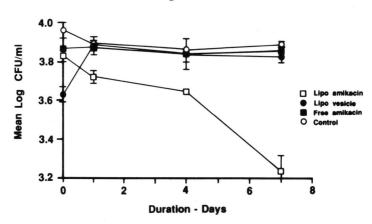

The effect of free amikacin is much less pronounced, and the liposome encapsulated form showed marked inhibitory activity when the drugs were given 48 hours prior to the phagocytosis by the bacteria (Figure 11).

In contrast to the in vitro studies discussed above, when the macrophages were harvested from the animals previously treated with either liposome encapsulated amikacin or free amikacin, there was negligible difference between the two groups (Figure 12).

Figure 12

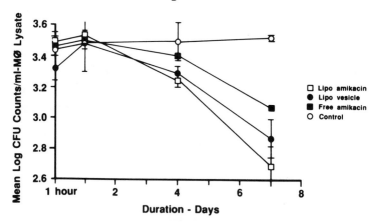

The above studies were repeated wherein such adherent macrophages had further addition of the drug along with the bacteria showed greater inhibition compared to those of the free amikacin group (Figure 13).

Figure 13

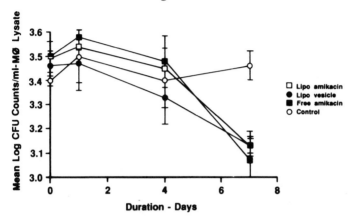

Likewise, free and liposome encapsualted forms showed similar inhalation of MAC inside J-774 A.1 cell lines.

In conclusion, liposome encapsulated amikacin showed enhanced in vivo activity in the beige mouse model as well as in the macrophage system against MAC. This is encouraging in that the marked efficacy of this drug which was shown by us and others in in vitro and animal studies (6,7), can be further simplified for clinical application by reducing the amount of dose and number of injections. While confirming the advantage of liposome encapsulation of aminoglycoside antibiotics for application of effective chemotherapy against mycobacterial infections, these studies pave the way for further approaches in similar situations. Besides our studies, there are only two or three reports dealing with experimental chemotherapy of mycobacterial diseases using liposome encapsulation formulations (15,16). While aminoglycoside antibiotics have been of great use in the treatment of mycobacterial diseases, their application to chemotherapy of MAC disease, a stubborn mycobacterial infection with liposome encapsulated forms is encouraging.

ACKNOWLEDGEMENTS

The authors thank Ms. Kishori Parikh for technical assistance, Mr. Barry Silverstein for illustrations.

REFERENCES

1.   Horsburgh CR, Mason VG III, Farhi DC and Iseman MD (1985). Disseminated infection with Mycobacterium avium complex. Medicine 64: 36-48.

2. Wong B, Edwards FF, Kiehn TE, Whimbey H, Donnely, Bernard EM, Gold JWM and Armstrong D (1985). Continuous high-grade Mycobacterium avium complex bacteremia in patients with the acquired immune deficiency syndrome. Am J Med 78:35-40.

3. L.S. Young (1986). Management of opportunistic infections complicating the acquired immunodeficiency syndrome. J Med Clin North Amer 70:677-692.

4. Gangadharam PRJ, Edwards CK III, Murthy PS and Pratt PF (1983). An acute infection model for Mycobacterium intracellulare disease using beige mice: Preliminary results. Am Rev Respir Dis 127:648-649.

5. Gangadharam PRJ and Lindholm-Levy PJ (1984). Radiometric and conventional drug susceptibility studies of different serovars of Mycobacterium intracellulare. Am Rev Respir Dis 129:A186 (abstract).

6. Gangadharam PRJ, Kesavalu L, Podapati NR, Perumal VK and Iseman MD (1988). Activity of amikacin against Mycobacterium avium complex under simulated in vivo condition. Antimicrob. Agents Chemother 32:483-87.

7. Gangadharam PRJ, Perumal VK, Podapati NR, Kesavalu L and Iseman MD. In vivo chemotherapeutic activity of amikacin alone or in combination with clofazimine or rifabutin or both against acute experimental Mycobacterium avium complex (MAC) infections in beige mice. Antimicrob. Agents Chemother., (In press).

8. Bertram MA, Inderleid CB, Yadegar S, Kolanski P, Yamada JK and Young LS (1986). Confirmation of the beige mouse model for study of disseminated infection with Mycobacterium avium complex. J Inf Dis 154:194-198.

9. Gangadharam PRJ, Pratt PF (1983). In vitro response of murine alveolar and peritoneal macrophages to Mycobacterium intracellulare. Am Rev Respir Dis 128:1044-7.

10. Gangadharam PRJ and Edwards CK III (1984). Release of superoxide anion (O_2^-) from resident and activated mouse peritoneal macrophages infected with Mycobacterium intracellulare. Am Rev Respir Dis 130:834-838.

11. Duzgunes N, Wilschut K, Hong K, Fraley R, Perry C, Friend DS James TL and Papahadjopoulos D (1983). Physiochemical characterization of large unilamellar phospholipid vesicles prepared by reverse-phase evaporation. Biochem Biophys Acta 732:289-299.

12. Szoka F, Olson F, Heath T, Vail W, Mayhew E and Papahadjopoulos (1980). Preparation of unilamellar liposomes of intermediate size (0.1 - 0.2 um) by a combination of reverse phase evaporation and extrusion through polycarbonate membranes. Biochem Biophys Acta 601:559-571.

13. Bartlett Gr (1959) Phosphorus assay in column chromatography. J Bio Chem 234:466-468.

14. Gangadharam PRJ, Perumal VK and Kesavalu L. Unpublished Observation.

15. Orozco LCC, Quintana FO, Beltran RM, de Moreno I, Wasserman M and Rodriquez G (1986). The use of rifampicin and isoniazid entrapped in liposomes for the treatment of murine tuberculosis. Tubercle 67:91:97.

Liposomes in the Therapy of Infectious Diseases and Cancer, pages 191–203
© 1989 Alan R. Liss, Inc.

COMPARISON OF FREE AND LIPOSOMAL MTP-PE:
PHARMACOLOGICAL, TOXICOLOGICAL AND PHARMACOKINETIC ASPECTS

G. Schumann, P. van Hoogevest, P. Fankhauser,
A. Probst, A. Peil, M. Court, J.-C. Schaffner, M. Fischer,
T. Skripsky, and P. Graepel

Research and Development Laboratories,
Pharmaceuticals Division, CIBA-GEIGY Limited,
Basle, Switzerland

ABSTRACT   When   compared   with   MTP-PE   solubilized   in
buffer,   MTP-PE   encapsulated   in   multilamellar   liposomes   composed   of   the   synthetic   phospholipids   POPC
and   OOPS   (MLV)   given   intravenously   showed   a   10   times
higher   efficacy   in   eradicating   lung   and   lymph   node
metastases   in   mice   bearing   the   B16/BL6   melanoma   (0.1
mg/kg MTP-PE/MLV versus 1 mg/kg MTP-PE in free form).
In   two   weeks   to   3   months   intravenous   toxicity   tests
in   dogs   and   rabbits,   the   MLV   formulation   was   less
toxic   than   the   free   form   (toxic-no-effect   level   0.1
mg/kg   MTP-PE/MLV   versus   0.01   mg/kg   MTP-PE   in   free
form)   indicating   an   increased   therapeutic   window   of
the liposomal formulation.
Pharmacokinetic   studies   show   that   30   minutes   and   6
hours   after   i.v.   injection   most   of   the   free   MTP-PE   is
located   in   blood   and   liver   while   MTP-PE/MLV   is   mainly
located in lung, liver and spleen.

INTRODUCTION

The   lipophilic   muramyl   peptide   MTP-PE   either   solubilized   in   buffer   or   encapsulated   in   liposomes   (multilamellar
vesicles,   MLV),   has   pronounced   immunomodulating   activities
in vitro   and   in vivo   particularly   characterized   by   beneficial   effects   in   various   experimental   tumor   and   viral
systems   (1 - 11;   for   additional   references   see   12   and   13).
Several   investigators   found   that   intravenously   applied

MTP-PE in MLV consisting of egg phosphatidyl choline and beef brain phosphatidyl serine in a 7:3 weight ratio resulted in site specific targeting thus increasing the efficacy and the therapeutic window of the MTP-PE. In vitro and in vivo, MTP-PE/MLV appeared to be a more effective and longer lasting macrophage activator than unencapsulated MTP-PE. It showed increased therapeutic or prophylactic efficacy in tumor and infection models (14, 15) and decreased toxicity (16).

Pharmacological, toxicological and pharmacokinetic experiments have been carried out using solubilized "free" MTP-PE and a fully synthetic liposomal formulation consisting of MTP-PE and the endogenous lipids palmitoyl-oleoyl phosphatidyl choline and dioleoyl phosphatidyl serine. The results of these experiments are reported here.

MATERIALS AND METHODS

Preparation of Free and Liposomal MTP-PE.

MTP-PE is a N-acetyl-muramyl-L-alanyl-D-isoglutaminyl-L-alanine-(1',-2'-dipalmitoyl-sn-glycero-3'-hydroxy-phosphoryloxy)-ethanolamine. Unless otherwise stated, it has been dissolved at a 1 % concentration in Dulbecco's Ca^{2+}- and Mg^{2+}-free phosphate buffered salt solution (PBS) by heating at 37° C for 5 min.

Liposomal MTP-PE was prepared in situ from a dry lyophlisate composed of 1 mg MTP-PE, 175 mg 1-palmitoyl,2-oleoyl phosphatidyl choline (POPC) and 75 mg 1,2-dioleoyl phosphatidyl serine (OOPS) by means of a standard constitution procedure. In one Figure also data with a liposomal formulation consisting of POPC and 1,2-dimiristoyl phosphatidyl serine (MMPS) are shown. Liposomal suspensions were prepared by shaking the lyophilisate with 2.5 ml of Ca^{2+}- and Mg^{2+}-free PBS. The manufacture of the dry lyophilisate as well as the detailed preparation of the in situ constitution of the suspension is described in this book (see P. van Hoogevest et al.).

Inhibition of B16/BL6 Melanoma Metastases in Mice.

To produce spontaneous metastases, C57B1/6 mice were given intra-footpad injections of 3×10^4 viable B16/BL6 melanoma cells in 0.02 ml PBS. When the primary tumors had reached a diameter of about 10 mm 29 days later, the mice were anaesthetized with Penthrane (Abbott Laboratories, North Chicago, Ill.) and the tumor-bearing leg was amputated at the mid-femur to include the draining popliteal lymph node. Mice treated by this surgical procedure are not cured of melanoma. Within 60 - 100 days after injection of the tumor cells, > 90 % of the mice die. The majority of the metastases are located in the lungs and lymph nodes but liver and kidney metastases are also developed at a low frequency (17,18).

Free MTP-PE and MTP-PE/MLV was injected intravenously twice weekly for four weeks (total 8 injections) starting one day after amputation of the primary tumor. The dose of MTP-PE was 0.01, 0.1 and 1 mg/kg. In experiments where MTP-PE/MLV was injected, the lipid content was 250 mg/kg for the three MTP-PE doses.

Dead mice were collected and necropsied to ascertain the presence of disseminated melanoma. The survival of drug-treated groups was statistically compared with that of the placebo-treated control group using the Fisher's exact test and Bonferroni correction as well as other statistical analyses (19).

Toxicity Studies in Dogs and Rabbits.

a)   Two-week toxicity study in dogs after intra-venous injections of free MTP-PE (see also Ref. 20).
Five groups of beagle dogs, 5 males and 5 females per group, were given daily intravenous injections of 0.001, 0.01, 0.1 and 1.0 mg MTP-PE/kg or 1 ml/kg vehicle (5.0 % aqueous mannitol solution) for two weeks. Three animals/sex/group were sacrificed after two weeks medication while 2 dogs/sex/group were allowed a six week recovery period. Signs, mortality and food consumption were monitored daily. Body weights were determined three times/week. Clinical laboratory determinations, ophthalmoscopic, neuro-logical, and cardiographic examinations were performed pretest, at the end of medication and at the

end of the six week recovery period. Gross and histopathologic examinations were conducted on all animals.

b)   Three-month toxicity study in dogs after intravenous injections of MTP-PE/MLV. Five   groups   of
beagle dogs, 3 males and 3 females per group, were
given daily intravenous injections of 0.001, 0.01 or
0.1 mg/kg body weight of MTP-PE encapsulated in 0.25,
2.5 or 25 mg/kg MLV respectively, or 25 mg/kg placebo
MLV or 0.25 ml/kg of suspension vehicle for 90 days.
In addition, 3 dogs per sex receiving the high dose
and 2 dogs per sex receiving placebo MLV were sacrificed   after   a   one   month   recovery   period.   Signs,
mortality and food consumption were monitored daily.
Body weights were determined three times per week.
Clinical   laboratory   determinations   were   performed
pretest and at weeks 2, 5, 9, and 13, and after the
recovery period. Additional examinations were also
conducted in vehicle control and high dose animals
during the first four days of treatment. Ophthalmoscopic, neurological, and cardiographic examinations
were performed pretest and during weeks 2 or 3, 9,
and 13, and at the end of recovery. Gross and histopathologic examinations were conducted on all animals.

c)   Two-week toxicity study in rabbits after intravenous injections of free MTP-PE (see also Ref. 20).
Groups of 5 male and 5 female CH:Chbb (SPF) rabbits
were administered intravenous doses of 0.001, 0.01,
0.1 and 1.0 mg MTP-PE/kg body weight for 14 consecutive days. MTP-PE was dissolved in 5 % aqueous mannitol solution and administered at a constant volume of
1 ml/kg. A control group of 10 animals received 1
ml/kg of mannitol solution. Three males and three
females per group were sacrificed at the end of
treatment while the remaining 2 males and 2 females
were observed for an additional six weeks before
being sacrificed. Symptoms, mortality, and body
weights were recorded daily. Blood chemistry, hematology, eye examinations, and hearing tests were conducted at various intervals. Gross pathology, histo-
pathology and bone marrow examinations were also
conducted.

d)   One-month toxicity study in rabbits after intravenous injections of MTP-PE/MLV. Five   groups   of
CH:Chbb (SPF) rabbits, 3 males and 3 females/group,
were injected intravenously with one of the following: 0.001, 0.01 or 0.1 mg/kg of MTP-PE encapsulated
in 0.25, 2.5, and 25 mg MLV/kg respectively; control
groups received 25 mg placebo MLV/kg or phosphate
buffer suspension vehicle. In all cases 1 ml/kg was
administered. Injections were made daily for one
month and animals were sacrificed at the end of the
treatment period. In addition, 2 males and 2 females
receiving intermediate and high doses, as well as the
placebo MLV, were allowed a recovery period of one
month following treatment before they were sacrificed. Mortality, signs, and body weights were recorded daily. Clinical laboratory parameters, electro-
cardiography, and ophthalmic examinations were conducted pretest, and at the end of the treatment and
recovery periods. Gross and histopathologic examinations were performed on all animals.

Organ Distribution Studies in Rats.

^{3}H-labelled MTP-PE (specific activity 115 µCi/mg) was
prepared as described earlier (24). ^{14}C-labelled MLV
(POPC/OOPS, 7:3 w:w, specific activity 0.048 µCi/mg lipid)
either "empty" or containing ^{3}H-labelled MTP-PE were
supplied by Pharmaceutical Development of CIBA-GEIGY Ltd.,
Basle, Switzerland.
0.4 ml PBS containing either 160 µg free ^{3}H-MTP-PE or
160 µg ^{3}H-MTP-PE encapsulated in 40 mg ^{14}C-MLV were injected intravenously into Tif:RAIf SPF rats. For each preparation 30 minutes and 6 hours after administrations two
animals were exsanguinated and blood samples were taken
for radiometry. The total blood content was assumed as 7 %
of the animal weight. Lung, liver, spleen and brain were
obtained by dissection. The weight of the whole organ was
determined and blood samples of 100 mg and organ samples
of 30 to 200 mg were prepared for simultaneously counting
^{3}H and ^{14}C and radiometry data analyzed for significance.

RESULTS AND DISCUSSION

Pharmacological Effects.

Fig. 1 shows the therapeutic effect of two synthetic liposome preparations (POPC/MMPS and POPC/OOPS) containing MTP-PE on metastases from B16/BL6 melanoma in C57B1/6 mice. About 70 - 80 % of the mice treated with these preparations survive day 200 of the experiment indicating that established micrometastases have been eradicated. Empty MLV's (POPC/MMPS, POPC) are ineffective. Interestingly, MTP-PE encapsulated in MLV's consisting only of POPC did not show significant effectiveness suggesting that the phosphatidyl serine content is essential. These data support earlier findings by Fidler and coworkers using liposomes consisting of natural PC and PS (22,23). That liposomal MTP-PE is 10 times more efficacious than free MTP-PE is demonstrated in Fig. 2. While a significant enhancement of survival could be obtained with 1 mg/kg free MTP-PE, MTP-PE/MLV was effective at a dose of 0.1 mg/kg.

Toxicological Effects.

Free MTP-PE: In a 2 weeks' toxicity study in rabbits no treatment-related mortality was seen in the doses tested. Adverse effects were generally confined to the 1.0 and 0.1 mg/kg/day dose levels and the severity of the changes was roughly dose-related. Effects included transient weight loss, reversible decreases in alkaline phosphatase and albumin, increase in globulin fractions and fibrinogen levels, slight decreases in erythrocyte parameters and monocytosis. Most prominent were the histopathologic changes in small and medium sized arteries which occurred with variable severity and unequal distribution in a wide range of organs from all rabbits treated with 1.0 and 0.1 mg/kg/day. The lesions were characterized by slight to marked cellular accumulations in the intima, and sometimes the media, while focal areas of inflammatory cells were present throughout the arterial wall and surrounding tissue. The changes were reversible after a 6-week recovery period at the 0.1 but not at the 1.0 mg/kg dose level. Liver changes, spleen weight increases, bone

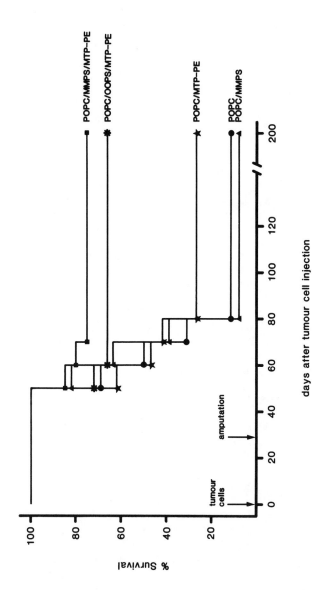

FIGURE 1. Treatment of spontaneous B16/BL6 melanoma metastases by the systemic administration of synthetic liposomes containing MTP–PE

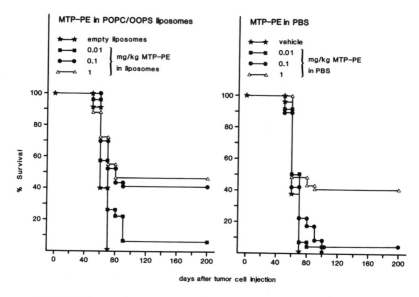

FIGURE 2.   Treatment of spontanoeous B16/BL6 melanoma
metastases by the systemic administration
of liposomal MTP-PE and free MTP-PE.

marrow hypercellularity and thymus atrophy were also
observed in the 1.0 mg/kg dose group. No changes of toxicological relevance were observed in the 0.001 and 0.01
mg/kg/day groups and it was concluded that 0.01 mg/kg/day
is the no-toxic-effect level for free MTP-PE in rabbits.
    Similar results were obtained in the 2 weeks toxicity
study in dogs. No mortality was produced. Adverse physical
signs, clinical pathology deviations and histopathologic
changes in small arteries, pericarditis and synovitis were
confined to the 0.1 and 1 mg/kg doses. After a 6 week
recovery period all changes except the arterial and peri-
cardial changes had been reversed.
    MTP-PE/MLV: In a one month study in rabbits MTP-PE/
MLV was tolerated at all dose levels without mortality,
major adverse physical signs or clinical laboratory deviations. Electrocardiographic and ophthalmoscopic examinations revealed no compound-related changes. Gross and
histopathologic changes occurred predominantly in the
lungs, spleen, bone marrow, heart and at the injection
sites. The changes in the lung, spleen and bone marrow

were predominantly of an inflammatory nature, featuring infiltration/accumulation of leukocytes/macrophages around blood vessels, which is probably compatible with the macrophage activating properties of MTP-PE/MLV. Intimal thickening and/or thrombus formation in pulmonary arteries was prominent in intermediate and high dose groups, although a tendency toward reversibility was observed at the end of the one month recovery period. It was concluded that the pulmonary arterial lesions were not specific for MTP-PE/MLV as seen in the studies with free MTP-PE and of uncertain etiology in rabbits that also have a background of spontaneous nodular pneumonitis. Therefore the no-toxic-effect dose of MTP-PE/MLV was considered to be 0.1 mg/kg/ day for this animal species.

In the 3-month toxicity study in dogs, in which i.v. doses of 0.001, 0.01 and 0.1 mg/kg/day were used, adverse effects were practically non-existent. A slight decrease in albumin, increases in alpha- and beta-globulins, decreases in gamma-globulins, and slight leucocytosis were the only major changes observed. There were no relevant gross or histological changes. Based on these findings, the i.v. no-toxic-effect level for MTP-PE/MLV was considered to be approximately 0.1 mg/kg in dogs.

In conclusion, the toxicological findings in rabbits and dogs demonstrate that the free MTP-PE is about 10 times more toxic than the liposomal formulation (toxic no-effect level 0.01 vs 0.1 mg/kg).

Organ Distribution Studies

That liposomal MTP-PE is pharmacologically more efficacious and less toxic than free MTP-PE, could be further elucidated by organ distribution studies. The distribution of radioactivity in rats after intravenous administration of ^{3}H-MTP-PE either as free drug or entrapped in MLV containing a ^{14}C-labelled phospholipid is shown in Table 1. Thirty minutes after administration of free ^{3}H-MTP-PE radioactivity was present mainly in blood and liver. Six hours after administration radioactivity was located almost completely in the liver. The body distribution of ^{3}H radioactivity after administration of liposome-entrapped ^{3}H-MTP-PE was significantly different from that obtained with free ^{3}H-MTP-PE. After 30 minutes the ^{3}H concentrations in liver, lung and spleen were distinctly

TABLE 1

PERCENTAGE OF ADMINISTERED RADIOACTIVITY IN BLOOD AND ORGANS OF RATS AFTER INTRAVENOUS ADMINISTRATION OF ^{3}H-LABELLED MTP-PE AS FREE SUBSTANCE OR ENCAPSULATED IN ^{14}C-LABELLED LIPOSOMES (MLV)

Percentage of Administered Radioactivity

Organ	MTP-PE (^{3}H) 0.5 h	6 h	MTP-PE/MLV (^{3}H) 0.5 h	6 h	MLV (^{14}C) 0.5 h	6 h
Blood	35.48	1.40	11.68	0.78	11.40	1.90
Lung	0.81	0.10	18.68	3.39	18.47	3.56
Liver	22.33	25.45	54.54	40.34	55.53	35.63
Spleen	0.38	0.14	15.47	15.78	13.71	6.69
Brain	0.10	0.06	0.13	0.10	0.14	0.13

higher and in blood significantly lower than after dosing free ^{3}H-MTP-PE. The lung contained ~ 20 % of the administered ^{3}H radioactivity. Our data support earlier findings of Fogler et al. (21) where organ distribution studies have been carried out in mice using MTP-PE and MLV consisting of natural lipids.

The data demonstrate that the encapsulation of MTP-PE in MLV changes its organ distribution. Free MTP-PE is concentrated in the blood stream where major toxicological effects (vascular lesions) can be observed, while MTP-PE/MLV avoids excessive exposure of the vasculature and accumulates in lung, spleen and liver. The 10-fold increased therapeutic effect of liposomal MTP-PE could be explained by this phenomenon.

In summary, our data show that encapsulation of MTP-PE in liposomes results in better pharmacological activity and lower toxicity thus increasing the therapeutic window of this drug.

REFERENCES

1. Fidler IJ (1986). Optimization and limitations of systemic treatment of murine melanoma metastases with liposomes containing muramyl tripeptide phosphatidylethanolamine. Cancer Immunol Immunother 21:169.

2. Fidler IJ, Jessup JM, Fogler WE, Staerkel R, Mazumder A (1986). Activation of tumoricidal properties in peripheral blood monocytes of patients with colorectal carcinoma. Cancer Res 46:994.

3. Fidler IJ, Fogler WE, Brownbill AF, Schumann G (1987). Systemic activation of tumoricidal properties in mouse macrophages and inhibition of melanoma metastases by the oral administration of MTP-PE, a lipophilic muramyl dipeptide. J Immunol 138:4509.

4. Fogler WE, Fidler IJ (1985). Nonselective destruction of murine neoplastic cells by syngeneic tumoricidal macrophages. Cancer Res 45:14.

5. Le Grue SJ, Saiki I, Romerdahl CA Fidler IJ (1986). Systemic macrophage activation by liposomes containing MTP-PE in mice immunosuppressed with cyclosporin-A. Transplantation 43:584.

6. Saiki I, Milas L, Hunter N, Fidler IJ (1986). Treatment of experimental metastasis with local thoracic irradiation followed by systemic macrophage

activation with liposomes containing muramyl tripeptide. Cancer Res 46:4966.

7. Sone S, Tandon P, Utsugi T, Ogawara M, Shimizu E, Nu A, Ogura T (1986). Synergism of recombinant human interferon gamma with liposome-encapsulated muramyl tripeptide in activation of the tumoricidal properties of human monocytes. Int J Cancer 38:495.

8. Talmadge JE, Lenz BF, Klabansky R, Simon R, Riggs C, Guo S, Oldham RK, Fidler IJ (1986). Therapy of autochthonous skin cancers in mice with intravenously injected liposomes containing muramyltripeptide. Cancer Res 46:1160.

9. Yamagami S, Brownbill AF, Schumann G (1987). Induction of tumouricidal macrophages by MTP-PE: its enhancement by a factor produced spontaneously by tumor cells. Cell Biol Int Rep 11:465.

10. Dietrich FM, Hochkeppel HK, Lukas B (1986). Enhancement of host resistance against virus infections by MTP-PE, a synthetic lipophilic muramyl peptide. I. Increased survival in mice and guinea pigs after single drug administration prior to infection, and the effect of MTP-PE on interferon levels in sera and lungs. Int J Immunopharmacol 8:931.

11. Gangemi JD, Nachtigal M, Barnhart D, Krech L, Jani P (1987). Therapeutic efficacy of liposome-encapsulated ribavirin and muramyl tripeptide in experimental infection with influenza or herpes simplex virus. J Infect Dis 155:510.

12. Schumann G (1986). Antiviral and antitumor effects of liposome-entrapped MTP-PE, a lipophilic muramylpeptide. In Seidl PH, Schleiffer KH (eds): "Biological Properties of Peptidoglycan" Walter der Gruyter and Co., Berlin/ New York: p 255.

13. Schumann G (1987). Biological activities of a lipophilic muramylpeptide (MTP-PE). In Azuma I, Jolles G (eds): "Immunostimulants: Now and Tomorrow" Japan Sci. Soc. Press, Tokyo/Springer-Verlag, Berlin: p 71.

14. Koff WC, Showalter SD, Hampar B, Fidler IJ (1983). Protection of mice against fatal Herpes simplex type 2 infection by liposomes containing muramyl tripeptide. Science 228:495.

15. Schumann G, Brownbill AF, Dukor P, Tarcsay LZ, Braun DG (1985). MTP-PE, a synthetic lipophilic muramyl-peptide that stimulates host defence mechanisms

against tumor metastases. Proc. 14th Int. Congress of Chemotherapy, (ed. J. Ishigami), University of Tokyo Press: p 55.

16. Fidler IJ, Brown NO, Hart IR (1985). Species variability for toxicity of free and liposome-encapsulated muramyl peptides administered intravenously. J Biol Resp Modif 4:298.

17. Fidler IJ, Sone S, Fogler WE, Barnes ZL (1981). Eradication of spontaneous metastases and activation of alveolar macrophages by intravenous injections of liposomes containing muramyl dipeptide. Proc Natl Acad Sci USA 78:1680.

18. Hart IR (1979). The selective characterization of an invasive variant of the B16 melanoma. Am J Pathol 97:587.

19. Schoenfeld D (1981). The asymptotic properties of nonparametric tests for comparing survival distributions. Biometrics 68:316.

20. Braun DG, Dukor P, Lukas B, Schumann G, Tarcsay L, Court M, Schaffner JC, Skripsky T, Fischer M, Graepel P (1987). MTP-PE, a synthetic lipophilic muramyl-tripeptide: Biological and toxicological properties. In Berlin A et al. (eds): "Immunotoxicology" M. Nijhoff Publishers, Dordrecht/Boston/Lancater: p 219.

21. Fogler WE, Wade R, Brundish DE, Fidler IJ (1985). Distribution and fate of free and liposome-encapsulated (^{3}H) nor-muramyl dipeptide and (^{3}H) muramyl tripeptide phosphatidylethanolamine in mice. J Immunol 135:1372.

22. Fidler IJ, Raz A, Fogler WE, Kirsh R, Bugelski P, Poste G (1980). Design of liposomes to improve delivery of macrophage-augmenting agent to alveolar macrophages. Cancer Res 40:4460.

23. Schroit AJ, Galligioni E, Fidler IJ (1983). Factors influencing the in situ activation of macrophages by liposomes containing muramyl dipeptide. Biol Cell 47:87.

24. Brundish DE, and Wade R (1985). Synthesis of N-[2-^{3}H]-Acetyl-D-muramyl-L-alanyl-D-iso-glutaminyl-L-alanyl-2-(1',2'-dipalmitoyl-sn-glycero-3'-phosphoryl) ethylamide of high specific radioactivity. J of Labelled Comp and Radiopharmac 22:29.

Liposomes in the Therapy of Infectious Diseases and Cancer, pages 205–214
© 1989 Alan R. Liss, Inc.

THE IMPACT OF LIPOSOME ENCAPSULATION OF GENTAMICIN
ON THE TREATMENT OF EXTRACELLULAR GRAM-NEGATIVE
BACTERIAL INFECTIONS

Richard S. Ginsberg, George M. Mitilenes, Robert P. Lenk,
Jo-Ann Jedrusiak, Kathy Savage, Christine E. Swenson

The Liposome Company, Inc., One Research Way,
Princeton, New Jersey 08540

ABSTRACT The impact of liposome encapsulation of
gentamicin was evaluated in two murine models of
gram-negative extracellular infection: Klebsiella
pneumonia and a neutropenic mouse thigh infection
with Klebsiella. Greater activity, measured in terms
of survival and bacterial killing, was seen when
liposome-encapsulated gentamicin was used to treat
a model of Klebsiella pneumonia. Gentamicin levels
in infected lungs were found to be significantly
increased and prolonged in animals given liposome-
encapsulated gentamicin. Enhanced bacterial killing
was noted in treatment of a neutropenic mouse thigh
infection model with liposome-encapsulated
gentamicin. These experiments demonstrate the
possible utility of liposome encapsulation of
antibacterials in treatment of infections caused by
both intracellular and extracellular pathogens.

INTRODUCTION

The published work on the use of liposome-
encapsulated antibiotics in discriminative animal models
of bacterial infection has almost exclusively involved
treatment of diseases caused by facilitative intracellular
bacteria (1). These studies have generally involved
infections where the predominant sites of bacterial
localization are the fixed macrophages of the liver and
spleen, thus taking advantage of the organ specific and

possibly cellular and subcellular targeting of liposomes. Exceptions to this approach have been reported. Liposomes coated with palmitoylamylopectin were used to direct kanamycin-containing vesicles to the lung to successfully treat a model of Legionnaires disease (2). We report on the use of liposome-encapsulated gentamicin (LEG) in the treatment of two models of gram-negative extracellular infection in mice--_Klebsiella_ pneumonia and a _Klebsiella_ thigh infection in neutropenic animals.

METHODS

Liposome Preparation

Stable plurilamellar vesicles containing gentamicin were prepared essentially as described previously (3). Large liposomes were removed by passage through a 3 micron Nucleopore filter. LEG was appropriately diluted in saline to achieve a volume of .3 ml per dose in each animal.

Analysis

Spectrophotometric. The concentration of gentamicin in liposome suspension was determined by adding trinitrobenzenesulfonic acid (TNBS) under appropriate conditions. TNBS reacts with amino groups on aminoglycosides to form a yellow amine compound which is then quantitated by comparison of the absorption of the sample at 410 nm with known standards.
Microbiological assay. The antibacterial activity of the liposome suspension was determined after disruption of the lipid membranes with 0.4% Triton X-100 using a standard well agar diffusion assay with _Bacillus_ _subtilis_ (ATCC #6633) as the indicator organism. Microbiological assay was used to analyze blood and tissue samples for gentamicin activity.
Lipid concentration. Lipid concentration was determined using Bartlett's phosphorus assay (4).
Vesicle sizing. Vesicle size was determined by electron microscopy, as reported previously (3).

Efficacy Models

Klebsiella pneumonia model. The method of Nishi
and Tsuchiya (5), using an aerosolized suspension of
Klebsiella pneumoniae DTS (minimum inhibitory concentration of gentamicin 0.08 mcg/ml), was used to induce
pneumonia in CD-1 male mice. Intravenous injection of the
appropriate test article was begun 30 to 36 hours after
initiation of infection, during the log phase growth
period of the organism in the lung. High doses of free
gentamicin (FG) (40 and 80 mg/kg) were given by
intramuscular injection due to acute toxicity from
intravenous dosing. In multiple dose experiments, a total
of three injections were administered 18 hours apart.
Efficacy was measured either by daily mortality counts
or bacterial time-kill experiments. For survival
experiments, 10 animals were entered into each group.
In bacterial time-kill studies, at various times post
treatment, 5 animals per point were sacrificed, lungs
aseptically removed, homogenized, and quantitative
bacterial cultures done. Statistical analysis was done
by an analysis of variance and Newman-Keuls test (6).
Neutropenic mouse thigh infection model. Efficacy
was also tested in the neutropenic mouse thigh model (7),
using Klebsiella pneumoniae DTS as the infecting organism,
as previously reported. On day 0, mice were injected in
the left thigh muscle with 1x10^6 CFU of Klebsiella
pneumoniae DTS. At two hours post infection, mice were
treated with a single IV dose of FG or LEG. Mice were
sacrificed 24 hours or 48 hours post infection, left thigh
removed, homogenized, and quantitative bacterial culture
performed. Cultures with no growth were reported as
containing 100 organisms, the lowest detectable number of
organisms per thigh.

Blood and Tissue Concentrations

Mice with respiratory infection were injected with a
dose of 20 mg/kg of LEG or FG. At serial intervals post
treatment, animals were anesthetized, bled by cardiac
puncture, sacrificed by cervical dislocation, and organs
harvested. Organs were weighed, diluted with peptone
broth, and homogenized. Gentamicin activity was
determined by bioassay.

RESULTS

Liposome Characterization

Gentamicin to lipid weight ratios ranged from 1:5 to 1:10. The percent of starting drug entrapped ranged from 9.8 to 23. Mean vesicle size was between 50–500 nanometers.

Treatment of <u>Klebsiella</u> Pneumonia

Survival studies done after a single intravenous treatment showed greater effect of gentamicin when administered in a liposome (Figure 1). When compared with untreated controls, both preparations of gentamicin prolonged survival of infected animals. Enhanced potency and greater efficacy was noted with LEG when compared to

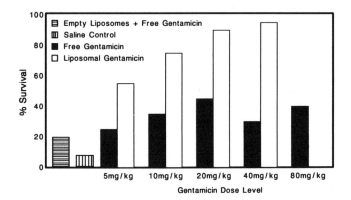

FIGURE 1. Summary of single dose treatment studies of <u>Klebsiella</u> pneumonia. Data represent the percentage of animals from three consecutive experiments surviving 10 days after infection.

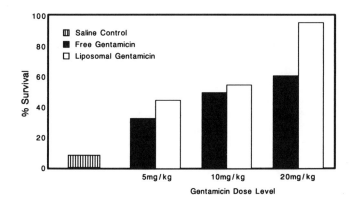

FIGURE 2. Summary of multiple dose treatment studies of <u>Klebsiella</u> pneumonia. Data represent the percentage of animals from three consecutive experiments surviving 12 days after infection .

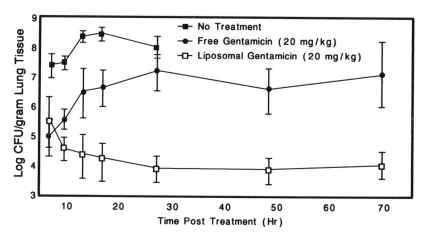

FIGURE 3. Bacterial time-kill studies of <u>Klebsiella</u> pneumonia. Data represent the mean ± S.E.M. for 5 animals. CFU = Colony Forming Units.

maximal doses of intravenous FG and when compared to large intramuscular doses (80 mg/kg) of FG. Preparations of empty liposomes and FG showed activity equivalent to that of FG in saline. In multiple dose studies, differences between free and liposomal drug were seen only at the 20 mg/kg dose level (Figure 2). Bacterial time-kill experiments (Figure 3) demonstrated rapid bacterial killing with both FG and LEG; however, regrowth of lung bacteria was noted at 8 hours post treatment in the FG group, while prolonged bacterial suppression was observed for up to 72 hours after treatment with LEG (p less than .05 for LEG group at 12, 24, 48 and 72 hour time points).

Neutropenic Mouse Thigh Model (Figure 4)

        Both FG and LEG showed increased bacterial killing with increasing dose. At higher doses of LEG, organisms were not recovered from any of the thighs 24 and 48 hours after infection, suggesting that LEG may have eliminated the organism in some of the infected thighs. With FG, organisms were recovered from the thighs of mice in all dosage groups, and in most cases the mean number of organisms was greater at 48 hours than at 24 hours, indicating re-growth of residual bacteria.

Blood and Tissue Concentrations

        Higher and prolonged gentamicin concentrations were found in the lung when gentamicin was liposome-encapsulated (Figure 5). Peak lung levels for liposome-treated animals were five times higher than for those animals given FG. Detectable levels of gentamicin were present up to 96 hours after treatment for LEG, as compared to 4 hours for FG. Higher and prolonged blood levels were also noted with LEG. Data from the spleen and liver demonstrated high levels of gentamicin after dosing with liposomal drug. Slightly decreased concentrations of gentamicin in the kidney were seen with LEG.

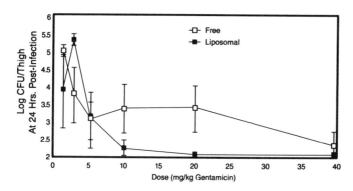

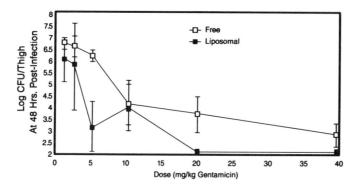

FIGURE 4. Dose-response curves for FG and LEG in the neutropenic mouse thigh model at 24 and 48 hours after infection. Data represent mean ± S.D. for 3 animals. CFU = Colony Forming Units.

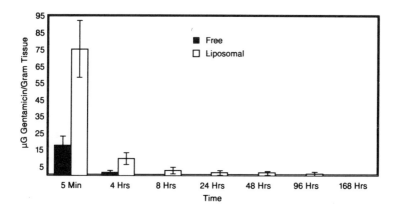

FIGURE 5. Gentamicin levels in lungs of infected animals receiving either FG or LEG. Data represents the mean ± S.D. of 5 organs.

DISCUSSION

The leading rationale for use of liposomes in treatment of infections is based on the uptake of liposomes by macrophages and other phagocytic cells where certain intracellular pathogens predominantly reside. Additionally, the vascular endothelial barrier limits the egress of liposomes from the vascular compartment, except at sites of sinusoidal capillaries; thus, liposome delivery of antimicrobial agents has been exploited to improve therapy in a variety of experimental bacterial, viral, protozoan, and fungal infections, primarily involving tissue macrophages located in the liver and spleen (1,8).

In these studies we have observed enhanced therapy with the use of LEG in two predominantly extracellular infections occurring in extravascular sites of the lung and thigh. The mechanism by which liposome-encapsulation of gentamicin improves the therapeutic effect in extra-cellular infections is not clear. One explanation for these observations is that liposomes are capable of transcapillary migration at sites of inflammation in spite of the presence of a continuous capillary bed that is found in the lung and in muscle; however, Poste et al. (9) found no evidence that even small unilamellar vesicles (600 angstroms) will traverse normal pulmonary endothelia to reach the interstitium, or that extravasation of liposomes occurs in areas of inflammation.

A second explanation is that circulating phagocytic cells might act as secondary carriers of liposomes to sites of inflammation; thus, the entrapped drug would be concentrated at the site of infection; however, this explanation is not consistent with the observations of therapeutic benefit with LEG in the neutropenic mouse thigh model.

A third possibility may be related to the altered in vivo fate of gentamicin when liposome-encapsulated, resulting in significant pharmacokinetic differences. There has been an increasing awareness of the importance of pharmacokinetic and pharmacodynamic parameters in the successful therapy of extracellular bacterial infections (10). For aminoglycosides, killing of gram-negative bacilli is primarily dependent on the area under the curve of the drug in serum, and/or the peak concentration levels

of drug relative to the minimum inhibitory concentration
of the infecting organism. Aminoglycosides also exert a
post antibiotic inhibition of bacterial regrowth. In our
experiments, the altered pharmacokinetic profile of LEG
in the blood and lungs with single bolus dosing are
consistent with greater antibacterial effect, assuming
that the measured tissue concentrations represent active
(non-entrapped) drug. That differences, in effect, are
lessened by a multiple dosing regimen in the Klebsiella
pneumonia model is consistent with this hypothesis, as
pharmacokinetic differences between FG and LEG will be
lessened with this dosing schedule.

Higher and prolonged levels at the site of infection
could be achieved by leakage of drug from circulating
liposomes in the vascular compartment. In pulmonary
infections, liposomes may be transiently constrained
within the low-pressure capillary bed of the arterial
capillary network, thus resulting in high local
concentrations of gentamicin in the lung. Further
research will be necessary to define the underlying
mechanism(s) for the enhanced antibacterial effect we
have seen with LEG in extracellular infection.

ACKNOWLEDGMENTS

We wish to thank Scott Schultz for his able
technical assistance, Lois Bolcsak for statistical help,
and Rita Chesterton for preparation of the manuscript.

REFERENCES

1. Popescu M, Swenson C, Ginsberg R (1987). Liposome-
    mediated treatment of viral, bacterial, and protozoal
    infections. In Ostro MJ (ed): "Liposomes from Bio-
    physics to Therapeutics," New York: Marcel Dekker,
    p 219.
2. Sunamoto J, Goto M, Iida T, Hara A, Tomonaga A
    (1983). Unexpected tissue distribution of liposomes
    coated with amylopectin derivatives and successful
    use in the treatment of experimental Legionnaires
    disease. In Gregioriadis G, Poste G, Senior J,
    Trouet A (eds): "Receptor-Mediated Targeting of
    Drugs," New York: Plenum Press, 359.

3. Gruner S, Lenk R, Janoff A, Ostro M (1985). Novel
    multilayered lipid vesicles: comparison of physical
    characteristics of multilamellar liposomes and stable
    plurilamellar vesicles. Biochemistry 24:2833.
4. Kates, M (1986). "Techniques of Lipidology:
    Isolation Analysis and Identification of Lipids,"
    New York: Elsevier, pg 113.
5. Nishi T, Tsuchiya K (1980). Experimental respiratory
    tract infection with Klebsiella pneumonia DTS;
    chemotherapy with kanamycin. Antimicrob Agents
    Chemother 17:494.
6. Zar J (1974). "Biostatistical Analysis,"
    Englewood-Cliffs: Prentice-Hall, pg. 151.
7. Gerber A, Craig W, Brugger H, Feller C, Vastola A,
    Brandel J (1983). Impact of dosing intervals on
    activity of gentamicin and ticarcillin against
    pseudomonas aeruginosa in granulocytopenic mice.
    J Inf Dis 147:910.
8. Lopez-Berestein G, Juliano, R (1987). Applications
    of liposomes to the delivery of antifungal agents.
    In Ostro MJ (ed): "Liposomes from Biophysics to
    Therapeutics," New York: Marcel Dekker, p 253.
9. Poste G (1983). Liposome targeting in vivo: problems
    and opportunities. Biol Cell 47:19.
10. Drusano G (1988). Role of pharmacokinetics in the
    outcome of infections. Antimic Agents Chemother
    32:289.

Liposomes in the Therapy of Infectious Diseases and Cancer, pages 215–226
© 1989 Alan R. Liss, Inc.

The limitations of carrier mediated sodium stibogluconate chemotherapy in a BALB/c mouse model of visceral leishmaniaisis

K.C. Carter[1,2], Dolan T.F.[1], Baillie A.J.[1], and Alexander J.[2].

[1]PHARMACY DEPT. [2]IMMUNOLOGY DIV., UNIVERSITY OF STRATHCYLDE, GLASGOW, SCOTLAND, U.K.

ABSTRACT   A comparison of the anti-parasitic effect of the free and vesicular forms of sodium stibogluconate in a BALB/c mouse model of visceral leishmaniasis was carried out. Mice were treated with free drug, or large or small drug loaded vesicles (niosomes and liposomes) and the % suppression in parasite numbers in the spleen, liver and bone marrow calculated. Treatment with a total dose of 44.4 mg Sb[V]/kg free stibogluconate caused a 100% suppression in liver parasite burdens but caused a <20% reduction in spleen and bone marrow burdens. The highest free drug dose, 1776 mg Sb[V]/kg, suppressed parasite burdens in these two sites by ↓80% but was associated with acute toxicity. Treatment with large drug loaded niosomes also revealed an organ dependent parasite susceptibility to stibogluconate. In this form, a total antimony dose of 14.4 mg Sb[V]/kg caused a 100% reduction in liver burdens and the highest dose, 36 mg Sb[V]/kg, ↓80% reduction in spleen burdens, with no suppression of bone marrow parasite numbers. Drug loaded into small vesicles (niosomes or liposomes) had greater efficacy against bone marrow parasites.

In this case the highest drug dose, 36 mg Sb^V/kg, gave >50% suppression of bone marrow parasite numbers and >70% suppression of spleen burdens. With small vesicles, 100% reduction in liver burdens was achieved at 14.4 mg Sb^V/kg.

INTRODUCTION

Visceral leishmaniasis is a disease caused by the intracellular parasite *Leishmania donovani* which resides within macrophages of the reticuloendothelial system (RES), predominantly in the liver, spleen and bone marrow. Present treatment of the disease involves a multidose regimen (1) which is associated with patient compliance problems and phlebitis if the drug is given intravenously. There is a perceived need for more efffective new antileishmanial drugs or improved methods of administering existing drugs so that either the number of doses, or the total drug dose, could be significantly decreased. As a disease of the RES, visceral leishmaniasis is frequently described as the archetypal disease state the therapy of which would benefit greatly from the use of a drug carrier system such as liposomes. Various workers using animal models of the disease (2,3,4,5) have shown that treatment with drug loaded vesicles is significantly more effective than with free drug in reducing parasite burdens. However, in all these studies the efficacy of the carrier mediated therapy was based on liver parasite burdens before and after treatment even though *Leishmania* parasites are known to occur in other parts of the RES. Using an experimental protocol described by Baillie *et al.* (5), which is similar to that used in other studies of experimental leishmaniasis and was known to cause 100% suppression of

liver parasite numbers, we have shown that a corresponding
decrease in spleen and bone marrow parasites numbers is not
readily acheived (6), with either free or carrier forms of
sodium stibogluconate. It would appear that it is difficult to
deliver or maintain parasiticidal concentrations of
stibogluconate at either of these latter sites. Therefore in this
study we have investigated various factors which may
influence the anti-parasitic activity of the free or vesicular
forms of sodium stibogluconate at all three sites in the RES.

MATERIALS AND METHODS

Materials

Sodium stibogluconate (Pentostam) equivalent to 0.32 mg Sb
mg^{-1} was obtained from the Wellcome Foundation, UK.,
synthetic (>99% pure). L-α- phosphatidylcholine (DPPC) and ash
free cholestrol (CHOL) were obtained from Sigma. The single
chain non-ionic surfactant I (7) was obtained from L'Oreal,
France. Liposomes and niosomes comprised 70% amphiphile
(DPPC or non-ionic surfactant) and 30% CHOL, on a molar basis.
The method of producing niosomes and liposomes has already
been described (7). Briefly large multilamellar liposomes were
produced by dissolving 150μmol of DPPC/CHOL mixture in 10ml
chloroform in a 50ml round-bottomed flask. The solvent was
removed at room temperature (20^0C), under reduced pressure
and the resulting film hydrated with 5ml drug solution at
$50-60^0C$ with gentle agitation. Sonicated liposomes were
produced by probe sonicating the multilamellar preparation at
60^0C for 3 minutes using an M.S.E. 150W sonicator, fitted with
a titanium probe, set at approximately 10-15% of maximum
power output. Large niosomes were produced by dissolving
450μmol surfactant/CHOL in 20ml diethyl ether and injecting
the mixture slowly (0.25ml min^{-1}) through a 14 G needle into

4ml of drug solution maintained at 60⁰C. Sonicated niosomes were produced by sonication of a suspension of large niosomes as described for liposomes above.

Animals

In house bred 8-10 week-old female BALB/c mice (wt. 20-25g) were used throughout experiments. In house bred Golden syrian hamsters (*Mesocricetus auratus*) which originated from the Bantim and Kingman colony (The Field Station, Aldborough, Hull) were used to maintain the parasite.

Parasite

Leishmania donovani, strain LV9, was harvested and maintained as described by Carter *et. al.*(8). Mice were injected via the tail vein (without anaesthetic) with 1-2 x 10⁷ *L.donovani* amastigote parasites in 0.2ml.

Parasite distribution

The method of determining parasite burdens (numbers/1000 host cell nuclei) in the liver, spleen and bone marrow has been described by Carter *et. al.*(6). The number of Leishman-Donovan units (LDU) was calculated per organ for the liver and spleen using the formula: LDU = number of amastigotes per 1000 host cell nuclei x the organ weight (g) (9).

Parasite suppression

In a typical experiment infected mice were treated via the tail vein (without anaesthetic) on days 7 and 8 post-infection with 0.2ml of one of the following: water (controls); sodium

stibogluconate solution (5, 45 or 100 mg antimony/ml);
liposomal or niosomal drug (0.8mg antimony/ml). At various
time intervals, day 6, 29 or 50 post-drug treatment, parasite
numbers in the spleen, liver and bone marrow of control and
drug treated mice were determined. In some experiments, mice
were treated with 2, 3, 4 or 5 daily doses (44.4 mg
Sb^V/kg/day, free drug and 7.2 mg Sb^V/kg/day, vesicular drug),
starting on day 7 post-infection, and killed for determination
of parasite burdens 6 days after the last injection.

Presentation of data

The parasite burden for the spleen and liver is the log_{10}
LDU/organ and for bone marrow the mean number of
parasites/1000 host cell nuclei. The % parasite suppression
was calculated relative to the mean parasite burden of an
appropriate untreated control group. The data is presented as
the mean % parasite suppression obtained ± standard error in
each organ for a given total antimony dose.

RESULTS

Free drug

The dose response curve (Fig.1) for the three organs shows
that parasites residing in the spleen and bone marrow are
equally susceptible to stibogluconate treatment but are
apparently less susceptible than those in the liver. A total
antimony dose of 44.4 mg Sb^V/kg, which gave 100%
suppression of liver parasite burden acheived only a 0-20%
suppression of spleen and bone marrow parasites. By
extrapolation, 100% parasite suppression in the spleen and bone

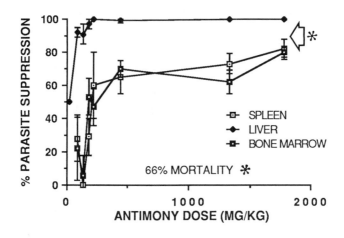

Figure 1. Suppression (%) of *L.donovani* parasite burdens in the liver, spleen and bone marrow acheived by treatment of infected BALB/c mice with free sodium stibogluconate. Mice were treated on days 7 and 8 post-infection with i.v. stibogluconate solution, equivalent to the total antimony dose shown. Parasite burdens were determined 6 days after the last dose of drug. The mean suppression values the shown (n ≮ 5 ± standard error) were calculated relative to the parasite burdens of infected, untreated control groups.

marrow would require in excess of 2000 mg Sb^V /kg, although the highest total dose of 1776mg Sb^V/kg used here caused a 66% mortality.

The suppressive effects of treatment with free drug were time dependent (Fig. 2) so that although the suppressive effects observed at day 6 post-treatment were maintained out to day 29, assessment at day 50 post-treatment revealed a significant decrease in suppression at all three sites which was most pronounced in bone marrow and spleen.

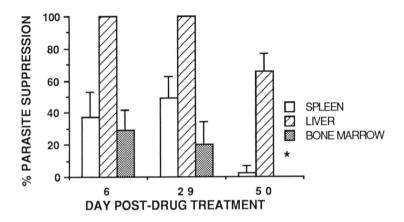

Figure 2.   The time course of the suppression (%) of
L.donovani parasite burdens in the liver, spleen and bone
marrow acheived by treatment of infected BALB/c mice with
free sodium stibogluconate.   Mice were treated on days 7 and 8
post-infection with i.v. stibogluconate solution, equivalent to a
total antimony dose of 88.8 mg Sb^V/kg.   Mean parasite
suppression, determined 6, 29 and 50 days post-treatment, is
shown (n ≬ 5 ± standard error).   * no suppression observed.

Drug loaded vesicles

Treatment with large (400 nm mean diameter) drug loaded
niosomes also revealed a site dependent parasite susceptibility
to drug treatment, with liver parasites being the most and bone
marrow parasites the least susceptible (Fig.3). In this case
100% suppression of liver parasites was obtained at a total
dose of 14.4 mg Sb^V/kg which gave no significant reduction in
bone marrow parasite numbers and some 30% mean suppression
of spleen parasite numbers.

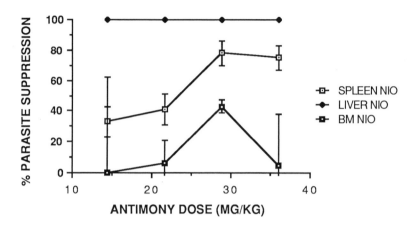

Figure 3. Suppression (%) of *L.donovani* parasite burdens in
the liver, spleen and bone marrow acheived by treatment of
infected BALB/c mice with large sodium stibogluconate loaded
niosomes. Mice were treated i.v. with the niosomal suspension
(equivalent to7.2 mg Sb^V/kg/day) on days 7 and 8, days 7, 8 and
9, days 7, 8, 9 and10 and days 7, 8, 9, 10 and 11 post-infection
to give the total equivalent antimony doses shown. Parasite
burdens were determined 6 days after the last dose of drug.
The mean parasite suppression (n { 5 ± standard error) is
shown. NIO = niosomes; BM = bone marrow.

Reducing the size of the niosomes or liposomes increased
the efficacy of the drug loaded vesicles against bone marrow
parasites and a total dose of 36 mg Sb^V/kg which caused a 58%
suppression (niosomes) when administered as a sonicated
vesicle suspension, caused only a 5% suppression in the form
of large niosomes (Figs. 3 and 4). In addition the apparent
difference in suceptibility between spleen and bone marrow
parasites observed when animals were treated with large
niosomes (Fig. 3) was less marked when animals were treated
with similar stibogluconate doses delivered in small vesicles
(Fig. 4). Administering the drug dose in either small or large
vesicles had no effect on the dose response curve obtained for
liver parasites.

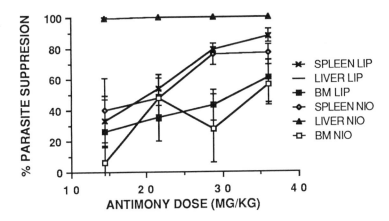

Figure 4. Suppression (%) of *L.donovani* parasite burdens in the liver, spleen and bone marrow acheived by treatment of infected BALB/c mice with small sodium stibogluconate loaded vesicles. Legend as Figure 3. LIP = liposomes.

DISCUSSION

The results obtained in this study clearly demonstrate that parasites residing in the spleen, liver and bone marrow have either different susceptibilities to sodium stibogluconate therapy or the access of the drug to each site is different. The parasites in the spleen and bone marrow are not more resistant to chemotherapy since liver parasites of animals, infected with amastigotes harvested from the spleens of drug treated mice, were susceptible to drug therapy, suggesting that the resistance was based on anatomical barriers (8). The highest total dose of 1776mg Sb^V/kg in the form of free stibogluconate gave a 100% reduction in liver parasite burdens but only <20% inhibition of spleen and bone marrow parasite numbers and caused a 66% mortality so that this, or any higher dose, is impractically toxic. It is certainly very high by present treatment guidelines, which for patients with visceral leishmaniais are 20mg Sb^V/kg, up to a maximum of 850mg Sb^V/kg (10). This discrepancy is a further illustration of the low activity of free stibogluconate against spleen and bone marrow parasites in the BALB/c mouse.

The failure to completely remove parasites from all three sites provides the probable explanation for the relapse observed by day 50 post-drug treatment, when parasites could again be recovered from the liver. Presumably spleen and bone marrow parasites surviving drug treatment simply multiply and recolonise the liver. Relapse after chemotherapy also occurs in man (10) possibly because of similar organ dependent antileishmanial effects. A recent study has shown that parasites can be recovered from bone marrow aspirates of patients who have completed a course of drug therapy (11).

Although it was possible to reduce parasite numbers in both liver and spleen by multiple dosing with large drug loaded niosomes, only multiple dosing with small drug loaded liposomes or niosomes reduced bone marrow parasite burdens. The inhibitory effect of the small drug loaded vesicles (<100nm) in the spleen was not a surprise since the fenestrations in the sinusoidal epithelium are an effective barrier to larger particles (12). Suppression of spleen parasite numbers by multiple dosing with large drug loaded niosomes (>100nm) suggests that RES blockade was also involved since it can alter the relative biodistribution of liposomes within the RES (13,14,15). Only small drug loaded vesicles were capable of reducing parasite numbers in the bone marrow implying that either, large particles are unable to gain access to the bone marrow or, that blockade of the spleen is more pronounced with small vesicles. Different binding sites for small and large liposomes have been shown to exist in the liver (14), and the results of this study would suggest that similar sites for large and small drug loaded niosomes become saturated at the same time since both caused a reduction in spleen parasite burdens. The differential effect of small niosomes in the bone marrow would suggest that binding sites for small particles in the spleen are more easily saturated.

The results suggest that the use of small vesicles would benefit similar liposomal therapy in man.

ACKNOWLEDGEMENTS

This study was supported by the Medical Research Council. J. Alexander is a Wellcome Trust Lecturer and T.F. Dolan is supported by SERC. The donations of Pentostam and the non-ionic surfactant are gratefully acknowledged.

REFERENCES

1.   Bryceson A (1987). Therapy in man. In Peters W, Killick-Kendrick R (eds)."Leishmaniases in Biology, and Medicine" Academic Press, p 847.

2.   Black CDV, Watson GJ, Ward RJ (1977). The use of pentostam liposomes in the chemotherapy of experimental leishmaniaisis. Trans Roy Soc Trop Med Hyg 30 : 550.

3.   Adinolfi LE, Bonventre PF, Vander Pas M, Eppstein DA (1985). Synergistic effect of glucantime and a liposome-encapsulated muramyl dipeptide analog in therapy of experimental visceral leishmaniaisis. Infection and Immunity 48 : 409.

4.   Alving CR (1986). Liposomes as drug carriers in Leishmaiasis and Malaria. Parasitology Today 2 : 101.

5.   Baillie AJ, Coombs GH, Dolan TF, Hunter CA, Laakso T, Sjoholm I, Stjarnkvist P (1987). Biodegradable microspheres: polyacryl starch microparticles as a delivery system for the antileishmanial drug, sodium stibogluconate. J Pharm Pharmacol 39 : 832.

6.   Carter KC, Baillie AJ, Alexander J, Dolan TF (1988). The therapeutic effect of sodium stibogluconate in BALB/c mice infected with *L.donovani* is organ dependent J Pharm Pharmacol 40 : 370.

7.   Baillie A J, Florence A T, Hume L R, Muirhead G T, Rogerson A (1985). The preparation and properties of niosomes – non-ionic surfactant vesicles. J Pharm Pharmacol 37 : 863.
8.   Carter KC, Dolan TF, Alexander J, Baillie AJ, McColgan C (1988). Visceral leishmaniaisis: drug carrier system characteristics and the ability to clear parasites from the liver, spleen and bone marrow in *Leishmania donovani* infected BALB/c mice. J Pharm Pharmacol (In press).
9.   Bradley D J, Kirkley J (1977). Regulation of Leishmania populations within the host. 1. The variable course of Leishmania donovani infections in mice. Clin E Immunol 30 :119.
10.   WHO (1984) The leishmaniasis. Technical report series 701. World Health Organisation, Geneva.
11.   Wickramasinghe SN, Abdalla SH, Kaisili EG (1987). Ultrastructure of bone marrow in patients with visceral leishmaniaisis. J Clin Path 40 : 267.
12.   Scherphof GL (1982). Interaction of liposomes with biological fluids and fate of liposomes *in vivo*. In Leserman LD , Bardet J (eds) "Liposome Methodology" Inserm, Paris. p79.
13.   Abra RM, Bosworth ME, Hunt CA (1980). Liposome deposition *in vivo* effects of predosing with liposomes. Res Comm Chem Pathol Pharmacol 29 : 349.
14.   Abra RM, Hunt CA (1982). Liposomes deposition *in vivo*: IV The interaction of sequential doses of liposomes having different diameters. Res Comm Chem Pathol Pharmacol 36 : 17.
15.   Proffitt RT, Williams LE, Presant CA, Tin GW, Uliana JA, Gamble RC (1983). Liposomal blockade of the reticuloendothelial system: improved tumour imaging with small unilamellar vesicles. Science 220 : 502.

IV. LIPOSOMES IN INFECTIOUS DISEASES–II

Liposomes in the Therapy of Infectious Diseases and Cancer, pages 229–238
© **1989 Alan R. Liss, Inc.**

LIPOSOMES AS CARRIERS OF ENVIROXIME FOR USE IN AEROSOL THERAPY OF RHINOVIRUS INFECTIONS[1]

Howard R. Six, Brian E. Gilbert, Philip R. Wyde, Sam Z. Wilson, and Vernon Knight

Department of Microbiology and Immunology, Baylor College of Medicine, One Baylor Plaza, Houston, Texas 77030

ABSTRACT Mixtures of enviroxime (E), a potent antiviral compound active against rhinoviruses, and egg yolk phosphatidylcholine were shown to form liposomes. Formation of a permeability barrier was confirmed by entrapment of markers known to reside in the aqueous compartments of liposomes. E, however, was shown to associate with the lipid bilayer. Liposomes containing E were prepared in lyophilized form and were used for laboratory and clinical studies. E in liposomes retained full anti-rhinovirus activity in tissue culture. Small particle aerosols of liposomes generated by Collison nebulizer had an aerodynamic mass median diameter (AMMD) of 2.1 μm (GSD about 2.8 μ). While those generated by a Puritan Bennett had an AMMD of 3.1 (SD about 3.1).

INTRODUCTION

We believe that earlier failure to demonstrate appreciable antiviral effects of enviroxime in rhinovirus infections in man with an aerosol produced from a pressurized container was due to failure to deliver sufficient drug to the surface of infected cells in the respiratory tract (1). This was due to the low dosage administered and to deposition of drug sprayed principally to the nasopharynx where it was promptly swallowed.

---

[1]This work was supported by funds from the Clayton Foundation for Research, 3 Riverway, Suite 1625, Houston, Texas 77056.

Administration of drug in small particle aerosol will lead to its deposition throughout the respiratory tract, and its presence in a liposome will lead to its presentation at the cell surface at higher concentrations than previously delivered and in a form that can be absorbed efficiently.

The present studies were undertaken to prepare E in liposomes suitable for use in small particle aerosol and to determine the feasibility of the use of this preparation for treatment of rhinovirus infections in man.

MATERIALS AND METHODS

Preparation of Liposomes

Multilamellar liposomes were initially prepared from egg yolk phosphatidylcholine (EYPC, Avanti Polar Lipids, Pelhan, AL) as previously described (2). When enviroxime (E, Eli Lilly and Company, Indianapolis, IN) was to be included the appropriate quantities of drug, a micronized powder, was added to EYPC in chloroform solution. The solvent was removed on a rotovap under vacuum. The dried lipid film was dissolved in t-butanol and again dried under vacuum; this process was repeated a second time. The liposomes were then formed by mechanical shaking of the dried residue in sterile water or saline.

Liposome batches intended for use in humans were prepared by a similar procedure with the following modifications: first, prior to use the EYPC was required to be free of detectable endotoxin by the limulus lysate assay; second, the final t-butanol solution was filtered, dispensed into sterile 50 ml serum bottles and lyophilized. Bottles containing the dried powder were flushed with argon, sealed with injectable stoppers and the bottles stored at -12°C. These batches were prepared at Avanti Polar Lipids (Pelhan, AL) to our specifications. As needed, liposomes were prepared by injection of 30 ml of sterile, pyrogen-free water and shaken for approximately one minute. Analysis of more than 10 bottles over a three-month interval showed that liposomes prepared from these bottles contained 14.2 mg of EYPC/ml and 5.3 mg of E/ml, were free of endotoxin and were sterile.

Quantitation of Enviroxime

Enviroxime concentrations were determined by high
performance liquid chromatography (HPLC) using a Microsorb
C18 stainless steel column and the effluent was monitored
at 215 nm (Waters, Milford, MA). This method and the procedures used for separation of enviroxime from liposomes
and biological fluids are described in detail elsewhere
(3).

Antiviral Assays

Inhibition of rhinovirus 1A and 13 replication in KB
cells was used to assess enviroxime activity. The method
has been described in detail elsewhere (4). Briefly, solutions to be tested for antiviral activity were serially
diluted in 96-well plates (Flow Laboratories). Approximately 100 50% tissue culture infectious doses (TCID$_{50}$)
were then added to each well, followed by the addition of
2 x 10^4 KB cells. Virus growth was assessed by CPE and
antiviral titers expressed as the highest dilution that
inhibited virus replication by 50% when compared to controls without added drugs.

RESULTS

Preparation of Liposomes Containing Enviroxime

To determine whether liposomes were formed in the
presence of enviroxime, dried lipid films composed of EYPC
and varying concentrations of drug were dispersed in aqueous solutions. Construction of a functional permeability
barrier was used as a criterion for liposome formation.
Umbelliferone phosphate (UMP), a marker known to be entrapped in the aqueous compartments was used to assess this
property (5). As shown in Table 1, liposome formation was
confirmed at drug concentrations as high as 5 mg/ml and
low levels of entrapped UMP were observed at 7.5 mg/ml of
drug. Liposomes were apparently not formed with 10 mg/ml
of drug. Other experiments with UMP and ^{125}I-labeled
proteins (bovine serum albumin and goat IgG) have repeatedly confirmed the formation of liposomes at drug concentrations up to 5 mg/ml. Entrapment was inconsistent at con-

centrations of 6 to 7.5 mg/ml and did not occur at concentrations of 8 mg/ml and above.

TABLE 1

EFFECT OF ENVIROXIME CONCENTRATION ON LIPOSOME FORMATION

Enviroxime mg/ml	Ratio enviroxime to phospholipid[a]	Percentage UMP entrapped[b]
0.0	–	2.5
0.1	1:150	3.4
0.5	1:30	3.2
1.0	1:15	3.8
2.5	1:6	3.8
5.0	1:3	3.4
7.5	1:2	0.5
10.0	1:1.5	0.0

[a]Phosphatidylcholine (lecithin) purified from egg yolk was used at final concentration of 15 mg/ml.
[b]Liposomes were swollen in 100 mM umbelliferone phosphate.

Radiolabeled (^{14}C) enviroxime was added to the drug-lipid mixtures to determine the quantities associated with the final liposome preparations (Table 2). Varying concentrations of enviroxime were added to EYPC and after swelling in water the liposomes were separated by centrifugation (or in other experiments by molecular sieve chromatograhy). High amounts of enviroxime were recovered with the liposomes at all concentrations tested. Quantitative association occurred even when the amounts of drug exceeded the phospholipid concentration and functional lipid bilayers were apparently not formed. Similar results were obtained when enviroxime concentrations were determined by the HPLC assay.

TABLE 2
INCORPORATION OF ENVIROXIME INTO EGG YOLK
PHOSPHATIDYLCHOLINE LIPOSOMES[a]

Enviroxime (mg/ml[b])	Percentage ^{14}C-enviroxime recovered in liposomes
2	75
4	76
5	86
6	96
8	93
10	93
20	96

[a]Liposomes were prepared with EYPC at a final concentration of 15 mg/ml and the indicated concentrations of enviroxime.
[b]Enviroxime contained 1.3×10^6 cpm of ^{14}C-enviroxime. Number indicates the drug concentrations present at the time of liposome formation.

Antiviral Activity of Liposomes Containing Enviroxime

Enviroxime carried by liposomes was found to be equally active at inhibiting rhinovirus replication as free enviroxime (Table 3). A series of experiments were performed in which liposomes containing varying concentrations of enviroxime ranging from 0.025 to 2 mg/ml (1:300 to 1:4 ratios by weight) were tested for their antiviral activity. The minimum inhibitory concentrations for EYPC liposomes containing the lowest and highest concentrations of enviroxime were 20 and 38 ng/ml, respectively. The values were comparable to those obtained with liposomes containing a positive (PE) or a negative (PA) charge. The activity of all the enviroxime containing liposome preparations was comparable to the free drug. In other experiments (data not shown) we failed to observe a difference in antiviral activity with single lamellar liposomes containing enviroxime. Liposomes without drug did not inhibit virus replication and they did not produce cytopathic effect in these cells. Of particular interest, enviroxime carried by liposomes was much less toxic to the cells than was free

drug. This result has also been observed in another human
cell line, as well as, mouse and canine cells (4).

TABLE 3
INHIBITION OF RHINOVIRUS 13 REPLICATION IN KB CELLS BY
ENVIROXIME AND ENVIROXIME CARRIED BY LIPOSOMES OF
DIFFERENT COMPOSITION

Liposome composition (charge)[a]	Ratio enviroxime to phospholipid (mg/mg)[b]	Minimum inhibitory concentration (ng/ml[c])
E:EYPC	1:300	20
	1:4	38
E:EYPC:PE (+)	1:300	24
	1:4	61
E:EYPC:PA (-)	1:300	49
	1:4	61
E (control)	—	20

[a]E = enviroxime; EYPC = egg yolk phosphatidylcholine;
PE = phosphatidylethanolamine, PA = phosphatidic acid.
[b]Liposomes were prepared at a concentration of 7.5
mg/ml of EYPC. PA or PE were present at a concentration of 0.7 mg/ml when added. At least 7 different
ratios for each liposome composition were tested.
Only the highest and lowest ratios are presented
here, as all preparations were comparable.
[c]Minimum concentration required to inhibit virus replication by 50%. Rhinovirus 13 challenge doses of
100 to 320 $TCID_{50}$ were used.

Properties of Small Particle Aerosols of Phosphatidylcholine
Liposome Preparations

Liposomes consisting of phosphatidylcholine without
enviroxime (control liposomes) were tested in the Collison
aerosol generator used for administration of ribavirin
treatment of respiratory syncytial virus infections (6) and
in the Puritan-Bennett, model 1920, nebulizer. The quantity
of liposomes and the particle size distribution of aerosol
produced by these devices is shown in Table 4. The Puritan-

Bennett nebulizer produces a more heterogenous aerosol than the Collison because of the larger number of particles with an AMMD greater than 4.7 µm. The output of particles less than this diameter is very similar, 5700 and 5300 µg for the Collison and Puritan Bennett device, respectively. If the usual dosage of enviroxime was contained in these particles the aerosol particles in the smaller size range would contain about 20 µg of E/l of air (3). Particles above 5 µm in diameter are increasingly deposited in the nasopharynx and are promptly swallowed. Below 5 µm there is a substantial penetration of particles to the lower respiratory tract (7). By analogy with estimated deposition of ribavirin aerosol in the respiratory tract the average adult would deposit about 7-10 mg of E/hr. The regional deposition of these particles has not been determined.

TABLE 4

PARTICLE SIZE DISTRIBUTION AND QUANTITY OF PHOSPHATIDYL-CHOLINE RECOVERED FROM LIPOSOME AEROSOLS

Impaction range of plate (µm)	Plate no.	Collison	Puritan Bennett Model no. 1920 (diluting air aperture closed)
4.7->9.0	1[a]	1440[b]	3880[b]
3.3-4.7	2	1185	1230
2.1-3.3	3	1545	1395
1.1-2.1	4	1680	1365
0.7-1.1	5	600	570
0.4-0.7	6	250	375
0.0-0.4	7	400	390
TOTAL		7100	9205
Aerodynamic mass median diameter		2.4 µm	3.1 µm
Geometric standard deviation		2.8	3.1
Phospholipid output		113 µg/l	147 µg/l
Aerosol flow rate		12.13 l/min	12-13 l/min

[a]Anderson cascade sampler plates, 5 min. sample.
[b]Phostidylcholine, µg, calculated from phosphate determinations.

Larger multilamellar liposomes were processed in the small particle aerosol (SPA) generator to smaller particles. Using a Coulter counter we observed a marked decrease (>80%) in the number of liposomes more than 2 μm in diameter after one hour in either type of nebulizer. Examination by electron microscope of samples obtained from the reservoir and of the SPA after one hour of aerosolization showed the liposomes to be multilamellar but most were less than 100 nm in diameter (3).

Aerosol Exposure of Adult Volunteers

In studies described elsewhere (3), five adult males were exposed to SPA of liposomes containing enviroxime (5.3 mg/ml) for one hour. Nasal wash specimens collected 5 to 60 minutes after exposure showed enviroxime levels ranging from 84 to 750 μg. None of the volunteers noted any untoward reactions to the treatment and the only comment noted was a minor nasal drip that occurred late in the treatment and that ceased when aerosol inhalation was stopped.

DISCUSSION

The present studies have shown that enviroxime can be incorporated into the lipid bilayers of liposomes prepared with EYPC. Enviroxime carried by liposomes retained full antiviral activity. These liposomes could be successfully delivered as a small particle aerosol using commercially available nebulizers. Aerosol thus generated was capable of delivering 7-10 mg/hour of enviroxime to an adult respiratory tract with no apparent side effects.

Liposomes composed of 15 mg/ml of EYPC incorporated enviroxime quantitatively at all concentrations tested and formation of functional lipid bilayers was confirmed at concentrations up to 6 mg/ml of drug, a molar ratio of 0.9 to 1.0 (E:EYPC). Above this concentration liposome formation could not be confirmed although vesicles that could be collected by centrifugation were formed. A similar phenomenon has been observed with cholesterol where the transition from liposomes to vesicles occurred at nearly the same molar ratio. Also, both cholesterol and enviroxime stabilized the permeability properties of EYPC when present at a molar ratio of 0.75 to 1.0 (E:EYPC) or less. More-

over, recent experiments have shown that cholesterol and
enviroxime compete for the same binding sites in EYPC
liposomes (Garcon and Six, unpublished data). Thus, several
lines of evidence suggest that enviroxime becomes an inte-
gral component of the liposomes possibly binding to the
fatty acids of EYPC in the bilayers.

Incorporation of enviroxime into liposomes over a wide
range of concentrations did not alter its antiviral activity. Also we observed no increase or decrease in antiviral
activity when the drug was carried by negatively or positively charged liposomes. In this regard, it was interesting that aggregation of liposomes containing both enviroxime
and phosphatidic acid was not observed. While enviroxime
carries a positively charged amino group which could extend
from the liposome bilayers, it apparently did not interact
with neighboring liposomes bearing phosphatidic acid as a
negative charge. It seems possible that the amino group of
enviroxime is sufficiently deep in the bilayer that it is
protected by the EYPC head groups. Nonetheless, such
interactions did not seem to affect antiviral activity.

Liposome size also did not affect antiviral activity
as single lamellar vesicles (approximately 30 nm diameter)
were comparable in antiviral activity to multilamellar vesicles (diameter range 30 nm to >5 μm) when they contained
the same drug concentration. While liposomes did not increase the potency of the drug against rhinoviruses, our
present data suggest that they decrease the toxicity of
enviroxime to a number of tissue culture cells. Such an
effect has been observed previously with the polyene antibiotics, streptomycin, adriamycin and a number of other
drugs discussed at this meeting.

In experiments highlighted here and described in detail elsewhere (3), we have demonstrated that liposomes
are an effective vehicle for delivery of water insoluble
drugs by SPA. As previously reported by Farr (8), we
confirmed that the size of the liposomes was reduced during
passage through the nebulizer system. In this regard the
size of the liposomes (<250 nm) in the SPA was always much
smaller than the AMMD ($\bar{3}$.1 μM) of the particles. Thus,
it is probable that several liposomes were carried by each
aerosol droplet. Direct sampling of the aerosol indicated
that the concentrations of enviroxime delivered to the
patient should be in excess of that necessary to inhibit
rhinovirus replication in the nasopharynx. Our results
with a few volunteers indicated that the drug levels detected in nasal wash specimens were in excess of the con-

centrations required. While additional studies in humans
are needed to establish the efficacy and safety of liposomal
delivery, the lack of any significant reaction in our preliminary study is encouraging. Moreover, we believe that
the liposome SPA methodology may have wide applicability to
a variety of water insoluble drugs.

ACKNOWLEDGEMENTS

We thank Kay Brown for typing the manuscript.

REFERENCES

1. DeLong DC (1984). Effects of enviroxime on rhinovirus
   infections in humans. In Leive L, Schlessinger P (eds):
   "Respiratory virus infections and antiviral agents,"
   Washington: ASM, p 431.
2. Kinsky SC (1974). Preparation of liposomes and a
   spectrophotometric assay for release of trapped glucose
   marker. Methods Enzymol 32:501.
3. Gilbert BE, Six HR, Wilson SZ, Wyde PR, Knight V (1988).
   Small particle aerosols of enviroxime-containing
   liposomes. Antiviral Res (submitted).
4. Wyde PR, Six HR, Wilson SZ, Gilbert BE, Knight V (1988).
   Enviroxime in liposomes: toxicity, anti-rhinovirus
   efficacy and delivery by small particle aerosol.
   Antimicrob Agents Chemother (submitted).
5. Six HR, Young WW, Uemura K, Kinsky SC (1974). Effect
   of antibody-complement on multiple vs single compartment liposomes: application of a fluorometric assay
   for following charges in liposomal permeability.
   Biochem 13:4050.
6. Taber LH, Knight V, Gilbert BE, McClung HW, Wilson SZ,
   Norton HJ, Thurston JM, Gordon WH, Atmar RL, Schlaudt WR
   (1983). Ribavirin treatment of bronchiolitis associated with respiratory syncytial virus infection in
   infants. Pediatrics 72:613,
7. Knight V, Yu CP, Gilbert BE, Divine GW (1988). Ribavirin aerosol dosage according to age of patient and
   other variables. J Infect Dis (in press).
8. Farr SJ, Kellaway IW, Parry-Jones DR, Woodfrey SG
   (1985). 99M-Technetium as a marker of liposomal
   deposition and clearance in the human lung. Intl J
   Pharmaceut 26:303.

Liposomes in the Therapy of Infectious Diseases and Cancer, pages 239–248
© 1989 Alan R. Liss, Inc.

TREATMENT OF MICE INFECTED ORALLY WITH SALMONELLA dublin USING A STABLE GENTAMICIN LIPOSOME FORMULATION[1]

Annie Yau-Young[2], Loren Hatlin[3], Jan-Ping Lin[2], Rick Hogue[2], Daniel Estrella[2], and Joshua Fierer[3]

[2]Liposome Technology Inc., Menlo Park, CA 94025
[3]U.C. San Diego School of Medicine,
V.A. Medical Center, San Diego, CA 92161

ABSTRACT   Systemic intracellular infections within the reticulo-endothelial system (RES) are difficult to treat because the pathogens are intracellular and so protected from many antibiotics. Since the RES takes up particulate matter with high efficiency, it is advantageous to encapsulate the appropriate anti-biotic in liposomes for intravenous administration targeted to the intracellular compartment. We have designed a gentamicin liposome formulation which has stability characteristics potentially suitable for a commercial product and tested its efficacy against a Salmonella infection model in mice. It was found that after a single intravenous injection of genta-micin liposomes, the formulation was very effective against the infection, whereas free gentamicin solution and placebo liposomes were not effective at all. Sterilization of the spleen and liver could be accomplished after a single dose of gentamicin liposomes at 20 mg/kg. At this relatively high dose, the free-drug treated mice suffered from neuromus-cular toxicity while the gentamicin liposome treated group did not. However, the gentamicin liposomes were only partially effective against the pathogen in the lymphoid tissues. The clinical relevance of the persistence of the pathogen at low numbers in the lymphoid tissues remains to be investigated.

---

[1]This work was supported by NIH SBIR Grant No. N44-AI-62600 to Liposome Technology, Inc. and the V.A., M.R.S.

INTRODUCTION

The aminoglycosides are potent bactericidal antibiotics against many Gram-negative pathogens. Although
they are effective in killing many pathogens in culture,
aminoglycosides are often less effective or ineffective
against intracellular infections by pathogens which are
sensitive to the drugs in vitro. This phenomenon is
presumably due to the poor permeability of the drug into
the intracellular compartment where the pathogens reside.
The problem of poor permeability is compounded by the
narrow therapeutic ranges of aminoglycosides, which cause
oto- and renal toxicities: high doses cannot be
administered in the hope that adequate amounts of the drug
will be able to penetrate into the infected cells to kill
the pathogen.

Macrophages constitute a primary line of natural
defense against many infections. One of their major
functions is to phagocytize and digest foreign invaders
and cellular debris. Intracellular infections are caused
by organisms which are capable of surviving inside the
cells. In some cases, they are capable of multiplying in
the extracellular environment as well; these organisms
are known as facultative intracellular parasites. A
number of these infections, such as salmonellosis,
brucellosis, various Mycobacterium infections, listeriosis
and plague are of clinical importance. These infections
are often localized in organs that have large numbers of
tissue macrophages.

By virtue of their particulate nature, the major
route of clearance of liposomes after intravenous
injection is phagocytosis by macrophages of the liver and
spleen. Liposomes containing drugs are thus delivered to
the intracellular compartment in which these pathogens
reside. Hence, it may be possible to achieve efficacy
which is not easily attainable with free drug alone.
Another advantage is that the overall toxicity of the drug
may be reduced since the drug is delivered more
preferentially to the site of infection rather than
distributed throughout the body to affect sensitive
organs. This application of liposome technology has been
demonstrated to improve therapeutic indices of several
drugs in a number of infectious models. These studies
have been reviewed recently by Emmen and Storm (1) and
Popescu, et. al.(2).

In this study, we report on the efficacy and the stability performance of a gentamicin liposome formulation.

METHOD

Liposome Formulation

Oligolamellar gentamicin liposomes composed of partially hydrogenated egg phosphatidylcholine, egg phosphatidylglycerol, cholesterol and alpha-tocopherol were prepared aseptically by a solvent injection method developed by Liposome Technology, Inc.(3). The liposomes were extruded through a one micron pore size polycarbonate filter. Unencapsulated gentamicin was removed by washing the gentamicin liposomes in isotonic buffer by centrifugation. Gentamicin concentration in the final liposome formulation was 3 mg/mL. Greater than 97% of the total drug was liposome associated as determined by the method described below. The mean diameter (number average) of the particles in the liposome formulation was determined to be 1.1 micron by using the Coulter Multichannel Counter (Model TAII). The gentamicin liposomes and the control samples were shown to be negative in the Limulus Amebocyte Lysate assay (Assoc. of Cape Cod, Inc., Woods Hole, MA) for endotoxin.

Treatment Protocol of Infection Model

Normal female BALB/c mice (approximate body weight = 20 g) were infected with 1-2 x 10^7 Salmonella dublin in 0.1 M $NaHCO_3$ by oral gavage. Infections of this type typically start at the ileum, and spread to the regional lymph nodes, liver and spleen (4). The infected mice usually died by 10 days after infection. The test samples (0.16 mL) were injected intravenously on day 4 after infection. The mice were observed daily, and at the appropriate time points the surviving mice were sacrificed. The spleens, mesenteric lymph nodes and Peyer's patches in the ileum were removed aseptically. Each organ was weighed, homogenized and cultured to determine the number of viable bacteria (4). The pH of the agar was adjusted to 5.7 to decrease the antibacterial activity of gentamicin without affecting the growth of S.

dublin. Random colonies were picked and confirmed to be S. dublin.

Stability Study

Two mL samples of gentamicin liposomes, gentamicin solution, placebo liposomes and buffer were aliquoted into sterile amber serum vials and stored in the dark at $4^{\circ}C$ and $25^{\circ}C$. At the appropriate time points, duplicate vials at each temperature were assayed. Total gentamicin was determined using the stability indicating EMIT assay for gentamicin (5) after the liposome samples were lysed by mild detergent treatment. The distribution of the gentamicin as free drug solution in the external compartment of the liposomes versus the drug associated within or on the surface of the liposomes was determined by quantitative centrifugation; the gentamicin liposomes were subjected to centrifugation in isotonic buffer and the drug concentration in the supernatant and in the pellet was assayed by the EMIT assay. The particle size and size distribution were measured by the Coulter Multichannel Counter Model TAII. Total phospholipid and phospholipid subclasses of fractions from silica gel thin layer chromatography were analyzed by the Bartlett method (6) as modified by Marinetti (7) from each of the four samples.

RESULTS

Efficacy Testing

By day 4 after infection with S. dublin, the mice appeared very ill: they were anorexic, inactive and their hair appeared "rough". The mice which received buffer, control liposomes or free gentamicin at all doses eventually died between 8 and 11 days. The mice which had received free gentamicin at 20 mg/kg immediately became flaccid, and two of the mice died within a few minutes after injection. These two mice were excluded from the study and two additional infected mice were added to this group. Gentamicin injected at the lower doses (2 and 10 mg/kg) did not produce any signs of paralysis. There was no immediate toxicity in the mice which had received gentamicin liposomes at all doses, and they recovered from the infection in less than three days. Eighty to a

TABLE 1
Therapeutic Effect of Gentamicin Liposomes on the Prolongation
of Survival of Salmonella dublin Infected Mice

Sample	Dose (mg/kg)	No. of Survivors/No. of Mice Tested on Days After Infection									
		(days) 1-5	6	7	8	9	10	11	13	21	25
Gentamicin Liposome	2	10/10	10/10	10/10	9/10	9/10	9/10	9/10	9/10	8/10	8/10
	10	10/10	10/10	10/10	10/10	10/10	10/10	10/10	9/10	9/10	9/10
	20	10/10	10/10	10/10	10/10	10/10	10/10	10/10	10/10	10/10	10/10
Gentamicin	2	10/10	8/10	4/10	4/10	0/10					
	10	10/10	9/10	7/10	1/10	1/10	1/10	0/10			
	20	10/10	9/10	6/10	6/10	2/10	2/10	0/10			
Placebo Liposome	0	10/10	10/10	5/10	5/10	3/10	0/10				
Buffer Control	0	10/10	10/10	6/10	2/10	0/10					

BALB/C mice were infected orally with 1-2 x 10^7 S. dublin on day 0. Mice were treated with the test sample intravenously on day 4.

hundred percent of the mice survived and appeared normal
in their appetite, level of activity and hair appearance.
Survival data is shown in Table 1. On day 25, i.e., 21
days after treatment, viable Salmonella were enumerated in
the spleens, mesenteric lymph nodes and Peyer's patches of
three randomly selected mice which had received intravenous doses of gentamicin liposomes (Table 2). In the
gentamicin liposome treated group at 2 mg/kg, there were
low but significant numbers of S. dublin in the spleen,
lymph nodes and Peyer's patches. The intermediate dose of
10 mg/kg gentamicin liposomes treatment left a lower
number of surviving organisms. At the high dose of 20
mg/kg, the spleen and the Peyer's patches were practically
free of S. dublin but there was still a low number of
surviving pathogens in the mesenteric lymph nodes.

TABLE 2
NUMBER OF VIABLE S. dublin 24 DAYS AFTER I.V. INJECTION
OF VARYING DOSES OF GENTAMICIN LIPOSOMES

	Dose (mg/kg)		
Organ	2	10	20
Spleen	1.5×10^3 $(0.1\text{-}3.7 \times 10^3)$	8×10^2 $(0.1\text{-}2 \times 10^3)$	$<1 \times 10^1$ $(<1 \times 10^1)$
Nodes	3×10^6 $(0.00003\text{-}1 \times 10^7)$	4×10^2 (1.8×10^2)	3.5×10^2 $(0.2\text{-}6.6 \times 10^2)$
Peyer's Patches	5.3×10^2 $(2\text{-}7 \times 10^2)$	* (9.1×10^2)	4.7×10^1 $(2\text{-}9 \times 10^1)$

Three of the surviving mice from each treatment group
were sacrificed and the number of viable S. dublin
enumerated. The numbers represent the mean of three
organs and the range is indicated in parentheses.
*There was only one mouse in this group.

The efficacy of gentamicin liposomes was tested at
the 10 mg/kg dose on another set of infected animals with

free gentamicin and placebo liposomes as controls. On day 6, i.e., 3 days after treatment, three mice of each treatment group were sacrificed and the surviving organisms in the organs determined. The gentamicin and placebo liposomes treated groups had similar number of viable $\underline{S.}$ $\underline{dublin}$: 5 x 10^6 in the spleen, 1 x 10^5 in the mesenteric lymph nodes, and 1 x 10^4 in the Peyer's patches. The gentamicin liposomes treated mice had 1 x 10^3, 1 x 10^4 and 5 x 10^3 surviving $\underline{S. dublin}$ in the spleen, lymph nodes and Peyer's patches respectively. Thus, the efficacy of gentamicin liposomes was again more pronounced in the spleen (a reduction of 3.5 log in the number of surviving $\underline{S. dublin}$), and less pronounced in the lymphoid tissues (a one log reduction in the number of viable $\underline{S. dublin}$). Continued monitoring of the number of pathogens in these organs showed that the $\underline{S. dublin}$ continued to decrease in the spleen in the two weeks following treatment while the number of $\underline{S. dublin}$ in mesenteric lymph nodes and the Peyer's patches remained constant. Administering another dose of gentamicin liposomes did not have any significant effect on the number of organisms in the lymphoid tissues. A more thorough report of this study is in preparation.

Stability Data

The stability of gentamicin liposomes, placebo liposomes and gentamicin solution was monitored at 4^oC and at 25^oC. The pH and particle size were monitored. Total drug concentration and percent free drug not associated with the liposomes were determined. Finally, phospholipid stability with respect to extent of hydrolysis into lyso-compounds, and fatty acyl composition were measured. The stability data for the drug concentration, percent free drug, mean particle size and phospholipid hydrolysis of the gentamicin liposomes are shown in Figure 1. In summary, the following can be concluded from the 9 month study:

o   The drug concentrations remained constant as measured by the immunoassay employed.

o   There was no increase in the percent free drug in the gentamicin liposomes, i.e., about 97% of the gentamicin remained in the liposomes.

o   There was no detectable hydrolysis of the phospholipids into lyso-compounds at 4^oC. There appeared to be a small amount of phospholipid hydrolysis at 25^oC.

No significant change in the fatty acyl composition was observed (data not shown).
o   The mean particle size and size distribution profile of the gentamicin liposomes at 4°C were unchanged. There was a slight decrease in the mean particle size and a small shift to smaller particles in the particle size distribution profile of the samples at 25°C.
o   The pH of the formulations remained unchanged (data not shown).
The data indicate that gentamicin liposomes were stable over the study period at 4°C and may potentially have a shelf life suitable for a commercial product.

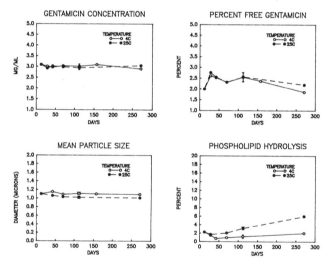

FIGURE I: STABILITY DATA OF GENTAMICIN LIPOSOMES STORED AT 4°C AND 25°C

Each point represents the average of the duplicate samples at each temperature. Error bar is shown for one of the points to illustrate the typical range of the parameter.

DISCUSSION

Success in using liposomes to deliver drugs to the RES for the treatment of diseases involving the RES has been documented by a number of studies (8,9). Due to the different drugs and infection models used in these studies, only qualitative comparisons can be made. In all cases the improvement in the therapeutic value was remarkable and a reduction in toxicity relative to a comparable dose of free drug was noted. In this study, it is demonstrated that a single intravenous dose of gentamicin liposomes is efficacious against <u>Salmonella</u> infection in mice, whereas a comparable dose of free gentamicin is not. At 20 mg/kg, gentamicin liposomes have no observable neuromuscular toxicity, while the free drug approaches lethality in the infected mice. At high doses (10 to 20 mg/kg), gentamicin liposomes can rid the spleen of invading <u>S. dublin</u>, but are only partially effective against the pathogen in lymphoid tissues. It should be noted that this animal infection model uses BALB/c mice which are easily susceptible to <u>Salmonella</u> infection. Thus the remaining <u>S. dublin</u> in the mice which had received gentamicin liposomes may be the worst case to be expected. Since the surviving <u>S. dublin</u> in the lymphoid tissues were not growing in these mice even three weeks after receiving the treatment, the infection is apparently under control. Whether the <u>S. dublin</u> infection will recur months later remains to be seen. It is also possible that the remaining organisms will be killed by the host's immune system, so that the infection will not recur.

Based on the results of this efficacy study, it is quite possible that if gentamicin liposomes are tested in patients infected with similar infections, the total dose of gentamicin given in liposome formulation will be much lower than that of the free drug. The dose interval of gentamicin liposomes will likely be much longer than that of the free drug to achieve improved efficacy against intracellular infection of the RES.

The stability of liposome formulations has been a potential area of concern from the product development perspective. Preliminary stability data for the gentamicin liposomes showed that the formulation appeared physically and chemically stable. If the formulation design takes into account the stability requirements of the liposomes as well as the drug, it is possible to have a liposome-based formulation stable enough to be a commercial product. In the case of aminoglycosides the stability in the liposome formulations is readily demonstrable due to their stability in aqueous solutions over a wide range of pH and their impermeability through a stable lipid bilayer. Thus, it is possible to design a priori a stable drug containing liposome formulation. On the other hand, if the stability requirement of the drug is not compatible with the stability requirement of the lipids, dried formulations or alternate bilayer forming components may be developed.

ACKNOWLEDGEMENTS

We would like to thank Drs. J. Ryan and F. Szoka for helpful discussions.   We gratefully acknowledge the excellent technical assistance of J. Czaple and E. Dvorsky and the expert assistance of Ms. M. Tamony in typing this manuscript.

REFERENCES

1.   Emmen F, Storm G (1987).   Liposomes in treatment of infectious diseases.   Pharma Weekbl Scientific Ed, 9:162.
2.   Popescu MC, Swenson CE, Ginsberg RS (1987). Liposome-mediated treatment of viral, bacterial, and protozoal infections.   In Ostro MJ (ed):   "Liposomes from Biophysics to Therapeutics."   New York: Elsevier/North Holland Biomedical Press, p 219.
3.   Martin FJ, West G (1986).   Patent application pending.
4.   Hefferman EJ, Fierer J, Chikami G, Guiney D (1987). Natural history of oral Salmonella dublin infection in Balb/c mice: Effect of an 80-kilobase-pair plasmid on virulence. J Inf Dis 155:1254.
5.   de Porceri-Morton C, Chang J, Specker M, Bastiani R, Gotcher S (1979).   Clinical Study No. 64 Summary Report: Performance Evaluation of the EMIT Gentamicin Assay. SYVA, Palo Alto, CA.
6.   Bartlett GH (1959).   Phosphorous assay in column chromatography. J Biol Chem 234:466.
7.   Marinetti GV (1962).   Chromatographic separation, identification, and analysis of phosphatides.   J Lipid Res 3:1.
8.   Desiderio JV, Campbell SG (1983).   Liposome-encapsulated cephalothin in the treatment of experimental murine salmonellosis.   RES: J of the Reticulothelial Soc 34:279.
9.   Tadakuma T, Ikewaki N, Yasuda T, Tsutsumi M, Saito S, Saito K (1985).   Treatment of experimental salmonellosis in mice with streptomycin entrapped in liposomes. Antimicrob Agents and Chemoth 28:28.

Liposomes in the Therapy of Infectious Diseases and Cancer, pages 249–262
© 1989 Alan R. Liss, Inc.

RETROVIRUS-INDUCED LYMPHOMATOUS MICE WITH SUBSEQUENT
CANDIDIASIS :TREATMENT WITH FREE AND LIPOSOME-ENCAPSULATED
DAUNORUBICIN AND AMPHOTERICIN B[1]

Bijay K. Pal, Jill P. Adler, Daniel A. Guerra,
and Jim S. Pieratos

Department of Biological Sciences,
California State Polytechnic University,
Pomona, California 91768

ABSTRACT   Wild mouse retroviruses produce splenic lymphoma and cause splenomegaly in wild as well as susceptible inbred mice. We standardized a wild mouse
retrovirus (10A1)-induced splenic lymphoma model in NIH-
Swiss mice and studied therapeutic efficacy of the anti-
cancer drug, Daunorubicin (DN) in this system. The lymphomatous mice (5-7 mo.old) were treated for 3 weeks by
i.v.injections of DN every 3 days at 5 and 15mg/kg dose
levels. Our results showed that DN was effective in reducing lymphomatous spleen weight and viral antigen
titer in spleen indicating successful lymphoma therapy.
However, DN appeared to show some cardiac damage. To al-
leviate inherent cardiotoxicity of free DN, it was encapsulated in multilamellar liposomes composed of phosphatidylserine, phosphatidylcholine and cholesterol
(3:7:10 molar ratio). Our results showed that, at both
therapeutic dose levels, the liposome-encapsulated DN
was more effective , compared to the free drug, in
treating the splenic lymphoma. Since a frequent compli-
cation of patients with lymphoma is susceptibility to
the opportunistic fungal infection, Candidiasis, we established the conditions for producing a lethal systemic
Candidiasis in retrovirus-induced lymphomatous mice. One
day post infection mice were treated (1x/day for 3 days)
with 0.3mg/kg Amphotericin B (AmB) or 0.9 to 3.4 mg/kg
AmB multilamellar liposomes (phosphatidylglycerol :
phosphatidylcholine: AmB, 7:3:1 molar ratio). Two weeks
post infection, the surviving mice were sacrificed and
their kidneys assayed for colony forming units (CFU) /mg
kidney. The results showed that the non-toxic dose
(0.9 mg/kg) of AmB liposomes reduced CFU significantly

---

[1] This work was supported by PHS grant CA 41713

more than the non-toxic dose (0.3mg/kg) of free AmB; 3.4mg/ kg dose reduced the CFU to <1.0 and was also non-toxic. Additional treatment with immunostimulating mycoviral dsRNA liposomes did not improve treatment efficacy in these mice. In conclusion, the data showed that non-toxic doses of AmB liposomes alone could be used to very effectively treat established systemic candidiasis in these mice.

INTRODUCTION

Type C retroviruses are indigenous to the wild mice (*Mus musculus domesticus*) trapped at various locations in Southern California(1-4). These retroviruses of wild mice consist of a mixture of related but distinct virus classes, called amphotropic (A-tropic) and ecotropic(E-tropic) (5,6). Natural history, biology and experimental transmission studies of the wild mouse retroviruses suggest that the A-tropic type C viruses are more prevalent and that they cause splenic lymphoma in wild as well as in susceptible inbred mice (such as NIH Swiss mice or SWR/J mice) (4). The E-tropic wild mouse viruses also produce lymphoma and a neurogenic paralytic disease under appropriate experimental conditions (4,7).In the experimental induction of lymphoma in NIH Swiss mice by A-tropic wild mouse retroviruses, one of the most important parameters is inoculation of high titer virus in new-born mice (<4 days old) . We described a highly oncogenic strain of A-tropic wild mouse retrovirus (10A1) which induced splenic lymphoma in NIH - Swiss mice in about three months with 90 - 100% disease incidence (8,9). The experimentally induced splenic lymphomas by 10A1 virus are histopathologically very similar to the retrovirus-induced natural lymphomas in wild mice which involve poorly differentiated B-lymphocytes (10,11) and simulates acute lymphoblastic leukemia in man.

Of the various cancer chemotherapeutic agents, the anthracycline antibiotics appear to be effective in the treatment of a variety of neoplasms including leukemia and lymphoma (12). In the first part of this investigation we have studied the therapeutic efficacy of the potent antitumor agent,Daunorubicin (an anthracycline antibiotic) using the mouse lymphoma model for possible application to human neoplasm. The major side effect of Daunorubicin (Dn) and related drugs is the accumulation of the drug in the heart tissue with inherent cardiotoxicity (12-15). This problem of cardiotoxicity of Dn may be solved and the antineoplastic effectiveness of the drug may be enhanced if Dn distribution can be reduced in the heart tissue and increased in the spleen tissue using an alternate drug delivery system. This has been investigated by using Dn encapsulated in multilamellar lipid vesicles or liposomes.

When individuals have leukemia or lymphoma, the likelihood of their contracting systemic fungal infection markedly increases because they are often on chemotherapeutic-immunosuppressive and/ or anti-bacterial regimens (16). In the second part of this study, we systemically infected our lymphomatous mice with Candida albicans and used them to study the therapeutic efficacy of different liposomal Amphotericin B (AmB) treatments, including the use of the immunostimulant, mycoviral double-stranded RNA (dsRNA). Although at the present time, the drug of choice for most systemic fungal infections is AmB, its effectiveness is limited by its acute and chronic toxicity at therapeutic dose levels. Encapsulating AmB into liposomes has been shown to significantly reduce this toxicity(17).

METHODS AND MATERIALS

I. Virus Propagation and Infection of Mice

Wild mouse retrovirus 10A1 was grown in the human bladder carcinoma cell line HT 1080 (18). Newborn NIH Swiss mice were infected by intraperitoneal injection of fresh tissue culture supernatant containing 10A1 virus. Lymphomas were produced within 3-4 months. When these mice were between 5-10 months old and had well-established splenic lymphoma, they were either treated with Dn preparations or challenged with fungus for subsequent treatment with AmB preparations. Uninfected NIH Swiss mice of similar ages were also used in this investigation.

II. Determination of Daunorubicin (Dn) Concentration

Dn concentration was determined by spectrofluorimetric assay following published procedures (19). All samples were diluted in acidified ethanol and read at 490 nm as excitation wavelength and 590 nm as emission wavelength.

III. Dn-Liposome Preparation

Multilamellar Dn-liposomes were made by using dipalmitoyl phosphatidylserine, distearoyl phosphatidylcholine and cholesterol in a 3:7:10 molar ratio (19). Lipids were vacuum evaporated into a thin film and resuspended in phosphate buffered saline(PBS) containing Dn (5mg/ml). The drug incorporation was determined and doses prepared accordingly.

IV. Dn Pharmacokinetics

Dn in its free form and liposome encapsulated form were injected into normal NIH Swiss mice in doses of 5mg/kg. Spleen, heart, liver, kidney, brain and blood were removed at various times (up to 48hrs) and the Dn concentration in each tissue was determined in relation to time.

V. Treatment of Lymphomatous Mice with Free- and Liposome-Dn

Mice were injected with liposome-encapsulated or free Dn in doses of 5mg/kg and 15mg/kg every 3 days for a period of 3 weeks. After treatment, heart and spleen tissues were removed, weighed, and assayed for Dn. Virus content was also determined in these tissues by an enzyme linked immunoassay method (20). Some lymphomatous mice were also held for one month following treatment with free- or liposome-Dn and virus content and Dn were monitored in the heart and spleen tissues of these animals. Heart tissue samples were also examined by transmission electron microscopy for cardiac damage.

VI. Preparation of Amphotericin B Liposomes (AmBL)

The AmBL formulation was dimyristoyl phosphatidylglycerol, dimyristoyl phosphatidylcholine , and AmB in a 3:7:1 molar ratio. Multilamellar liposomes were prepared from lipid films resuspended in PBS (pH 7.2). AmB concentration was determined spectrophotometrically (405nm) using linear regression analysis after extraction of the AmB from the AmBL with chloroform and methanol (17).

VII. Preparation of Free AmB Solution

When mice were treated with free AmB, the AmB (8mg) was dissolved in 1ml of dimethylsulfoxide, and diluted in PBS to the appropriate concentration for inoculation into the mice (0.3mg/kg).

VIII. Preparation of Mycoviral dsRNA

The term "mycovirus" refers to the dsRNA containing viruses that infect various species of fungi (21). The mycoviral dsRNA used as an immunostimulant in this study was extracted from Penicillium chrysogenum by a single phase phenol procedure (22) and encapsulated in multilamellar liposomes(dsRNAL) similar to those described above without the AmB (23).

IX. Treatment of Mice with Yeast Infection

Candida albicans (Cal Poly laboratory strain # 39) was maintained in Sabouraud's dextrose broth, and subcultured daily for 3 days prior to preparation of the experimental inoculum. NIH Swiss mice were inoculated IV with a lethal dose of a 24 hour old broth culture of Candida albicans(3 X 10^5 cells for lymphomatous mice and 3 X 10^6 cells for non-lymphomatous mice). One day post-infection, treatment was begun, and mice (5/group) were given daily IV inoculations with free AmB (0.3mg/kg) or AmBL (0.7, 0.9, 1.7, or 3.4mg/kg) on days 1,2 and 3. On the fourth day post-infection, some groups of mice were given dsRNAL(3.4mg/kg). Mice were examined daily for mortality and survivors were sacrificed 2 weeks post-infection. Kidneys were removed, weighed and macro-scopic observations of kidney pathology noted. Colony forming units(CFU) of each pair of mouse kidneys were determined by homogenizing, diluting and plating each homogenate dilution in duplicate on Sabouraud's dextrose agar plates incubated at room temperature. After 3-4 days, the CFU on each plate were deter-mined.

RESULTS

The first part of our study shows the effect of free- and liposome - encapsulated Dn in the treatment of wildmouse retrovirus- induced splenic lymphoma in NIH Swiss mice. Our results on distribution of free- and liposome - Dn in normal NIH Swiss mice are shown in Fig.1 and 2, respectively. Fig. 1 shows the pharmacokinetics of free Dn in spleen, heart, liver, kidney and blood following a single tail vein injection of the drug into mice. The results indicate that highest initial levels of the drug were attained in kidney and liver within 2-4 hrs after injection, followed by rapid decrease within 8 - 24 hrs. The level of Dn in the heart reached a peak at 4 hours post injection , underwent a slow decline and maintained a significant level up to 48 hrs. The lowest drug levels were detected in the spleen and blood. On the other hand, pharmacokinetics of liposome-Dn (Fig.2) showed that the drug attained and maintained a high level in the spleen and liver tissues while the concentration of the drug in the kidney and blood rapidly dropped to background level within 24 hrs. This study also showed that very little drug was detectable in the heart tissue when the drug was administered in liposome-encapsulated form.

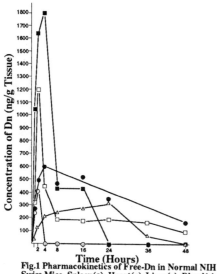

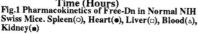

Fig.1 Pharmacokinetics of Free-Dn in Normal NIH Swiss Mice. Spleen(o), Heart(•), Liver(□), Blood(Δ), Kidney(■)

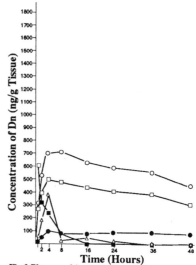

Fig.2 Pharmacokinetics of Liposome-Dn in Normal NIH Swiss Mice. Spleen(o), Heart(•), Liver(□), Blood(Δ), Kidney(■)

In the retrovirus - induced splenic lymphoma model, the major parameters of the progression of the disease included spleenomegaly and increased viral antigen titer in the spleen tissue. Our results on the treatment of these lymphomatous mice with free- and liposome-Dn show that the mice treated with liposome - Dn (both at 5mg/ kg and 15mg/ kg) had significantly lower spleen weight and viral antigen titers in the spleen ($P \leq$ 0.05) after 3 weeks of treatment and maintained such low levels even one month following the 3 weeks treatment (Fig. 3, 4). Treatment of such lymphomatous mice with free- Dn (5mg and 15mg/ kg) did not significantly reduce the spleen weights compared to the untreated mice. Although a significantly low level of viral antigen was detected only in mice treated with 15mg/ kg of free Dn, this low viral antigen level was not maintained one month following the treatment (Fig. 4).

Since one of the major side effects of Dn is cardiotoxicity, we investigated the concentration of the drug in the heart and spleen tissues of the mice treated with free- and liposome-Dn (Fig. 5 ,6). Our results show that while significantly higher levels of Dn were detected in the heart tissue of animals treated with free Dn compared to those treated with liposome Dn, the drug level in the spleen was higher in the animals treated with liposome-Dn. It appears that encapsulation of Dn in the lipid vesicles altered the drug distribution in the spleen and heart tissues (i.e.liposome-Dn localized more in the spleen and less

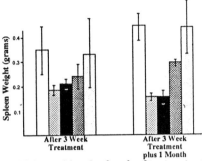

Fig.3 Spleen weights after 3 weeks of treatment and 1 month following 3 weeks of treatment, ☐ Control, ▨15 mg/kg liposome-Dn, ■ 5mg/kg Liposome-Dn, ▨ 15mg/kg free-Dn, ☐ 5mg/kg free-Dn

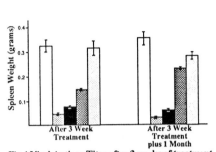

Fig.4 Viral Antigen Titer after 3 weeks of treatment and 1 month following 3 weeks of treatment, ☐ Control, ▨ 15 mg/kg liposome-Dn, ■ 5mg/kg Liposome-Dn, ▨15mg/kg free-Dn, ☐ 5mg/kg free-Dn

in the heart, compared to the free drug), enhanced the therapeutic effectiveness (Fig.3 and Fig.4) and may reduce the cardiotoxic side effects of the drug as indicated by preliminary transmission electron microscopic studies (data not shown).

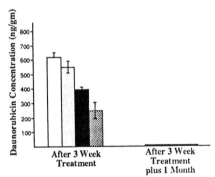

Fig.5 Dn concentration in the spleen after 3 weeks of treatment and 1 month following 3 weeks of treatment, ☐15 mg/kg liposome-Dn, ☐5mg/kg Liposome-Dn, ■ 15mg/kg free-Dn, ▨5mg/kg free-Dn

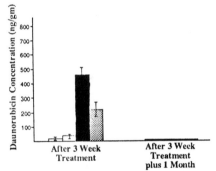

Fig.6 Dn concentration in the heart after 3 weeks of treatment and 1 month following 3 weeks of treatment, ☐15 mg/kg liposome-Dn, ☐5mg/kg Liposome-Dn, ■ 15mg/kg free-Dn, ▨5mg/kg free-Dn

The second part of this study shows the results of the treatment of Candida-infected lymphomatous mice with free- and liposome-encapsulated AmB. Lymphomatous mice with established systemic Candidiasis, treated with 0.9, or 3.4 mg/kg AmBL , show a statistically significant reduction (P=.025 and P=.005,respectively) in CFU compared with PBS (untreated) and free-AmB(0.3mg/kg) treated mice (Figures 7-9). This dose of free AmB was chosen since higher doses produced some deaths due to acute drug toxicity. AmBL treated lymphomatous mice even at the highest dose of AmB show no acute toxicity. At 3.4mg/kg AmBL, the reduction in CFU was the greatest and some mice were completely cured (Figure 9).

When the immunostimulant dsRNAL was used in lymphomatous mice following AmBL treatment, there was no additional therapeu-

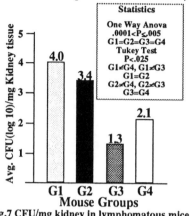

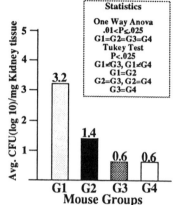

Fig.7 CFU/mg kidney in lymphomatous mice
G1=PBS
G2=0.3 mg/kg Free AmB
G3=0.9 mg/kg AmBL
G4=0.9 mg/kg AmBL and 3.4 mg/kg dsRNAL

Fig.8 CFU/mg kidney in lymphomatous mice
G1=PBS
G2=0.3 mg/kg free AmB
G3=1.7 mg/kg AmBL
G4=1.7 mg/kg AmBL and 3.4 mg/kg dsRNAL

tic effect seen at any of the doses tested (Figures 7-9). When non-lymphomatous NIH Swiss mice were treated with a combination of AmBL(0.7mg/kg) followed by dsRNAL(3.4mg/kg), however, there was a statistically significant reduction in CFU ($P= 0.05$) compared with those mice given just AmBL(0.7mg/kg)(Figure 10).

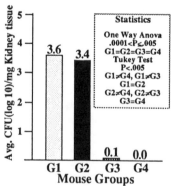

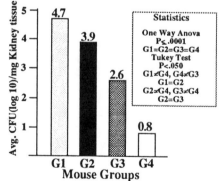

Fig.9 CFU/mg kidney in lymphomatous mice
G1=PBS
G2=0.3 mg/kg free AmB
G3=3.4 mg/kg AmBL
G4=3.4 mg/kg AmBL and 3.4 mg/kg dsRNAL

Fig.10 CFU/mg kidney in nonlymphomatous mice
G1=PBS
G2=0.3 mg/kg free AmB
G3=0.7 mg/kg AmBL
G4=0.7 mg/kg AmBL and 3.4 mg/kg dsRNAL

Furthermore, treatment with 0.7mg/kg of AmBL alone was not very effective in reducing the CFU in the kidneys. The data indicate that the lymphomatous condition in the mice interfered with the immunostimulating effect of the dsRNAL seen in the normal NIH Swiss mice.

Although there was no correlation between kidney weight and degree of severity of the infection, gross kidney pathology at the time of sacrifice did correlate with the number of CFU/mg kidney. The highest CFU were observed in the groups having the most number of pale kidneys(Table 1).

DISCUSSION

Our data on the pharmacokinetics of Dn in various tissues of normal NIH Swiss mice suggest that very small amounts of the free drug can be detected in spleen which is eliminated within 4 hrs, while a significant amount of the free drug tends to accumulate in the cardiac tissue (Fig.1). It is possible that such accumulation of free Dn in heart tissue is the cause of cardiac damage. Similar observations were also made by other investigators (12-15,24). Encapsulation of Dn in multilameller lipid vesicles composed of distearyl phosphatidylcholine, dipalmitoyl phosphatidylserine and cholesterol (7:3:10 molar ratio) altered the distribution pattern of the drug in normal NIH Swiss mice following a single tail vein injection (Fig.2). Liposome Dn localized primarily in the spleen and liver and very low levels of the liposomal drug accumulated in the heart tissue. Liposome-Dn is presumably removed very rapidly from the bloodstream into the organs of the reticuloendothelial system, such as spleen and liver, avoiding its accumulation and subsequent injury to the cardiac tissue. A similar pharmacokinetic pattern has also been noted with liposome encapsulated adriamycin and other anthracycline antibiotics (19,25-27).

Treatment of 10A1 retrovirus-induced splenic lymphoma in NIH Swiss mice with free and liposome-Dn suggest that encapsulation of the drug in lipid vescicles enhanced the therapeutic index of the drug by directing higher levels of the drug at the target site (spleen), compared with the free drug. Moreover, such encapsulation of the drug inhibited the accumulation of Dn in the heart tissue, probably avoiding the major long term side-effect of the free drug , viz. cardiac injury. Compared to the treatment with free Dn, a significant reduction of lymphomatous spleen weight and virus titer in the spleen after three weeks of treatment with liposome-Dn and one month following the treatment period, is indicative of successful lymphoma therapy. Thus, it appears that encapsulation of Dn in liposome has improved its therapeutic

Mouse Groups	N[a]	S.P.[b]	P.[c]	P.L.[d]	D.[e]
Experiment 1[f]					
G1	1		1	3	
G2			4	1	
G3	3	2			
G4	2	3			
Experiment 2[f]					
G1	1		3	1	
G2		3		2	
G3	5				
G4	3		2		
Experiment 3[f]					
G1				4	
G2		1	1	2	
G3	2	2			
G4	2			2	
Experiment 4[g]					
G1				2	3
G2		2	1		2
G3	1	4			
G4	4	1			

Table 1
Macroscopic Observations of Kidney Pathology

a=Normal b=slightly pale c=Pale d=Pale with lesions e=died

f=NIH Swiss lymphomatous mice were inoculated IV with 3×10^5 cells of *Candida albicans* treated 1,2 and 3 days post infection with PBS, free AmB or AmBL; 4 days post infection some mice were given dsRNAL. Mouse groups (Ex 1&2 had 5 mice/group, Ex 3 had 4 mice/group) include, G1:PBS (0.20 ml all Ex), G2: Free AmB (0.3mg/kg all Ex), G3: AmBL (3.4mg/kg Ex 1, 1.7mg/kg Ex 2, and 0.9 mg/kg Ex 3) and G4: dsRNAL (3.4 mg/kg all Ex) and AmBL (3.4mg/kg Ex1, 1.7mg/kg Ex2, 0.9 mg/kg Ex 3).

g= NIH Swiss non-lymphomatous mice were inoculated IV with 3×10^6 cells of *Candida albicans* treated 1,2 and 3 days post infection with PBS, free AmB, or AmBL; 4 days post infection some mice were given dsRNAL. Mouse groups (5 mice/group) include: G1: PBS (0.20 ml), G2: Free AmB (0.3 mg/kg), G3: AmBL (0.7 mg/kg) and G4: dsRNAL (3.4mg/kg) and AmBL (0.7mg/kg) efficacy by specific targeting of the drug to the tumor site.

The results of the experiments on lymphomatous mice with Candidiasis showed that AmBL could be used to treat systemic fungal infection in mice with a well-developed tumor of the immune system. Although the mice were immunocompromised by this condition, they were still able to respond effectively to the AmBL therapy, even at low doses (0.9mg/kg). This is significant since these liposomes were multilamellar, and their effectiveness is probably related to their ability to be readily phagocytized by macrophages (28). The data also showed that although increased treatment efficacy in immunologically competent NIH Swiss mice could be obtained with low doses of AmB and the immunostimulant, dsRNAL, this was not true in lymphomatous mice. The dsRNAL, a macrophage activating agent (29) was not effective in the latter mice, and it suggests that macrophages in these mice may have been able to phagocytize liposomes but they could not perform all of their normal functions.

Previous studies in our laboratory showed that immunostimulation by dsRNAL could only be demonstrated in immunocompetent mice given low doses of AmBL (0.9mg/kg); higher doses of AmB, alone, markedly reduced CFU in the kidneys and masked any contribution of the dsRNAL (unpublished data). Furthermore, when dsRNAL was given to immunocompetent mice prior to AmBL treatment, several of the mice died before AmBL treatment could be completed (unpublished data). These results indicate that effective immunotherapy in this model requires initial administration of the antifungal agent to lower the numbers of yeast cells in the host prior to immunotherapy. Use of other types of immunostimulants in these Candida infected lymphomatous mice will help to determine the feasibility of using any type of immunotherapy for these mice.

ACKNOWLEDGEMENTS

We would like to thank Mr. Tarquinus Bunch for his assistance on the graphics in this paper and Ms. Joanna Watson for preparing the dsRNA liposomes.

REFERENCES

1. Gardner MB, Henderson BE, Estes JD, Casagrande J, Pike M, Huebner RJ (1976). The epidemiology and virology of C-type virus-associated hematological cancers and related diseases in wild mice. Cancer Res. 36:574.

2. Gardner MB, Henderson BE, Officer JE, Rongey RW, Parker JC, Oliver C, Estes JD, Huebner RJ (1973). A spontaneous lower motor neuron disease apparently caused by indigenous type-C RNA virus in wild mice. J. Natl. Cancer Inst. 51:1243.

3. Gardner MB, Officer JE, Rongey RW, Charman HP, Hartley JW, Estes JD, Huebner RJ (1973). C-type RNA tumor virus in wild house mice (*Mus musculus*). In : Unifying concepts of leukemia. Bibl. Haematol. 39:335.

4. Gardner MB (1978). Type-C viruses of wild mice: Characterization and natural history of amphotropic, ecotropic and xenotropic MuLV. Current Topics Microbiol. Immunol. 79:215.

5. Hartley JW, Rowe WP (1976). Naturally occurring murine leukemia viruses in wild mice: Characterization of a new "amphotropic" class. J. Virol. 19:19.

6. Rasheed S, Gardner MB, Chan E (1976). Amphotropic host range of naturally occurring Wild mouse leukemia viruses. J. Virol. 19:13.

7. Pal BK, Mohan S, Nimo R, Gardner MB (1983). Wild mouse retrovirus-induced neurogenic paralysis in laboratory mice I. Virus replication and expression in central nervous system. Arch. Virol. 77:239.

8. Rasheed S, Pal BK, Gardner MB (1982). Characterization of a highly oncogenic murine leukemia virus from wild mice. Int. J. Cancer 29:345.

9. Lai MMC, Shimizu CS, Rasheed S, Pal BK, Gardner MB(1982). Genomic characterization of a highly oncogenic *env*. recombinant between amphotropic retrovirus of Wild mouse, and endogenous xenotropic virus of NIH Swiss mouse. J. Virol. 41:606.

10. Bryant ML, Scott JL, Pal BK, Estes JD, Gardner MB(1981). Immunopathology of natural and experimental lymphomas induced by wild mouse leukemia virus. Am. J. Pathol. 104:272.

11. Pal BK, Cooper RE (1984). Methylation, virogene expression and stages of differentiation of B-cells transformed by wild mouse retrovirus. In : Cold Spring Harbor Meeting on RNA Tumor Viruses, p 121.

12. Goodman LS, Gillman A (1980). "The pharmacological basis of therapeutics."(6th. ed.) New York: Macmillan, p 1291.

13. LeFrak FA, Pitha FJ, Rosenheim J, Gottlieb J(1973). A Clinicopathological analysis of adriamycin cardiotoxicity. Cancer 32:302.

14. Doroshow JH, Locker GY, Myers CE(1979). Experimental animal models of adriamycin cardiotoxicity. Cancer Treat. Rep. 63:855.

15. Fichtner I, Arndt D, Elbe B, Reszka R (1984).
    Cardiotoxicity of free and liposomally encapsulated
    rubomycin (daunorubicin) in mice. Oncology 4:363.
16. Rippon JW (1982) Candidiasis and the pathogenic yeasts.
    In : "Medical Mycology: the pathogenic fungi and the
    pathogenic actinomycetes," Philadelphia: Saunders,
    p 484.
17. Lopez-Berestein G, Mehta R, Hopfer RL, Mills K, Kasi L,
    Mehta K, Fainstein V, Hersh EM, Juliano RL (1983).
    Treatment and prophylaxis of disseminated Candida
    albicans infections in mice with liposome encapsulated
    amphotericin B. J. Infect. Dis. 147:939.
18. Rasheed S, Nelson-Rees WA, Toth EM, Arnstein P, Gardner
    MB (1974) Characterization of a newly derived human
    sarcoma cell line (HT1080). Cancer 33:1027.
19. Gabizon A, Goren D, Fuks Z, Barenholz Y, Dagon A,
    Mesharer A (1983). Enhancement of adriamycin delivery to
    liver metastatic cells with increased tumoricidal effect
    using liposomes as drug carriers. Cancer Res. 43:4730.
20. Clark DP, Dougherty RM (1980). Detection of avian
    oncovirus-group specific antigens by the enzyme-linked
    immunosorbent assay. J. Gen. Virol. 47:283.
21. Bozarth RF (1979). The physico-chemical properties of
    mycoviruses. In Lemke PA (ed.):"Viruses and Plasmids in
    Fungi,"New York: Marcel Dekker, p 43.
22. Diener TO, Schneider IR (1968). Virus degradation and
    nucleic acid release in single-phase phenol. Arch.
    Biochem. Biophys. 124:401.
23. Guerra DA, Watson JM , Adler JP, Pieratos JS, Pal BK
    (1987). Treatment of murine candidiasis with liposome-
    amphotericin B and the immunostimulant, liposome-dsRNA
    Abstr. Annu. Meet. Am. Soc. Microbiol. p 394.
24. Bachur NR, Moore AL, Bernstein JG, Lio A (1970).
    Distribution and disposition of daunomycin in mice:
    Fluorimetric and isotopic methods. Cancer Chemotherap.
    Rep. 54:89.
25. Juliano RL, Stamp D (1975). The effects of particle size
    and charge on the clearence rates of liposome and
    liposome-encapsulated drugs. Biochem. Biophys. Res.
    Commun. 63:651.
26. Rahman A, Kessler A, More N, Sikii B, Rowden G, Wooley D,
    Schein D (1980). Liposomal protection of adriamycin-
    induced cardiotoxicity in mice. Cancer Res. 40:1532.
27. Olson F, Mayhew E, Maslow D, Rustums Y, Szoka F (1982)
    Characterization, toxicity, and therapeutic efficacy of
    ADM encapsulation in liposomes. Eur. J. Clin. Oncol.
    18:167.

28. Juliano RL (1981). Pharmacokinetics of liposome-
encapsulated drugs.In Knight CG (ed):."Liposomes: from
Physical Structure to Therapeutic Application,"
Amsterdam:Elsevier/North-Holland Biomedical Press,p 391.
29. Alexander P, Evans R(1971). Endotoxins and double-
stranded ribonucleic acid render macrophages cytotoxic.
Nature(New Biol). 232:76.

Liposomes in the Therapy of Infectious Diseases and Cancer, pages 263–273
© **1989 Alan R. Liss, Inc.**

EFFECT OF LIPOSOME ENCAPSULATION ON TOXICITY AND ANTIFUNGAL ACTIVITY OF POLYENE ANTIBIOTICS[1]

Reeta Taneja Mehta and Gabriel Lopez-Berestein

Section of Immunobiology and Drug Carriers, The University of Texas M. D. Anderson Cancer Center, Houston, Texas 77030

ABSTRACT   Polyene macrolide antibiotics are power-
ful but toxic antifungals. They exert an antibiotic
effect by binding to ergosterol in fungal cell membranes with a greater affinity than to cholesterol
in mammalian cell membranes; binding to cholesterol
is responsible for their toxicity. We used liposomes
to reduce toxicity and enhance the therapeutic
index of these drugs. Representatives from small
and large polyene groups were chosen for toxicity
and antifungal studies in vitro and in vivo. All
drugs had significant antifungal activity in vitro
both in their free and liposomal forms. Liposome
encapsulation protected human erythrocytes from the
toxic effects of large polyenes such as amphotericin B, nystatin, mepartricin and candidin but
provided little or no protection from the toxic
effects of small polyenes. We observed that liposomal forms of small polyenes, which are toxic in
vitro, are also toxic in vivo. Studies on the in
vivo toxicity of large polyenes showed different
behavior after liposome encapsulation. Liposomal
forms of amphotericin B, nystatin and candidin
showed a general pattern of protection in mice,
whereas liposomal mepartricin with the identical
lipid composition was more toxic than free drug.
Various lipid compositions were studied to obtain
an optimal formulation that could significantly
buffer the toxicity of mepartricin. Therapeutic
studies with free and liposomal forms of these
drugs showed that liposome encapsulation can

---

[1] This work was supported by NIH contract 72639.

improve the therapeutic index of large polyenes, in
general, although modifications may be required at
various steps of formulation to get significant
effects with different drugs.

INTRODUCTION

Polyenes are a group of macrolide lactones produced by
different species of <u>Streptomyces.</u> They differ in the number
of double bonds, the size of the conjugated ring and the
presence or absence of hexosamine, or aromatic moiety in the
molecule. All the polyenes interact with sterol-containing
membranes of eukaryotic cells to produce changes in membrane
permeability that lead to cell lysis (1). Based on their
mode of interaction with the biological membranes, they have
been divided into two groups, small and large polyenes (2).
In this study, we used representatives from groups of
tetraenes (nystatin and natamycin), pentaenes (filipin and
lagosin) and heptaenes (amphotericin B, mepartricin and
candidin) (Fig. 1). Nystatin is tetraene-diene (with six
double bonds) but has been included with tetraenes in the
literature (1). In general, small polyenes have been reported to cause more damage to the cell membranes than the larger
polyenes do. Differences in their relative affinity for cho-
lesterol- or ergosterol-containing membranes are responsible
for their usefulness as antifungal agents. Thus, amphotericin
B (AmB) and nystatin (Nys) are clinically useful because they
interact preferentially with ergosterol in fungal cell membranes; filipin is too toxic for use because it binds more
strongly to cholesterol in mammalian cell membranes (3). Our
earlier studies on AmB demonstrated that liposome encapsulation reduces the toxicity while maintaining the antifungal
activity, thereby improving the therapeutic index of the drug
(4-6). Recently, we reported that liposome encapsulation of
Nys could allow it to be administered intravenously Nys, rendering it active against systemic candidiasis (7, 8), perhaps
by targeting the drug to infected sites or stabilizing the
drug, which otherwise is unstable in aqeous milieu. In this
chapter, we compare the effect of liposome encapsulation on
toxicity and antifungal efficacy of large and small polyenes.

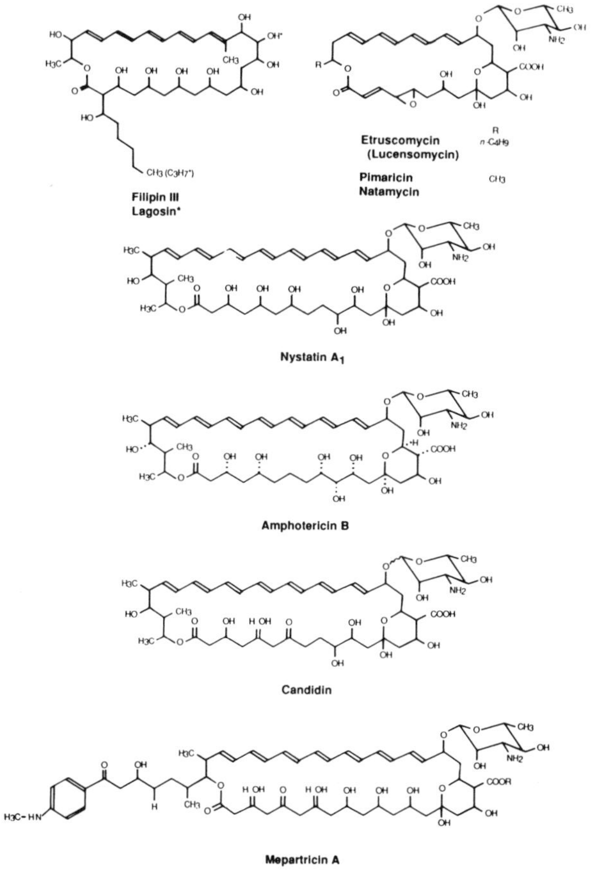

FIGURE 1. Structures of the polyenes studied.

RESULTS

Antifungal Activity In Vitro

The minimal inhibitory concentrations (MIC) of the free
and liposomal drugs used in this study (Table 1) show that
liposomal as well as free drugs had comparable antifungal
activity in vitro against Candida ablicans strain 336.

TABLE 1
ANTIFUNGAL ACTIVITY OF FREE VERSUS LIPOSOMAL POLYENES

Polyene	MIC (µg/ml)	
	Free	Liposomal
Small		
Filipin	8.0 - 16.0	16.0
Lagosin	4.0	3.0
Natamycin	4.0	8.0
Nystatin	1.0	1.0
Large		
Amphotericin B	0.4	0.4
Candidin	5.0	5.5
Mepartricin	2.0 - 4.0	2.0

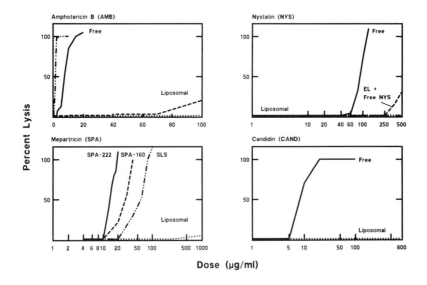

FIGURE 2.   In vitro toxicity of free versus liposome-encapsulated large polyenes.

In Vitro Toxicity

Liposome encapsulation of large polyenes protected RBC
from the toxicity of free drugs (Fig. 2). Free AmB (F-AmB)
caused a 100% lysis at 10 µg/ml, whereas liposomal AmB
(L-AmB) was not toxic up to 200 µg/ml, a concentration 20
times higher than the lytic concentration of free drug.
Liposomal Nys (L-Nys) showed no toxicity up to a concentration of 1 mg/ml which was eight times higher than 125 µg/ml,
the concentration at which free Nys (F-Nys) was 100% toxic.
Mepartricins used were of two types, lipophilic SPA-160 and
hydrosoluble SPA-222, which contained sodium lauryl sulphate
(SLS) with SPA-160 at a ratio of 2:1 (wt/wt). We observed
that SPA-222 was more toxic than SPA-160; this toxicity was
later found to be related to the SLS (Fig. 2). We compared
the toxicity of free SPA-160 to its liposomal form (L-SPA-
160) and observed that 30 times higher concentration of the
liposomal drug had no toxc effects, as compared with the free
drug. Similarly, liposomal candidin (L-Cand) was 40 times
less toxic than the free drug.

The incorporation of small polyenes in liposomes did not
significantly reduce RBC toxicity significantly (Fig. 3).

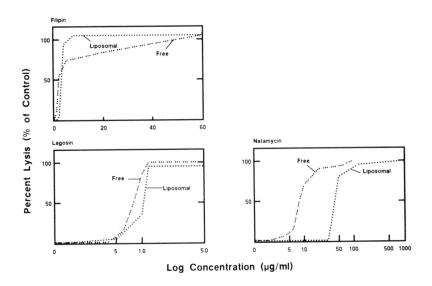

FIGURE 3. In vitro toxicity of free versus liposome-
encapsulated small poleyenes.

The toxicity pattern of filipin and lagosin did not change with liposome encapsulation, whereas liposome encapsulation of natamycin provided some protection at lower doses.

Toxicity in Mice

All small polyenes were as toxic in liposomal forms as free forms. Both free and liposomal forms of natamycin were not toxic in vivo at doses up to 40–80 mg/kg; however, no antifungal activity was observed in therapeutic experiments (data not shown). Liposome encapsulation of large polyenes, on the other hand, led to reduced toxicity as compared with the free drugs (Fig. 4). The maximal tolerated dose (MTD) of F-AmB was 0.8 mg/kg, with LD_{50} at 1 mg/kg. All the animals

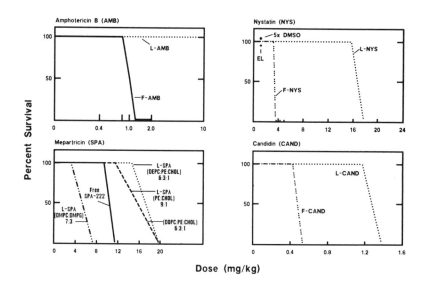

FIGURE 4.   Toxicity of free versus liposome-encapsulated large polyenes in mice.

died at a dose of 1.2 mg/kg. L-AmB, on the other hand, was not toxic up to the doses tested. The MTD of F-Nys and L-Nys were 4 mg/kg and 16 mg/kg, respectively. L-Cand showed a three-fold reduction in toxicity over the free form. However, it was surprising to note that liposomal mepartricin (DMPC:DMPG,

TABLE 2
IN VIVO TOXICITY OF LIPOSOMAL MEPARTRICIN
WITH DIFFERENT LIPID COMPOSITIONS

Lipid composition[b]	Immediate reaction[a] at 8 mg/kg dose	MTD (mg/kg) Normal mice	MTD (mg/kg) Infected mice
DMPC:DMPG (7:3)	Yes	<8.0	4.0
DMPC:DMPG:chol (6:3:1)	No	8.0	-
DMPC alone	Yes	<8.0	-
DMPC:chol (9:1)	No	12.0	-
Egg PC alone	Yes	<8.0	-
Egg PC:chol (9:1)	No	20.0	12.0
DPPC alone	No	<8.0	-
DPPC:chol (9:1)	No	8.0	-
DPPC :PE:chol (6.5:2.5:1)	No	16.0[c]	-
DSPC alone	No	<8.0	-
DSPC:chol (9:1)	No	10.0	-
DSPC:PE:chol (6.5:2.5:1)	No	20.0	10.0
DOPC alone	No	8.0	4.0
DOPC:chol (9:1)	No	14.0	-
DOPC:PE:chol (6:3:1)	No	20.0	12.0
DEPC alone	Yes	<8.0	-
DEPC:chol (9:1)	Yes	<8.0	-
DEPC:PE:chol (6.5:2.5:1)	No	14.0	-

[a] The animals that had immediate reactions died instantly after the intravenous injection.
[b] DMPC, dimyristoyl phosphatidyl choline; DMPG, dimyristoyl phosphatidyl glycerol: EGG PC, egg phosphatidyl choline; DPPC, dipalmitoyl phosphatidyl choline; PE, phospholatidyl ethanolamine; DSPC, distearoyl phosphatidyl choline; DOPC, dideoyl phosphatidyl choline; DEPC, dielaidyl phosphatidyl choline; chol, cholesterol.
[c] Mice died after 24 hours.

7:3) was more toxic than the free drug. This observation prompted us to change the liposome composition with this drug. The data on MTD of various liposomal mepartricin preparations in normal and infected mice is presented in Table 2. Of these, only three lipid compositions were found to buffer the toxicity significantly, PC:chol (9:1), DOPC:PE: chol (7:3:1) and DEPC:PE:chol (7:3:1) as shown in Fig. 4.

Therapeutic Studies

In general, compared with the free drugs at either equiv-alent or higher doses, liposomal drugs increased the survival

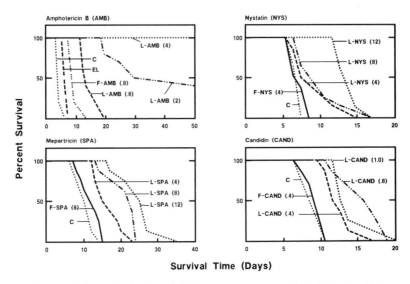

FIGURE 5. Effect of liposome encapsulation on the survival of mice infected with Candida albicans and treated with single doses of large polyenes.

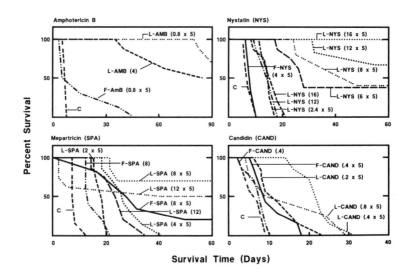

FIGURE 6. Survival of mice treated with multiple doses of free or liposome-encapsulated polyenes two days after infection with Candida albicans.

of mice (Fig. 5). Mice injected with single doses of 0.8 mg/kg L-AmB survived longer than those receiving equivalent doses of F-AmB. Furthermore, a dose-dependent increase in survival was observed with higher doses of L-AmB. Nys in free form did not show any antifungal activity in vivo. However, L-Nys significantly increased the survival of the infected animals. Single doses of L-SPA-160 also improved survival in a dose-dependent manner. Similarly, L-Cand increased survival at doses two times higher than those of the free drug; however, toxic effects were observed at the highest dose. Thus, large polyenes, including Nys, improved the survival of animals after liposome encapsulation, although the degrees of improvement varied.

Multiple doses of F-AmB at MTD were needed to improve survival, whereas a single 4 mg/kg dose of L-AmB increased the survival of mice significantly. Moreover, five daily doses of 0.8 mg/kg L-AmB were better than a single high dose. Five daily doses of F-Nys did not improve the survival. A single dose of L-Nys was as effective as the same amount split into five doses; higher doses of L-Nys significantly improved survival in a dose-dependent manner. A dose of 16 mg/kg L-Nys given five times resulted in 100% survival of mice up to 60 days. A dose-dependent increase in survival was also observed with L-SPA-160, although the highest dose, 12 mg/kg given five times, showed some toxicity. Similar results were obtained with L-Cand, which produced a better survival pattern with a medium dose, 0.4 mg/kg; doses higher than this were toxic.

DISCUSSION

These studies suggest that modulation of drug action by liposome encapsulation is a complex phenomenon. A variety of factors may be involved when a drug is encapsulated in liposomes. Even closely related drugs may behave differently after liposome encapsulation because of differences in their orientation within the phospholipid bilayers, the molecular interactions between the drug and phospholipids and the physicochemical characteristics of liposomes.

The toxicity of polyenes has been related to their affinity for cholesterol or ergosterol in biological membranes (3). Large polyenes have been reported to bind more avidly to ergosterol than to cholesterol, whereas the small polyenes have a greater affinity for cholesterol, with a few exceptions; i.e., natamycin, a small polyene, binds more strongly to ergosterol, and Nys has chemical characteristics of a tetraene but behaves biologically like a large polyene. Thus, large polyenes, including Nys, that had a weaker affinity for cholesterol showed reduced toxicity after liposome encapsulation. Filipin and lagosin, because of their different orientation in the bilayer and higher affinity for cholesterol, may be transferred more readily from liposomes to cholesterol-containing RBC membranes, leading to their lysis. Other reasons, such as conformational instability of small polyenes within liposomal membranes, may also be responsible for lack of protection with these liposome preparations. However, natamycin, which binds more strongly to ergosterol (9), showed some reduction of toxicity after liposome encapsulation. Moreover, we observed that the in vitro toxicity of drugs may or may not correlate with the in vivo situation. For example, L-SPA-160, a large polyene that significantly protected RBC from toxicity, was highly toxic in vivo using a liposome composition similar to that used with other drugs.

Overall, liposome encapsulation of large polyenes enhanced the therapeutic index of the drugs tested. The toxicities of AmB and candidin was reduced so that higher doses could be administered. Nys, which cannot be used intravenously, could be administered intravenously as L-Nys and targeted to the reticuloendothelial system where the candida infections reside (8). The toxicity of L-SPA-160 could be buffered by changing liposome composition, while the antifungal activity in vitro remained unchanged. Similar observations have been reported by Juliano et al. (10) using L-AmB of various lipid compositions in vitro. In conclusion, liposome encapsulation resulted in an improved therapeutic index of large polyenes when liposomes of appropriate lipid compositions were used. Small polyenes, on the other hand, were found to be poor candidates for antifungal therapy using DMPC:DMPG (7:3) liposomes. However, extensive modifications in liposome compositions may be useful in modifying the effects of these drugs.

ACKNOWLEDGMENTS

We thank T. McQueen for her technical assistance and Jennie Schreyer and Terry Punch for typing and editorial assistance.

REFERENCES

1. Omura S, Tanaka H (1984). Production, structure and antifungal activity of polyene macrolides. In Omura S (ed): "Macrolide Antibiotics: Chemistry, Biology, and Practice," New York: Academic Press, p 351.
2. Kotler-Bratburg J, Medoff G, Kobayashi GF, Boggs S, Schlessinger R, Pandey C, Rinehart Jr. KL (1979). Classification of polyene antibiotics according to chemical structure and biological effects. Antimicrob Agents Chemother 15:716.
3. Gale EF (1984). Mode of action and resistance mechanisms of polyene macrolides. In Omura S (ed): "Macrolide Antibiotics: Chemistry, Biology, and Practice," New York: Academic Press, p 425.
4. Lopez-Berestein G, Mehta R, Hopfer RL, Mill K, Kasi L, Mehta K, Fainstein V, Luna M, Hersh EM, Juliano RL (1983). Treatment and prophyhlaxis of disseminated infection due to Candida albicans in mice with liposome-encapsulated amphotericin B. J Inf Dis 147:939.
5. Mehta R, Lopez-Berestein G, Hopfer RL, Mills K, Juliano RL (1984). Liposomal amphotericin B is toxic to fungal cells but not to mammalian cells. Biochim Biophys Acta 77:230.
6. Lopez-Berestein G, Fainstein V, Hopfer R, Mehta K, Sullivan MP, Keating M, Rosenblum MG, Mehta R, Luna M, Hersh EM, Reuben J, Juliano RL, Bodey GP (1985). Liposomal amphotericin B for the treatment of systemic fungal infections in patients with cancer: A preliminary study. J Inf Dis 151:704.
7. Mehta RT, Hopfer RL, Gunner LA, Juliano RL, Lopez-Berestein G (1987). Formulation, toxicity and antifungal activity in vitro of liposome encapsulated nystatin as therapeutic agent for systemic candidiasis. Antimicrob Agents chemother 31:1897.
8. Mehta R T, Hopfer RL, McQueen T, Juliano RL, Lopez-Berestein G (1987). Toxicity and therapeutic effects in mice of liposome-encapsulated nystatin for systemic fungal infections. Antimicrob Agents Chemother 31:1901.
9. Teerlink, T, Dekruiff B, Demel RA (1980). The action of pimaricin, etruscomycin and amphotericin B on liposomes with varying sterol content. Biochim Biophys Acta 599:484.
10. Juliano RL, Grant CW, Barber KR, Kalp MA (1987). Mechanism of selective toxicity of amphotericin B incorporated into lipsomes. Mol Pharmacol 31:1.

Liposomes in the Therapy of Infectious Diseases and Cancer, pages 275–285
© 1989 Alan R. Liss, Inc.

LIPOSOME-ENCAPSULATED AMPICILLIN OR MURAMYL DIPEPTIDE
AGAINST *LISTERIA MONOCYTOGENES* IN VIVO AND IN VITRO

Irma A.J.M. Bakker-Woudenberg[1], A.F. Lokerse[1],
J.C. Vink[1], and F.H. Roerdink[2]

[1]Department of Clinical Microbiology, Erasmus University,
P.O.Box 1738, 3000 DR Rotterdam, The Netherlands
[2]Laboratory of Physiological Chemistry, State University,
Bloemsingel 10, 9712 KZ Groningen, The Netherlands

ABSTRACT The effect of liposomal encapsulation of the
antibiotic agent ampicillin or the immunostimulating
agent muramyl dipeptide on the antibacterial resistance
was studied. Liposomal encapsulation of ampicillin led
to a 90-fold increase in therapeutic activity in
experimental *Listeria monocytogenes* infection in mice,
resulting from delivery of the antibiotic to the site
of infection, i.e. the liver and spleen. The increased
antibacterial activity of liposome-encapsulated
ampicillin was also demonstrated in vitro in mouse
macrophages infected with *Listeria monocytogenes*. The
lipid composition of the liposomes appeared to be an
important determinant for the rate of intracellular
liposomal degradation and thus the rate at which
liposome-encapsulated ampicillin was released intracellularly. Exposure of mouse macrophages in vitro to
muramyl dipeptide resulted in an increased cellular
uptake of *Listeria monocytogenes*, and in addition in
intracellular bacterial killing. Liposomal encapsulation of muramyl dipeptide led to a 1000-fold reduction
in the amount of muramyl dipeptide to obtain these
effects.

INTRODUCTION

It is well-known from clinical experience that antibiotic treatment of severe infections is often not
successful. Several factors may contribute to the failure of

antimicrobial treatment (1). One involves the intracellular localization of some infectious organisms and the relative inefficiency of antimicrobial agents to penetrate infected cells. Another cause of unsuccessful antimicrobial treatment is the failure of the host defense system to provide adequate support to antibiotic therapy. In this experimental study it is investigated whether administration of the antibiotic agent ampicillin or the immunostimulating agent muramyl dipeptide (MDP) in the liposome-encapsulated form results in considerable enhancement of the antibacterial resistance against intracellular *Listeria monocytogenes* infection.

METHODS

In vivo *Listeria monocytogenes* infection. Infections were induced by intravenous injection of 5 x 10^3 bacteria into female C57Bl/Ka mice of 11-13 weeks old (2). The numbers of viable bacteria recovered from the liver, spleen and blood at different intervals after inoculation were used as indices of the severity of infection and as a parameter of therapeutic efficacy. The minimal bactericidal concentration of ampicillin for the bacterial strain is 0.16 mg/l.

In vitro *Listeria monocytogenes*-infected macrophages. Monolayers of peritoneal macrophages from C57Bl/Ka mice were cultured at 37°C in chamber/slides in medium containing D-MEM with 1% glutamine and 15% foetal bovine serum during 48 h before incubation with *Listeria monocytogenes* in a ratio of 30 bacteria per macrophage (3,4). In some experiments macrophages were exposed during 15 h prior to incubation with bacteria to various concentrations of muramyl dipeptide (MDP) either free or liposome-encapsulated (4). After a half hour period of bacterial uptake, the noningested bacteria were removed, and the infected macrophages were reincubated during 6 h. In some experiments infected macrophages were reincubated in the presence of various concentrations of ampicillin either free or liposome-encapsulated. At different time intervals during the periods of uptake and reincubation the macrophages were disrupted, and the numbers of viable bacteria were determined (3).

Liposome preparations were 0.4 μm multilamellar vesicles consisting of either cholesterol, egg phosphatidyl-choline and L-α-phosphatidyl-L-serine (Chol/PC/PS, molar ratio 5/4/1) ("fluid" liposomes with transition temperature below 37°C), or cholesterol, L-α-distearoylphosphatidyl-choline and L-α-dipalmitoylphosphatidylglycerol (Chol/DSPC/

DPPG, molar ratio 10/10/1) ("solid" liposomes with transition temperature above 37°C). Liposomes were prepared as described previously (2), with some modifications for the Chol/DSPC/DPPG liposomes that were prepared at 62°C. Tissue distribution of liposomes after intravenous injection into mice was determined as described previously using [^{14}C] Inulin as a marker (2). Uptake of liposomes by macrophages in monolayer was determined using [^{3}H]cholesteryl-hexadecyl-ether as a nondegradable marker. Intracellular degradation of liposomes was determined using cholesteryl-[^{14}C]-oleate as a marker.

RESULTS

Therapeutic effect of liposome-encapsulated ampicillin in *Listeria monocytogenes* infection in mice. Intravenous inoculation with 5 x 10^3 *Listeria monocytogenes* organisms resulted in a progressive increase in bacterial populations in the liver and spleen of untreated mice during the first days, followed by decreases in bacterial numbers and spontaneous cure at day 19 (TABLE 1). Free ampicillin at a total dose of 48 mg (8 doses of 6 mg each) cured mice of *Listeria monocytogenes* infection in terms of sterilization

TABLE 1
EFFECT OF LIPOSOME-ENCAPSULATED AMPICILLIN AGAINST
LISTERIA MONOCYTOGENES **INFECTION IN MICE**

Organ	Treatment	Log no. of bacteria at day after infection:				
		4	7	12	16	19
Liver	LE. Amp	5.3	0	0	0	0
	Amp + L	5.8	5.7	N.D.	1.3	0
	Amp	3.0	0	0	0	0
	Control	5.5	6.3	2.8	1.5	0
Spleen	LE.Amp	4.9	0	0	0	0
	Amp + L	5.9	5.1	N.D.	0.8	0
	Amp	3.5	0	0	0	0
	Control	6.4	5.3	2.6	0.7	0

Antibiotic was administered intravenously, starting 40 h after bacterial inoculation of mice:
LE.Amp   2 doses of 0.27 mg Ampi/mouse in 2 μmol lipid at 72-h interval
Amp + L   2 doses of 0.27 mg Ampi/mouse + 2 μmol lipid at 72-h interval
Amp   8 doses of 6 mg Ampi/mouse at 12-h interval
Liposomes composed of Chol/PC/PS, molar ratio 5/4/1.

of liver and spleen at the end of treatment (day 7). When encapsulated in Chol/PC/PS liposomes a total dose of 0.54 mg (2 doses of 0.27 mg each) of ampicillin sufficed to obtain a similar therapeutic effect, whereas a treatment with 0.54 mg of non-encapsulated ampicillin plus empty liposomes had no effect upon the course of infection. The mechanism by which encapsulation of ampicillin in liposomes led to this 90-fold enhancement in the therapeutic activity appeared to be an increased delivery of the antibiotic to the site of infection: 1 h after injection of liposomes 56% of the injected amount was recovered from the liver and 23% from the spleen; substantial amounts of liposome-encapsulated ampicillin could be recovered from isolated Kupffer cells, the target cell in the liver of *Listeria monocytogenes* after intravenous inoculation (data not shown).

   Effect of liposome-encapsulated ampicillin on intracellular survival of *Listeria monocytogenes* in macrophages in vitro. Incubation of macrophages in monolayer with *Listeria*

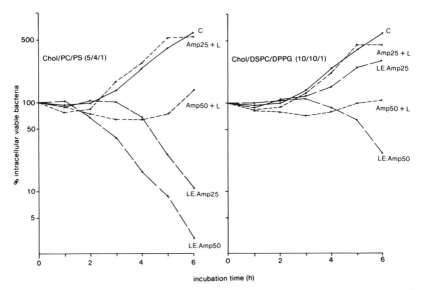

FIGURE 1. Effect of liposome-encapsulated ampicillin on intracellular survival of *Listeria monocytogenes* in vitro. Monolayers of macrophages with ingested bacteria were exposed to antibiotic:
LE.Amp   25 or 50 μg ampicillin in 1 μmol lipid per ml
Amp + L   25 or 50 μg ampicillin + 1 μmol lipid per ml
C   control incubations without ampicillin.
Two types of liposomes were used as indicated.

monocytogenes during a 2-h period resulted in bacterial uptake up to an average of 5 x 10^6 bacteria per 10^6 macrophages (100% at zero time, FIGURE 1). After removal of the noningested bacteria intracellular bacterial multiplication occurred up to 6-fold within 6 h. Incubation of infected macrophages in the presence of 25 μg of ampicillin per ml encapsulated in "fluid" Chol/PC/PS liposomes resulted in killing of 90% of the intracellular bacteria within 6 h. However when encapsulated in "solid" Chol/DSPC/DPPG liposomes 25 μg of ampicillin per ml did not result in bacterial killing: although significantly less as compared to controls multiplication of intracellular bacteria occurred up to 3-fold within 6 h. As shown for both types of liposomes 25 μg of free ampicillin plus empty liposomes had no significant effect upon the intracellular bacterial multiplication. Doubling the amount of ampicillin encapsulated in Chol/PC/PS liposomes to 50 μg per ml, led to a rapid killing of almost all (97%) of the intracellular bacteria. In contrast, when 50 μg of ampicillin was encapsulated in Chol/DSPC/DPPG liposomes, intracellular killing was delayed and less effective: only 70% of the

INTRACELLULAR DEGRADATION OF LIPOSOMES BY MACROPHAGES IN VITRO

Liposome composition	Incubation time (min)	cholesteryl-oleate (%)	oleate (%)	phospho-lipids (%)
Chol/PC/PS	0	100	0	0
(5/4/1)	2	91	7	2
	15	61	34	4
	30	37	53	9
	60	26	60	14
	120	16	50	33
Chol/DSPC/DPPG	0	100	0	0
(10/10/1)	2	96	2	2
	15	95	3	1
	30	91	7	1
	60	84	14	2
	120	75	20	5

Monolayers of macrophages were incubated with liposomes labeled with cholesteryl-[^{14}C]-oleate at 1 μmol liposomal lipid per ml. The amounts of radioactive-labeled cholesteryloleate, oleate and phospholipids are expressed as percent of total chloroform-soluble radioactivity in the cells.
Two types of liposomes were used as indicated.

intracellular bacteria were killed after 6 h. As shown for both types of liposomes, 50 µg of free ampicillin plus empty liposomes only inhibited intracellular bacterial multiplication but did not kill the bacteria.

The rates of uptake of both types of liposomes during 6 h of incubation by macrophages were found to be similar, and increased up to 11.9 nmol and 11.2 nmol liposomal lipid per 10^6 macrophages for Chol/PC/PS and Chol/DSPC/DPPG liposomes, respectively (data not shown). However, the rate of intracellular degradation of the liposomes appeared to be dependent on the lipid composition. As shown in TABLE 2 "fluid" Chol/PC/PS liposomes appeared to be much more sensitive to intracellular degradation than "solid" Chol/DSPC/DPPG liposomes. When incorporated in Chol/PC/PS liposomes cholesteryl-oleate was degraded very fast, resulting in a rapid increase in liberated oleate that was partly reutilized for synthesis of cellular phospholipids. When incorporated in Chol/DSPC/DPPG liposomes degradation of cholesteryl-oleate was relatively slow, which was also

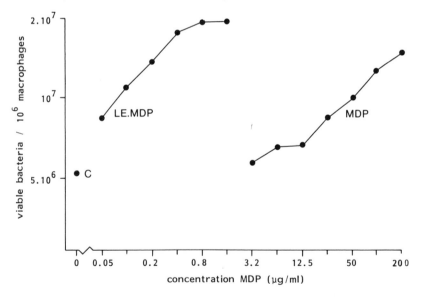

FIGURE 2. Effect of liposome-encapsulated MDP on uptake on *Listeria monocytogenes* by macrophages in vitro. Monolayers of macrophages were exposed during 15 hours before incubation with bacteria to muramyl dipeptide either free (MDP) or encapsulated within liposomes at 20 nmol per ml (LE.MDP). Uptake of bacteria was determined after 30 min. Liposomes composed of Chol/PC/PS, molar ratio 5/4/1.

reflected in a slow appearance of liberated oleate, and as a consequence incorporation of oleate into phospholipids was almost not detectable.

Effect of liposome-encapsulated muramyl dipeptide (MDP) on uptake and intracellular survival of Listeria monocytogenes by macrophages in vitro. The uptake of *Listeria monocytogenes* by macrophages that were exposed to various concentrations of free MDP or MDP encapsulated in Chol/PC/PS liposomes during 15 h prior to incubation with bacteria is shown in FIGURE 2. Whereas 5 x 10^6 bacteria were taken up by 10^6 macrophages not exposed to MDP, bacterial uptake was increased in MDP-exposed macrophages dependent on the concentration of MDP: bacterial uptake was 3-fold increased

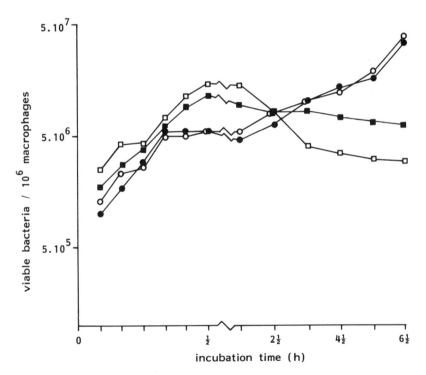

FIGURE 3. Effect of liposome-encapsulated MDP on uptake and intracellular survival of *Listeria monocytogenes* in macrophages in vitro. Monolayers of macrophages were exposed during 15 hours before incubation with bacteria at zero time to 200 μg of free MDP per ml (■), or 0.2 μg of liposome-encapsulated MDP per ml (LE.MDP) (□), or 0.2 μg of free MDP per ml plus empty liposomes (○). Macrophages not exposed to MDP (●). Liposomes composed of Chol/PC/PS, molar ratio 5/4/1.

when macrophages had been exposed to free MDP at a concentrations of 200 μg per ml or to liposome-encapsulated MDP at a concentration that was three orders of magnitude lower: 0.2 μg per ml.

In macrophages being exposed to 200 μg of free MDP or 0.2 μg of liposome-encapsulated MDP per ml, the uptake and intracellular survival of *Listeria monocytogenes* at different time intervals was studied (FIGURE 3). A gradual uptake of bacteria by macrophages not exposed to MDP to 5 x 10^6 bacteria per 10^6 macrophages after a half hour period was observed. When macrophages had been exposed to 200 μg of free MDP per ml, the bacterial uptake was increased from the first moment and resulted in 15 x 10^6 bacteria per 10^6 macrophages; after uptake, 50% of the intracellular bacteria were killed within 6 h, in contrast to the intracellular multiplication of bacteria up to 6-fold within 6 h in macrophages not exposed to MDP. In macrophages exposed to 0.2 μg of liposome-encapsulated MDP, again bacterial uptake was increased from the first moment, in addition 80% of the intracellular bacteria were killed within 6 h. Exposure of macrophages to 0.2 μg of free MDP mixed with empty liposomes had no effect upon the uptake or intracellular multiplication of *Listeria monocytogenes*, indicating that the effect of liposome-encapsulated MDP resulted exclusively from encapsulated MDP.

Free MDP at 200 μg per ml or 0.2 μg of liposome-encapsulated MDP in itself was not bactericidal for *Listeria monocytogenes* (data not shown).

DISCUSSION

Targeting of antimicrobial agents by means of liposomes may be of great value in the treatment of infections that prove refractory to conventional forms of antimicrobial therapy. In a clinical study Lopez-Berestein et al. demonstrated that liposome-encapsulated amphotericin B was beneficial in the treatment of fungal infections in eight out of twelve neutropenic and/or immunocompromised cancer patients who had previously failed to respond to treatment with the non-encapsulated drug (5). In experimental infection models in animals delivery of antimicrobial agents by means of liposomes was demonstrated. Studies were performed in parasitic infections such as leishmaniasis and malaria, in mycotic infections such as histoplasmosis, cryptococcosis and candidiasis, in viral infection caused by *Rift Valley* fever virus (for references, see ref. no 6), and in a limited number of experimental bacterial infections caused by *Mycobacterium tuberculosis* (7), *Legionella pneumophila* (8), *Salmonella enteritidis* (9) and *Brucella abortus* (10). The studies demonstrated an improved therapeutic index and reduced toxicity resulting from encapsulation of the antimicrobial drugs in liposomes. The present study, performed in a model of intracellular bacterial infection caused by *Listeria monocytogenes*, shows that liposomal encapsulation of ampicillin resulted in a considerable enhancement in its therapeutic activity by delivering the antibiotic in relatively high concentrations to the infected cells concerned, i.e. the macrophages of the liver and spleen. As demonstrated in vitro, intracellular *Listeria monocytogenes* in peritoneal mouse macrophages were effectively killed by ampicillin provided that the antibiotic was encapsulated in liposomes. Other investigators also observed the superiority of liposome-encapsulated antibiotics to non-encapsulated antibiotics in effecting intracellular killing of *Staphylococcus aureus*, *Escherichia coli* and *Salmonella typhimurium* in vitro (for references, see ref. no. 6). Although a substantial body of evidence supports the potential usefulness of liposomes as drug carriers, further studies are needed to establish optimal conditions for systemic therapy with liposome-encapsulated antimicrobial agents. The present study shows that by manipulating the lipid composition of the liposomes the intracellular degradation by macrophages could be influenced and thereby the rate at which the liposome-encapsulated ampicillin was released intracellularly and became available to exert its therapeutic action.

In spite of the improved therapeutic index of ampicillin in the liposome-encapsulated form as demonstrated in the present study in mice with intact host defense, in previous experiments liposomal ampicillin appeared to be ineffective in nude mice with impaired T cell-mediated immunity (2). As the ineffective antibiotic treatment in nude mice may be due to the failure of the host defense system to provide adequate support to antibiotic therapy, it is investigated whether immunostimulant agents are able to increase host resistance against intracellular *Listeria monocytogenes* infection. The present study shows that exposure of mouse macrophages in vitro to the immunostimulant agent MDP led to increased phagocytic and bactericidal activities against *Listeria monocytogenes*. Liposomal encapsulation of MDP resulted in a considerable enhancement of these effects. Whether administration of liposome-encapsulated MDP also results in a therapeutic effect in the treatment of *Listeria monocytogenes* infection in mice with intact or impaired host defense is under investigation. In experimental infections caused by *Candida albicans* or *Herpes simplex* virus in mice a therapeutic effect of liposome-encapsulated MDP or analogs was observed (11, 12).

REFERENCES

1. O'Grady F (1984). The second L.P. Garrod Lecture. Strategies for potentiating chemotherapy in severe sepsis: some experimental pointers. J Antimicrob Chemother 13:535.

2. Bakker-Woudenberg IAJM, Lokerse AF, Roerdink FH, Regts D. Michel MF (1985). Free versus liposome-entrapped ampicillin in treatment of infection due to *Listeria monocytogenes* in normal and athymic (nude) mice. J Infect Dis 151:917.

3. Bakker-Woudenberg IAJM, Lokerse AF, Vink-Van den Berg JC, Roerdink FH (1988). Liposome-encapsulated ampicillin against *Listeria monocytogenes* in vivo and in vitro. Infection 16 (Suppl. 2):164.

4. Bakker-Woudenberg IAJM, Lokerse AF, Vink JC, Roerdink FH (1988). Effect of free or lipsosome-encapsulated MDP on the uptake and intracellular survival of *Listeria monocytogenes* in peritoneal mouse macrophages in vitro. In Masihi KN, Lange W (eds): "Immunomodulators and nonspecific host defence mechanisms against microbial infections", Advances in the Biosciences vol. 68, New York:Pergamon press, p 21.

5. Lopez-Berestein G, Fainstein V, Hopfer R, Mehta K, Sullivan MP, Keating M, Rosenblum MG, Mehta R, Luna M, Hersh EM, Reuben J, Juliano RL, Bodey GP (1985). Liposomal amphotericin B for the treatment of systemic fungal infections in patients with cancer: a preliminary study. J Infect Dis 151:704.

6. Bakker-Woudenberg IAJM, Roerdink FH, Scherphof GL (1988). Drug-targeting in antimicrobial chemotherapy by means of liposomes. In Gregoriadis G (ed): "Liposomes as drug carriers", Sussex, England: John Wiley & Sons, p 325.

7. Vladimirsky MA, Ladigina GA (1982). Antibacterial activity of liposome-entrapped streptomycin in mice infected with *Mycobacterium tuberculosis*. Biomed Pharmacother 36:375.

8. Sunamoto J, Goto M, Iida T, Hara K, Saito A, Tomonaga A (1984). Unexpected tissue distribution of liposomes coated with amylopectin derivatives and succesful use in the treatment of experimental Legionaires' disease. In Gregoriadis G, Poste G, Senior J, Trouet A (eds): "Receptor-mediated targeting of drugs", New York: Plenum, p 359.

9. Tadakuma T, Ikewaki N, Yasuda T, Tsutsumi M, Saito S, Saito K (1985). Treatment of experimental Salmonellosis in mice with streptomycin entrapped in liposomes. Antimicrob Agents Chemother 28:28.

10. Dees C, Fountain MW, Taylor JR, Schultz RD (1985). Enhanced intraphagocytic killing of Brucella abortus in bovine mononuclear cells by liposomes containing gentamicin. Vet Immunol Immunopathol 8:171.

11. Fraser-Smith EB, Matthews TR (1981). Protective effect of muramyl dipeptide analogs against infections of Pseudomonas aeruginosa or Candida albicans in mice. Infect Immun 34:676.

12. Koff WC, Showalter SD, Hampar B, Fidler IJ (1985). Protection of mice against fatal Herpes simplex type 2 infection by liposomes containing muramyl tripeptide. Science 228:495.

Liposomes in the Therapy of Infectious Diseases and Cancer, pages 287–294
© 1989 Alan R. Liss, Inc.

TREATMENT OF MYCOBACTERIUM AVIUM COMPLEX INFECTIONS BY FREE AND LIPOSOME-ENCAPSULATED TUMOR NECROSIS FACTOR-ALPHA (CACHECTIN): STUDIES ON PERITONEAL MACROPHAGES AND THE BEIGE MOUSE MODEL[1]

N. Düzgüneş[a,b], V. K. Perumal[c], E. N. Brunette[a],
P. R. J. Gangadharam[c] and R. J. Debs[a]

Cancer Research Institute[a] and the Department of
Pharmaceutical Chemistry[b], University of California,
San Francisco, California 94143-0128;
Mycobacteriology Research Laboratory[c],
National Jewish Center for Immunology and Respiratory
Medicine, Denver, Colorado 80206

ABSTRACT *Mycobacterium avium-intracellulare* (MAC) is an opportunistic pathogen in AIDS and is resistant to antitubercle drugs. We have investigated the effect of tumor necrosis factor-alpha (TNF) on the growth of MAC in murine peritoneal macrophages and in the Beige mouse model of the disease. Both free and liposome-encapsulated TNF mediated the reduction of colony-forming units of MAC. Encapsulation in liposomes reduced drastically the toxic effects of TNF in the animal model, but was ineffective against MAC in the liver, spleen and lungs.

INTRODUCTION

Opportunistic infections are the major cause of morbidity and mortality in Advanced Immune Deficiency Syndrome (AIDS). *Mycobacterium avium-intracellulare* complex (MAC) is one of the most prevalent of these infections. The organism multiplies

[1]This work was supported by funds provided by a grant from the State of California, as recommended by the Universitywide Task Force on AIDS (ND and RJD), and by NIH Grant AI21897 and NIH Contract AI72636 (PRJG).

primarily in the resident macrophages of the lungs, spleen, liver and lymph nodes of infected individuals (1-3). Traditional antituberculosis therapy is not effective against MAC, and many drugs that have high *in vitro* activity against MAC have limited efficacy *in vivo*.

Tumor necrosis factor-alpha (TNF) is a cytokine secreted by macrophages stimulated with endotoxin and is a primary mediator of cachexia (hence the synonym, "cachectin") that accompanies disease states (4). It also activates monocytes to lyse tumor cells *in vitro* (5). It was of interest to determine whether TNF could activate macrophages to kill intracellular pathogens such as MAC. Since macrophage activation by cytokines *in vivo* is enhanced by encapsulation in liposomes (6), and natural targeting of cytokines to the marcophages in the liver and spleen can be achieved (7), the effect of liposome-encapsulated TNF was also determined. An additional advantage of liposome-encapsulated TNF *in vivo* would be its reduced toxicity compared to free TNF (8).

RESULTS

Thioglycollate-elicited peritoneal macrophages were incubated for 1 h with MAC strain 101, obtained from an AIDS patient, and treated with free or liposome-encapsulated TNF for 24 h. The cells were lysed after various times of incubation and the lysate plated on 7H11 agar. Colony-forming units (CFU) of MAC were counted after 2 weeks. Treatment of macrophages by 10 - 1000 units (U)/ml of recombinant human TNF, which is 78% homologous to murine TNF (4), caused the reduction of CFU counts over a 10-day period (Figure 1). Two days following infection, CFU of MAC in macrophages treated with 1000 U/ml TNF were reduced by an order of magnitude compared to untreated controls. At the 10-day point, all three concentrations of TNF appeared to be equally effective in reducing the CFU. Three days after the infection, 100 U/ml TNF caused a reduction of 0.5 log units in the CFU.

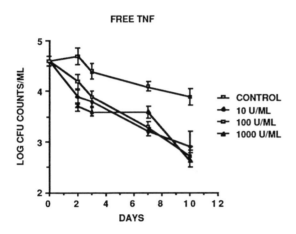

FIGURE 1. The effect of free TNF treatment on the time course of MAC CFU counts in peritoneal macrophages.

At this time point, the same concentration of TNF encapsulated in multilamellar phosphatidylserine (PS)/ cholesterol (2:1) liposomes mediated a further reduction of 0.9 log units in the CFU (Figure 2). However, at later

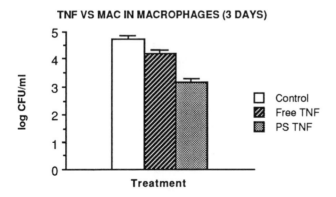

FIGURE 2. The reduction in MAC CFU counts in peritoneal macrophages 3 days after the onset of a 24 h incubation with 100 U/ml of TNF, free or encapsulated in PS/cholesterol (2:1) liposomes.

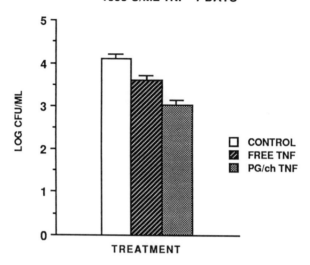

1000 U/ML TNF 7 DAYS

FIGURE 3. The effect of 1000 U/ml free or PG/cholesterol liposome-encapsulated TNF on the CFU of MAC in peritoneal macrophages, 7 days following infection.

time points, this difference between the effects of free and liposome-encapsulated TNF was diminished. At a higher dose (1000 U/ml), TNF was equally effective whether free or encapsulated in PS/cholesterol vesicles. On the other hand, the same dose of TNF in phosphatidylglycerol (PG)/cholesterol (2:1) liposomes exhibited a higher anti-MAC activity than free TNF 7 days following infection (Figure 3). By day 10, however, free TNF was more effective in reducing MAC CFU counts. The general trend over the course of the experiment was the reduction of CFU by about a factor 10, upon treatment of the macrophages by free or liposome-encapsulated TNF.

The effect of TNF was then tested on MAC infection in Beige mice, an established animal model of the disease (9). Free or liposome-encapsulated TNF was administered at a dose of 5 μg/mouse/week for 4 weeks. Controls included the injection of buffer (140 mM NaCl, 10 mM KCl, 10 mM Hepes), and buffer-loaded ("empty") liposomes. Forty percent of the animals receiving free TNF died within 12 hours of the first administration, but none of the animals receiving 4 weekly doses of TNF encapsulated in PG/cholesterol (2:1) liposomes died (10). The MAC CFU counts were determined in the lungs, spleen and liver of infected mice every two weeks. No significant effects of treatment on CFU counts were observed over an 8-week period. In the next series of experiments, the dose of TNF was reduced to 2.5 µg/mouse/injection, but the frequency was increased to twice a week. The mice receiving free TNF survived for two weeks, but all of them died within a few days thereafter. The animals that received liposomal TNF survived the 8-week experiment. The results of the experiment at the 4-week time point are shown in Table 1. Again, no significant effects of liposome-TNF on the CFU counts were observed (10).

TABLE 1
EFFECT OF LIPOSOME-ENCAPSULATED TNF
ON MAC IN BEIGE MICE

LOG CFU COUNTS/ML

ORGANS	1 DAY[a]	4 WEEKS CONTROL[b]	LIPOSOME-TNF[c]
Spleen	4.77	6.19	6.74
Lungs	4.00	5.00	5.40
Liver	5.75	6.71	6.84

[a] CFU counts within 1 day of infection with MAC strain 101
   Treatment was started at this point.
[b] No treatment. Animals received injections of buffer.
[c] Animals received 2 weekly injections of 2.5 µg TNF in
   PG/cholesterol liposomes for 4 weeks.

Since Beige mice are immunodeficient, particularly in NK cell activity (11), it was of interest to investigate whether the lack of effect of TNF in this animal model was due to this factor. Thus, similar experiments were performed with Black/6 mice. These animals survived the free TNF administration, but, again, no effect of TNF on MAC was observed in the spleen, lungs and liver (10).

DISCUSSION

TNF has been shown to activate neutrophils to degranulate and phagocytose, and eosinophils to kill extracellular *Shistosoma mansoni* (12-14), as well as activate macrophages to lyse tumor cells (5). Our results demonstrate that TNF can activate macrophages to kill the intracellular pathogen MAC. The mechanism by which the activated macrophages kill MAC remains to be investigated. The dose of TNF does not appear to have a definite effect, since the reduction in CFU by the three different doses varies as the incubation continues. Likewise, liposome encapsulation of TNF is more effective at certain times following the initial 24 h treatment period.

Despite the observations of the effect of TNF on MAC in macrophages in culture, the absence of any effectiveness of the cytokine *in vivo* is disappointing. Targeting of antibiotics to the liver and spleen by encapsulation in liposomes has an enhanced effect on MAC in these organs (15). It is possible that thioglycollate elicitation of the peritoneal macrophages primes them for the action of TNF. Perhaps the most significant finding of our *in vivo* experiments is the drastically reduced toxicity of TNF upon encapsulation in liposomes. The demonstration that the immunomodulatory functions of TNF are retained when encapsulated in liposomes (8) raises the possibility of the therapeutic use of such TNF preparations in selected cases.

REFERENCES

1.   Greene JB, Sidhu GS, Lewin S, Levine JF, Masur H, Simberkoff MS, Nichola P, Good RC, Zolla-Pazner SB, Pollock AA, Tapper ML, Holzman RS (1982). *Mycobacterium avium-intracellulare*: A cause of disseminated life-threatening infection in homosexuals and drug abusers. Ann Intern Med 97:539.

2. Wong B, Edwards FF, KiehnTE, Whimbey E, Donnely H, Bernard, EM, Gold JWM , Armstrong D (1985). Continuous high-grade *Mycobacterium avium-intracellulare* bactermia in patients with the acquired immune deficiency syndrome. Am J Med 78:35.
3. Young LS, Inderlied CB, Berlin OG, Gottlieb MS (1986). Mycobacterial infections in AIDS patients, with an emphasis on the *Mycobacterium avium* complex. Rev Infect Dis 8:1024.
4. Beutler B, Cerami A (1986). Cachectin and tumor necrosis factor as two sides of the same biological coin. Nature 320:584.
5. Philip R, Epstein LB (1986). Tumor necrosis factor as immunomodulator and mediator of monocyte cytotoxicity induced by itself, g-interferon and interleukin-1. Nature 323:86.
6. Poste G, Bucana C, Fidler IJ (1982). Stimulation of host response against metastatic tumours by liposome-encapsulated immunomodulators. In Gregoriadis G, Senior J, Trouet A (eds): "Targeting of Drugs." New York: Plenum Press, p. 261.
7. Roerdink F, Regts J, Daemen T, Bakker-Woudenberg I, Scherphof G (1986). Liposomes as drug carriers to liver macrophages: Fundamental and therapeutic aspects,. In: Gregoriadis G, SeniorJ, Poste G (eds) "Targeting of Drugs with Synthetic Systems," New York: Plenum Press, p. 193.
8. Debs RJ, Fuchs HJ, Philip R, Brunette EN, Düzgüneş N, Shellito JE, Liggitt D, Patton JS (1988). Immunomodulatory and toxic effects of free and liposome-encapsulated tumor necrosis factor-alpha in rats. J Immunol, submitted.
9. Gangadharam PR, Edwards CK III, Murthy PS, Pratt PF(1983). An acute infection model for *Mycobacterium intracellulare* disease using beige mice: Preliminary results. Am Rev Respir Dis 127:648.
10. Debs RJ, Perumal VK, Düzgüneş N, Brunette EN, and Gangadharam PRJ (1988). Manuscript in preparation.
11. Roder JC, Lohmann-Matthes ML, Domzig W, Wigzell HW (1979). The key mutation in the mouse. Selectivity of the natural killer (NK) cell defect. J Immunol 123:2174.

12. Gamble JR, Harlan JM, Klebanoff SJ, Lopez AF, Vadas MA (1985). Stimulation of the adherence of neutrophils to umbilical vein endothelium by human recombinant tumor necrosis factor. Proc Natl Acad Sci, USA 82:8667.
13. Silberstein DS, David JR (1986). Tumor necrosis factor enhances eosinophil toxicity to *Schistosoma mansoni* larvae. Proc Natl Acad Sci, USA 83:1055.
14. Shalaby MR, Agarwal BB, Rinderknecht E, Svedersky LP, Finkle BS, Palladino MA Jr (1985). Activation of human polymorphonuclear neutrophil functions by interferon-gamma and tumor necrosis factors. J Immunol 135:2069.
15. Düzgüneş N, Perumal VK, Kesavalu L, Debs RJ, Gangadharam PRJ (1988). Enhanced effect of liposome-encapsulated amikacin on *mycobacterium avium-intracellulare* complex infection in beige mice. Antimicrob Agents Chemother (submitted).

ACKNOWLEDGMENTS

We thank Dr. John Patton for providing the TNF used in our experiments; Dr. Demetrios Papahadjopoulos for discussions, his enthusiastic support and the use of his laboratory facilities; and Ms. Joanne Huddleston for preparation of the manuscript and editorial assistance.

V. CLINICAL TRIALS

Liposomes in the Therapy of Infectious Diseases and Cancer, pages 297–303
© 1989 Alan R. Liss, Inc.

INITIAL CLINICAL TRIAL OF MURAMYL TRIPEPTIDE DERIVATIVE
(MTP-PE) ENCAPSULATED IN LIPOSOMES: AN INTERIM REPORT

Patrick J. Creaven[1], Dean E. Brenner[1], J. Wayne
Cowens[1,2], Robert Huben[3], Constantine Karakousis[4], Tin
Han[5], Barbara Dadey[5], Kathe Adrejcio[6] and M. Kelli Cushman[1]

From the Departments of [1]Clinical Pharmacology and
Therapeutics, [2]Experimental Therapeutics, [3]Urologic
Oncology, [4]Soft Tissue Melanoma Service, [5]Medical Oncology,
Roswell Park Memorial Institute, New York State Department
of Health, Buffalo, New York, 14263 and [6]Ciba-Geigy
Corporation, Pharmaceuticals Division, Summit, New Jersey
07901.

INTRODUCTION

MTP-PE (CGP 19835A) encapsulated in liposomes
(liposomal MTP-PE) is a synthetic muramyl tripeptide,
coupled to dipalmitoylphosphatidyl-ethanolamine. It is
N-acetylmuramyl-L-alanyl-D-isoglutaminyl-L-alanine-2-
[(1,2-dipalmitoyl-sn-glycero-3-(hydroxyphosphoryloxy)]
ethylamide monosodium salt, encapsulated in a multilamellar
liposome formed from phosphatidylcholine and
phosphatidylserine in a molar ratio of 7:3 (1). The
material activates alvoelar macrophages to the tumoricidal
state in rodents (2). When given twice weekly for four
weeks the material is active in eradicating spontaneous
lung and lymph node metastases in mice bearing B-16/BL6
melanoma (3,4). In toxicology studies in dogs (5), the
major dose limiting toxicity was the production of infarcts
in the liver and lung which was seen at doses of 10 mg/m^2
and above. Arteritis was also seen at the higher doses.
The dose of 2 mg/m^2 was considered to be safe on daily
administration for 3 months. Mice were considerably less
sensitive to the drug than dogs. On the basis of its
ability to activate macrophages to the tumoricidal state
and its antitumor activity when given systemically, the
compound was introduced into phase I clinical trial.

MATERIALS AND METHODS

Patients:

Patients have solid tumors resistant to conventional therapy who give written informed consent to enter into the study. Entry requirements and exclusion criteria are listed in Table 1. The evaluations required for the study are listed in Table 2.

TABLE 1
ENTRY REQUIRMENTS AND EXCLUSION CRITERIA

Entry Requirements

Histologically proven malignant disease
Age: 18–70 years
Failure on conventional therapy or resistance to it
Normal bone marrow function (WBC $>$4,000/mm³ and platelet
  count ($>$100,000/mm³)
Normal hepatic and renal function (serum bilirubin $<$1.5
  mg/dl, SGOT $<$75 IU/L, serum creatinine $<$1.5 mg/dl)
Estimated survival of at least 2 months
Performance status of 0–2 (on a scale of 0–4) (ECOG)
At least three weeks since major surgery, radiotherapy or
  chemotherapy and recovery from all drug related toxicity
  (6 weeks for a nitrosourea and mitomycin C.)
Written informed consent for entry into the study

Exclusion Criteria

Pregnancy
Acute intercurrent complications such as sepsis
History of deep vein thrombosis
Bleeding diathesis (abnormal PT, APTT or bleeding time)
Uncontrolled hypertension: Systolic BP $>$180 mm Hg,
  diastolic BP $>$100 mm Hg
Diabetes
Documented coronary artery disease (angina pectoris,
  previous MI) or peripheral arterial vascular disease
Rheumatoid arthritis, SLE and other collagen vascular and
  autoimmune diseases

Table 2
REQUIRED EVALUATIONS

Pretreatment, 24h after doses 1,3,5, and 7 and off study:
    CBC with differential
    Chemistry profile[1]
    Coagulation profile[2]
    Antinuclear antibody
    Rheumatoid factor
    C reactive protein
    EKG
    Macrophage activation
Pretreatment and off study:
    Urinalysis
    Immunoglobulins

[1] BUN, serum creatinine sodium, potassium, chloride, CO_2, uric acid, bilirubin, alkaline phosphatase, SGOT, GGT, LDH, total protein, albumin, calcium, glucose, phosphorus, cholesterol
[2] PT,APTT, serum FDP, fibrin monomer, fibrinogen

The starting dose was 0.01 mg/m²/dose. This conservative starting dose was chosen because of the marked species variation in toxicity and the biological nature of the material. The drug is given by 1h infusion in 50 ml of isotonic saline through a safety filter twice a week for a total of 8 doses. In the presence of stable disease or tumor response, a further course or courses may be given. However, no intrapatient dose escalation is carried out.

Activation of peripheral blood monocytes is measured by the method of Kleinerman et al (6). Peripheral blood monocytes are isolated by adherence, incubated for 24h at 37°C in medium alone, or in medium containing lipopolysaccharide (positive control), and washed twice. Target cells (TC) (A375M human melanoma derived cell line) labelled with I^{125} are added to the monocyte cultures at a ratio of 1:20 (TC:monocyte). Labeled TC are also plated alone as a control. The cultures are incubated for 3 days at 37°C. The remaining radioactivity is measured after washing and the percentage cell kill (CK) is determined by:

$$CK = -\frac{CPM_{TC} - CPM_{TC+M}}{CPM_{TC}} \qquad Eq. \ 1$$

Where CPM_{TC} = counts/min of target cells

CPM_{TC+M} = counts/min of target cells + monocytes

RESULTS

The following dose levels (mg/m^2) have been evaluated: 0.01, 0.05, 0.1, 0.2, 0.4, 0.8, 1.2 and 1.8. Twenty five patients have been entered on the study. Their characteristics are given in Table 3.

Table 3
PATIENT CHARACTERISTICS

		Number	Percent
Patients entered		25	68
	Male	17	32
	Female	8	
Age (yrs)	Median	56	
	Range	18–75 yrs	
Diagnoses:			
	Renal cell carcinoma	10	40
	Melanoma	3	12
	Non-small cell broncho-genic carcinoma	2	8
	Colorectal carcinoma	2	8
	Soft tissue sarcoma	2	8
	Unknown primary	2	8
	Miscellaneous	4	16
Performance status (E.C.O.G.)			
	0	11	44
	1	13	52
	2	1	4
Prior therapy			
	Surgery	21	84
	Radiotherapy	11	44
	Chemotherapy	16	64
	Immunotherapy	5	20
	Hormonal therapy	1	4

A number of acute systemic toxicities have been seen of which fever and rigors are the most prominent (Table 4). There appears to be relatively little dose response relationship in these toxicities. However, toxicity is often more severe after the first than after subsequent doses. Thus, the median maximum temperature after dose 1 for all courses was 38.2° with a range of 37.3–40.4°. For dose 8, it was 37.3° (range 36.9°–38.1°).

Table 4
TOXICITY
(No. of Courses)

Toxicity	Grade[1]			Total[2]	Percent
	1	2	3		
Fever	12	9	2	23	68
Rigors	6	6	2	14	41
Tachycardia	7	4	0	11	32
Tachypnea	8	2	0	10	29
Nausea and vomiting	5	4	0	9	26
Hypertension	1	8	0	9	26
Hypotension	8	1	0	9	26
Headache	5	1	0	6	18
Fatigue	5	0	0	5	15
Vertigo	3	0	0	3	9
Anorexia	3	0	0	3	9
Skin rash	1	1	0	2	6
Cyanosis	2	0	0	2	6
Hypothermia	2	0	0	2	6

Misc: (each occuring on one course only) chest pain[3], diarrhea, muscle aches, leg cramps, pallor.

[1]Modified WHO Classification (see Appendix 1).
[2]From a total of 34 evaluable courses.
[3]Occurred after dose 1 only, EKG was normal.

Biochemical Changes

No alteration in hematological or biochemical parameters have been noted in any patient.

Macrophage Activation

Macrophage activation has been extremely variable from patient to patient, and from dose to dose in the same patient. In addition, the extent of pretreatment macrophage cytotoxicity has been variable, making the results difficult to interpret. A preliminary assessment of the data is shown in Table 5, in which the number of patients showing more than 10% increase in macrophage activation over the pretreatment sample is listed for doses 1, 3, 5 and 7, the denominator being the number of patients evaluable for macrophage activation at that dose level.

Table 5
MACROPHAGE ACTIVATION

Dose	1	3	5	7
0.05	0/2	0/1	0/1	–
0.1	0/3	0/2	1/1	1/2
0.2	0/2	1/2	1/2	0/2
0.4	2/4	1/2	1/3	1/4
0.8	1/6	2/4	2/5	1/3
1.2	0/4	1/2	1/4	0/3
1.8	1/2	0/1	0/1	0/1

*No of courses showing >10% increase at 24h in macrophage activation over pretreatment values (see Eq. 1).

Response

One patient with renal cell carcinoma with multiple small pulmonary metastases, showed a diminution in the size of the lesions after one course and further diminution after two courses. After three courses, the lesions could no longer be identified on CT scan.

SUMMARY AND CONCLUSIONS

This drug is well tolerated on a twice a week schedule for four weeks. The patient acceptance is high, and dose limiting toxicity has not been reached. The study is continuing.

ACKNOWLEDGEMENTS

The support of Ciba–Geigy Corporation, Pharmaceutical Division, Summit, New Jersey, for this study is gratefully acknowledged. The authors wish to acknowledge the expert assistance of Joan Solomon, R.N., April Proefrock, R.N. and Denise Traynor, R.N. in the performance of this study, of Marilyn Kuroski in the analysis of the data and Marty Courtney in preparation of the manuscript.

REFERENCES

1. Hanagan JR, Trunet P, LeSher D, Andrejcio K, Frost H (1988). Phase I development of CGP 19835A lipid (MTP–PE encapsulated in liposomes). in G. Lopez–Berestein G, Fidler I (eds): Liposomes in the Therapy of Infectious Diseases and Cancer. UCLA Symposia on Molecular and Cellular Biology, New Series Vol. 89, Alan R. Liss, Inc., New York, 1988.

2. Fidler IJ, Sone S, Fogler WE, Smith D, Braun DG, Tarcsay L, Gisler RH, Schroit AJ (1982). Efficacy of liposomes containing a lipophilic muramyl dipeptide derivative for activating the tumoricidal properties of alveolar macrophages in vivo. J. Biol. Resp. Modif. 1:43.

3. Key ME, Talmadge JE, Fogler WE, Bucana C, and Fidler IJ (1982). Isolation of tumoricidal macrophages from lung melanoma metastases of mice treated systemically with liposomes containing a lipophilic derivative of muramyl dipeptide. J. Nat. Cancer Inst. 69:1189.

4. Fidler IJ, Barner Z, Fogler WE, Kirsh R, Bugelski P, and Poste G (1982). Involvement of macrophages in the eradication of established metastases following intravenous injection of liposomes containing macrophage activators. Cancer Res. 42:496.

5. Kanter P. Personal communication.

6. Kleinermann ES, Erickson KL, Schroit AJ, Fogler WE, Fidler IJ (1983). Activation of tumoricidal properties in human blood monocytes by liposomes containing lipophilic muramyl tripeptide. Cancer Res. 43:2010.

Liposomes in the Therapy of Infectious Diseases and Cancer, pages 305–315
© 1989 Alan R. Liss, Inc.

PHASE I DEVELOPMENT OF CGP 19835A LIPID
(MTP-PE ENCAPSULATED IN LIPOSOMES).

J.R. Hanagan, P. Trunet,
D. LeSher, K. Andrejcio, H. Frost.

CIBA-GEIGY Corp.   Summit, N.J.
and
CIBA-GEIGY Ltd., Basle, Switzerland.

ABSTRACT   CGP 19835A Lipid is a synthetic muramyl
tripeptide encapsulated in liposomes that is believed
to exert its effects by activating monocytes.   Phase I
trials have been initiated at four clinical centers
involving patients with advanced malignancy and at one
center involving patients with AIDS-related Kaposi's
Sarcoma.   Drug is administered either once or twice
weekly intravenously on either an intra or inter
patient dose escalating schedule.   Ninety patients
have been enrolled to date exploring doses from
0.01-4.0 mg/m^2.   No serious adverse reactions have
been reported to date.   Acute reactions include fever
(79%) rigors (59%) and nausea (44%) (percent of
patients in parentheses).   Macrophage activation by
cytotoxicity assay is measured at various time points
pre and post-dosing.   To date no clear dose-response
or dose-duration trends are apparent for either clinical tolerability or macrophage activation.   The phase
I trials are continuing.

INTRODUCTION

CGP 19835A Lipid consists of a synthetic muramyl tripeptide encapsulated in liposomes.   In order to prepare CGP
19835A Lipid, the free drug is blended with phosphotidyl-
choline and phosphotidylserine in a molar ratio of 7:3.
This mixture is then lyophylized to obtain the dry lipid
preparation which is a white friable mass.   Reconstitution
is accomplished by adding a suspension medium to the lyophilized material and shaking according to a standard procedure.

The resulting liposome suspension is the dosage form utilized in the clinic. In order to prepare an IV infusion suspension, CGP 19835A Lipid is mixed with 50 cc. 0.9% NaCl solution. This infusion suspension is then administered over one hour by means of an automatic syringe pump through a safety filter.

The properties and activities of CGP 19835A Lipid were investigated in an extensive program of preclinical testing. The results of this program supported the following conclusions concerning the activity of this agent:

- mouse and rat alveolar macrophages can be activated to a tumoricidal state in vitro. (1, 2, 3)

- intravenous administration to mice leads to high levels of alveolar macrophage mediated cytotoxicity as measured by in vitro assay. (1, 4, 5)

- multiple systemic injections of the agent eradicated spontaneous lung and lymph node metastasis in the B16/BL6 melanoma system in mice. (4, 5, 6, 7, 8)

- human peripheral blood monocytes from normal donors can be activated in vitro to become tumoricidal. (9, 10, 11, 12)

- peripheral blood monocytes from colorectal carcinoma patients can be activated in vitro to become tumoricidal. (13)

CGP 19835A Lipid has been evaluated for safety in a number of test systems using intravenous administration and a multitude of dosing regimens. In the mouse, the least sensitive species tested, doses as high as 10 mg/kg were easily tolerated. In rabbits and dogs, the no-toxic-effect dose for daily repeated administration for up to three months was 0.1 mg/kg.

METHODS

Based on this preclinical and animal safety data base, design of a Phase I program began in 1985. The initial plans called for multiple studies in two different indications, advanced cancer and AIDS-related Kaposi's Sarcoma, in order to rapidly gain information on safety, immunopharmacologic activity and eventually efficacy using different dose schedules. The AIDS-related Kaposi's Sarcoma indication was included because of the different sensitivity of AIDS patients to many drugs and the complex immune dysfunction of AIDS patients as a target for immune modulation.

During the period June 1986 through March 1987, five clinical studies were initiated and these studies are continuing. Four studies involve treatment of patients with advanced cancer. All studies include dose escalation. Two studies employ a dosing frequency of twice per week and dose escalation is either within or between patients. Two studies employ a dosing frequency of once per week and dose escalation is either within or between patients. A single study treating patient with AIDS-related Kaposi's Sarcoma was initiated in February 1987 and is continuing. This study employs a once weekly dosing frequency with dose escalation between patients only.

All protocols included a detailed schedule of clinical surveillance including periodic history, physical examination, vital sign monitoring post-infusion and radiographic studies to assess disease status. Hematologic, biochemical and coagulation parameters were monitored as safety assessment. Toxicity was graded according to a modification of the World Health Organization toxicity scale. (14)

Immune system status was followed using a variable combination of parameters such as skin testing with recall antigens, measures of cell surface markers, and blood levels of immunoglobulin, interleuken 1 and interferon. The exact combination of such parameters varied among the study centers based on the availability of assays from center to center. In addition, all centers performed timed measurements of peripheral blood monocyte tumoricidal activity. (10)

Results

Ninety patients have been treated to date, data presented are based on interim analysis of approximately 60 of these patients. Patient distribution by age and sex is summarized in Table 1.

TABLE 1
PATIENT DISTRIBUTION BY AGE AND SEX

Protocol	# of Patients	Age Range	Mean Age	Sex M	F
1	23	18-75	57	16	7
2	20	18-71	51	11	9
3	11	23-70	54	8	3
4	3	40-56	50	1	2
5	2	31-39	35	2	0
Overall	59	18-75	53	38	21

The mean age of treated patients is 53 years with a broad range from 18 to 75 years. A slight male to female preponderance is present in the treated population. The majority of patients (84%) had received at least one form of anti-tumor therapy as noted in Table 2. Twenty-two percent (22%) had received chemotherapy and radiotherapy while eighteen percent (18%) had received some combination of chemotherapy, radiation therapy and immunotherapy.

TABLE 2
PRIOR THERAPY - NUMBER OF PATIENTS

	P01	P02	P03	P04	Total	%
CHEMOTHERAPY (CT)	6	2	3	2	13	24
RADIATION (RT)	2	2	0	0	4	7
IMMUNOTHERAPY (CT)	1	0	0	0	1	2
CT & RT	6	5	1	0	12	22
CT & IT	1	3	2	0	6	11
RT & IT	0	0	0	0	0	0
CT, RT & IT	2	4	3	1	10	18
NONE	5	2	2	0	9	16
TOTAL	23	18	11	3	55	

The patient population presented with a diversity of histologic tumor types as outlined in Table 3. The two most common histologies represented were renal cell carcinoma (21%) and colorectal carcinoma (20%).

TABLE 3
DISTRIBUTION OF TUMOR TYPES

Renal	13		
Colorectal	12		
Melanoma	6		
Lung	6		
		Adeno	4
		Small Cell	2
Breast	4		
Gastric	3		
Pancreas	3		
Sarcoma	4		
Osteosarcoma	2		
Kaposi's	2		
Gall Bladder	1		
Urinary Bladder	1		
Unknown Origin	3		
		Squamous	2
		Adeno	1

The majority of patients (70%) treated to date have received cumulative doses in milligrams which range from 0.1 to 9.9 (Table 4).

TABLE 4
CUMULATIVE DOSES RECEIVED

Dose Range (mg)	# of Patients
.01 - .09	2
.1 - .99	12
1 - 9.9	27
10 - 19	9
20 - 29	
30 - 39	1
40 - 49	
50 - 59	2
60 - 69	
70 - 79	1
80 - 89	1
90 - 99	
100 - 110	1

Adverse reactions which occurred in > 10% of patients analyzed and which were felt to be drug related (possible, probable, definite) in 61 patients are summarized in Table 5.

TABLE 5

DRUG RELATED (POSSIBLE, PROBABLE, DEFINITE)
ADVERSE REACTIONS REPORTED IN 61 PATIENTS

Reaction	# of PATIENTS	% of PATIENTS	# of EPISODES
FEVER	48	79	179
RIGORS	35	57	111
NAUSEA	27	44	60
TACHYCARDIA	23	38	54
VOMITING	17	28	39
FATIGUE	16	26	37
HYPERTENSION	15	25	24
HEADACHE	12	20	25
HYPOTENSION	11	18	18
MALAISE	11	18	86
ANOREXIA	10	16	12
RESP. DISORDER	10	16	15
PAIN (NOS)	6	10	6

Fever and rigors were overall the commonest adverse events noted occurring in seventy-nine percent (79%) and fifty-seven percent (57%) of patients respectively. Nausea, tachycardia, and vomiting occurred with less frequency. Of more interest are the adverse events listed by grade and displayed in relation to time of occurrence following dosing. Table 6 lists those events by grade that were observed/reported during the initial few hours after drug administration. Table 7 lists those events by grade that were observed/reported over the period of days intervening between drug doses.

TABLE 6

DRUG RELATED (POSSIBLE, PROBABLE, DEFINITE)
ADVERSE REACTIONS REPORTED IN 61 PATIENTS

DURING DRUG ADMINISTRATION

REACTION	# OF PATIENTS	# WITH GRADE 1	# WITH GRADE 2	# WITH GRADE 3	# WITH GRADE 4
FEVER	46	45	13	2	0
RIGORS	35	28	17	5	0
NAUSEA	20	11	7	0	0
TACHYCARDIA	23	23	0	0	0
VOMITING	9	4	6	0	0
FATIGUE	14	13	12	0	0
HYPERTENSION	15	10	8	0	0
HEADACHE	11	11	0	0	0
HYPOTENSION	11	9	2	0	0
MALAISE	9	8	6	0	0
ANOREXIA	6	6	0	0	0
RESP. DISORDER	10	10	0	0	0
PAIN (NOS)	2	0	2	0	0

TABLE 7

DRUG RELATED (POSSIBLE, PROBABLE, DEFINITE)
ADVERSE REACTIONS REPORTED IN 61 PATIENTS

POST DRUG ADMINISTRATION

REACTION	# OF PATIENTS	# WITH GRADE 1	# WITH GRADE 2	# WITH GRADE 3	# WITH GRADE 4
FEVER	3	3	0	0	0
RIGORS	1	1	0	0	0
NAUSEA	4	4	0	0	0
TACHYCARDIA	1	1	0	0	0
VOMITING	4	4	0	0	0
FATIGUE	1	1	0	0	0
HYPERTENSION	0	0	0	0	0
HEADACHE	0	0	0	0	0
HYPOTENSION	1	0	1	0	0
MALAISE	6	6	0	0	0
ANOREXIA	2	2	0	0	0
RESP. DISORDER	0	0	0	0	0
PAIN	1	1	0	0	0

In general, the majority of events occur within the first few hours following the infusion of the drug. The events which do occur during this period tend to be mild to moderate in intensity (Grade 1 or 2) with relatively few events of greater intensity noted (7 patients with Grade 3 events). In addition, the events tend to be self-limited as evidenced by both the marked decrease in number observed during the days between treatments and the decrease in grade of those events recorded (only one event > Grade 1).

Analysis of clinical laboratory parameters (hematology, biochemistry, coagulation factors) as measures of drug tolerability have shown no significant changes or trends to date. Abnormalities noted are felt to be related to the underlying disease and do not appear to change significantly in relationship to treatment.

Information regarding potential change in patient immune status in response to treatment is available only in a preliminary form on a subset of patients. Cell surface marker data (Table 8) and pre and post treatment immunoglobulin levels (Table 9) summarized in a global fashion do not demonstrate remarkable changes. Data from the monocyte tumoroidal activity assay is not yet available in sufficient volume at the various dosage levels across study centers to allow any statements regarding interpretation. Similarly, clinical efficacy across the Phase I program cannot yet be evaluated as patient numbers with adequate time under treatment at various dose levels remain small.

TABLE 8
CELL SURFACE MARKERS

	MEANS AND RANGES Cells/cubic mm Pre Treatment	Post Last Dose	N-# OF PATIENTS Percent Cells Pre Treatment	Post Last Dose
Lymphocytes	273 180-414	332 76-1002 N-12	23 14-35	25 14-41 N-16
T-Lymphocytes	1014 486-1703	1053 161-2081 N-12	83 71-91	82 66-90 N-16
Helper T-Lymphocytes	502 195-1025	500 49-1209 N-12	41 21-82	40 20-48 N-16
Suppressor T-Lymphocytes	323 130-552	333 67-701 N-12	31 19-54	29 19-39 N-16
Thymocytes & Thymic Stem Cells	405 165-922	473 102-1156 N-12	35 17-63	38 13-61 N-16
B Cells	83 24-177	104 22-273 N-12	8 2-18	10 4-17 N-16
Monocytes	327 31-1000	468 38-1932 N-11	5 2-9	5 1-14 N-11

TABLE 9

PRE AND POST TREATMENT IMMUNOBLOBULINS

MEAN AND RANGE OF VALUES ( ) OF 9 PATIENTS
mg/dl

	PRE	POST
IGG	1408 (777-2693)	1575 (576-3840)
IGA	254 (82-468)	271 (136-516)
IGM	172 (36-323)	170 (29-514)

DISCUSSION

The Phase I program with CGP 19835A Lipid represents
the initial step in an attempt to develop for clinical use
a totally synthetic immunomodulator with targetted delivery
to the effector cell of interest. Based on experience to
date in approximately ninety (90) patients, the drug appears to be well tolerated in doses up to 4.0 mg/m^2 given
twice weekly intravenously. No clinical events have
emerged at present which might threaten further development. The incidence of fever and rigors may well imply
biologic effect. Preliminary data indicate an effect on
monocyte activation which requires further definition. At
present, there is no apparent dose-response nor dose-duration relationship evident for either biologic effect nor
effect on monocyte activation. The task remains to evaluate data from multiple dose levels in a diverse patient
population in order to define dose, schedule, and appropri-
clinical indications. As the program has evolved, other
immune parameters and additional time points have been
added to the test battery. Neither the optimal immunomodulatory dose nor the maximal tolerated dose has been defined. The Phase I program is continuing toward definition
of these levels.

REFERENCES

1. Fidler IJ, Sone S, Fogler WE, Smith D, Braun DG, Tarcsay L, Gisler RH, Schroit AJ. Efficacy of liposomes containing a lipophlic muramyl dipeptide derivative for activating the tumoricidal properties of alveolar macrophages in vivo. J. Biol. Resp. Modif. 1:pp, 43-55, 1982.

2. Mutzuura S, Sone S, Tsubura K, Tachibana K, and Kishino Y,. Activation of antitumor properties in alveolar macrophages from protein-calorie malnourished rats. Cancer Immunol. Immunother. 21: pp. 63-68, 1986.

3. Schroit AJ, Fidler IJ. Effects of liposome structure and lipid composition on the activation of the tumoricidal properties of macrophages by liposomes containing muramyl dipeptide. Cancer Res. 42: pp. 161-167, 1982.

4. Fidler IJ, Fogler WE, Tarcsay L, Schumann G, Braun DG, and Schroit AJ. Systemic activation of macrophages and treatment of cancer metastases by liposomes containing hydrophilic or lipophilic muramyl dipeptide. Advances in Immunopharmacology 2, Eds. Hadden JW, et al., Pergamon Press, pp. 235-241, 1983.

5. Schroit A, Galligioni E, and Fidler IJ. Factors influencing the in situ activation of macrophages by liposomes containing muramyl dipeptide. Biol. Cell 47: pp. 87-94, 1983.

6. Key ME, Talmadge JE, Fogler WE, Bucana C, and Fidler IJ. Isolation of tumoricidal macrophages from lung melanoma metastases of mice treated systemically with liposomes containing a lipophilic derivative of muramyl dipeptide. J. Nat. Cancer Inst. 69: pp.1189-1198, 1982.

7. Talmadge E, Lenz BF, Collins MS, Uithoven KA, Schneider MA, Adams JS, Pearson JW, Agee WJ, Fox RE, and Oldham RK. Tumor models to investigate the therapeutic efficiency of immunomodulators. Behring Inst. Mitt. 74: pp. 219-229, 1984.

8. Fidler IJ. Optimization and limitations of systemic treatment of murine melanoma metastases with liposomes containing muramyl tripeptide phosphatidylethanolamine. Cancer Immunol. Immunother. 21: pp. 169-173, 1986.

9. Bucana CD, Hoyer LC, Schroit AJ, Kleinerman E, and Fidler IJ. Ultrastructural studies of the interaction between liposome-activated human blood monocytes and allogeneic tumor cells in vitro. Am. J. Pathol. 112: pp. 101-111, 1983.

10. Kleinermann, ES, Erickson KL, Schroit AJ, Fogler WE, Fidler IJ. Activation of tumoricidal properties in human blood monocytes by liposomes containing lipophilic muramyl tripeptide. Cancer Res. 43: pp. 2010-2014, 1983.

11. Sone S, Mutsuura S, Ogawara M, and Tsubura E. Potentiating effect of muramyl dipeptide and its lipophilic analog encapsulated in liposomes on tumor cell killing by human monocytes. J. Immunol. 132: pp. 2105-2110, 1984.

12. Sone S, Utsugi T, Tandon P, and Ogawara M. A dried preparation of liposomes containing muramyl tripeptide phosphatidylethanolamine as a potent activator of human blood monocytes to the antitumor state. Cancer Immunol. Immunother. 22: pp. 191-196, 1986.

13. Fidler IJ, Jessup JM, Fogler WE, Staerkel R, and Mazumder A. Activation of tumoricidal properties in peripheral blood monocytes of patients with colorectal carcinoma. Cancer Res. 46: pp. 994-998, 1986.

14. Miller AB, Hoogstraten B, Staquet M, Winkler A. Reporting Resulting of Cancer Treatment. Cancer 47: pp. 207-214, 1981.

Liposomes in the Therapy of Infectious Diseases and Cancer, pages 317–327
© 1989 Alan R. Liss, Inc.

TREATMENT OF SYSTEMIC FUNGAL INFECTIONS WITH
LIPOSOMAL-AMPHOTERICIN B

Gabriel Lopez-Berestein, M.D.

Immunobiology and Drug Carriers Section, The University of
Texas System Cancer Center, M. D. Anderson Hospital and
Tumor Institute at Houston, Houston, TX 77030

ABSTRACT   Liposomal amphotericin B (L-AmpB) was
shown to be less toxic and more active than free
AmpB in experimental candidiasis. L-AmpB, composed of dimyristoyl phosphatidyl choline (DMPC)
and dimyristoyl phosphatidyl glycerol (DMPG) in a
7:3 molar ratio, was shown to be more active in
vitro against a variety of fungi than positive,
neutral, or sterol-containing liposomes. Sixteen
patients with systemic fungal infections complicating their hematologic malignancies were
treated with L-AmpB.   All patients had failed to
respond to therapy with conventional AmpB and had
documented persistent or progressive fungal
infection.   Eleven patients showed a complete
response, and four failed to respond. No severe
acute or chronic renal toxicity was observed.
Phagocytic transport of liposomes may play an
important role in the enhanced therapeutic index
resulting from liposomal incorporation of AmpB.

INTRODUCTION

Amphotericin B (AmpB) has been in clinical use for
more than 30 years and still remains the most effective
antifungal drug available (1-3). Its intravenous administration, however, leads to severe acute and chronic side
effects such as renal tubular dysfunction, central nervous
system toxicity, rigors, and chills. Several new antifungals have been developed, but none have been shown to be as

effective as AmpB.   An alternative approach was to use
liposomes as carriers of AmpB. AmpB is a highly lipophilic
polyene antibiotic with a general structure consisting of a
mycosamine group and a series of seven carbon-to-carbon
double bonds, making AmpB compatible with incorporation
into a lipid carrier. Furthermore, the targeting of
liposomes to organs such as lung, liver and spleen that are
rich in macrophages and that are a frequent target of
systemic fungal infections made L-AmpB development
attractive.

Pre-clinical Studies

        Liposomes composed of dimyristoyl phosphatidyl choline
(DMPC) and dimyristoyl phosphatidyl glycerol (DMPG) were
used to incorporate AmpB. Negatively charged liposomes
were shown in earlier studies to be taken up avidly by
macrophages (4) and human monocytes (5) and to be nontoxic
when injected intravenously into mice (6) and man (7).
Further studies demonstrated this combination to be stable
for prolonged periods of time even after liposomal reconstitution. We first demonstrated that AmpB containing
liposomes composed of DMPC and DMPG in a 7:3 molar ratio
had an in vitro minimal fungicidal concentration (MFC)
similar to free AmpB. This preparation of liposomal AmpB
was far superior to those with neutral, positive or other
negatively charged compositions (Table 1). Furthermore,
the addition of ergosterol or cholesterol to the lipid
combinations led to lower in vitro antifungal efficacy (8).
A possible explanation for the lower efficacy observed with
sterol-containing liposomes is that they may reduce the
AmpB exchange from the liposome to the ergosterol-containing fungal membranes and thereby compete with binding of
the drug.
        When compared with AmpB, the in vitro antifungal effi-
cacy is maintained while its in vitro toxicity to mammalian
cells is markedly reduced (Fig. 1, left graph). AmpB leads
to a marked reduction of human peripheral blood NK cell
activity even at normally occurring plasma levels, while
L-AmpB even at several-fold higher concentrations is not
toxic (Fig. 1, right graph).
        We tested the toxicity of intravenously administered
L-AmpB (Fig. 2, left graph) (9). The maximal tolerated
dose (MTD) of a single intravenous dose of L-AmpB corres-
ponded to 12 mg AmpB/kg body weight, and the LD50 was 14 mg
AmpB/kg. For AmpB the MTD was 0.8 mg/kg and the LD50 was

TABLE 1
MIMINAL FUNGICIDAL CONCENTRATION RESULTS WITH A VARIETY
OF YEAST ISOLATES AND LIPOSOME PREPARATION CONTAINING
STEROLS

Organism and strain no.	MFC (µg AmpB/ml)			
	AmpB	L–AmpB	L–AmpB–C[a]	L–AmpB–E[b]
Candida albicans				
306	1.6	1.6	3	>25[c]
704	0.4	0.8	1.6[c]	>25[c]
Candida tropicalis				
251	3	6	12[c]	>25[c]
2463	1.6	1.6	3	6[c]
Candida parapsilosis				
139	3	>25[c]	>25[c]	>25[c]
1341	>25	>25	>25	>25
Torulopsis glabrata				
684	3	25[c]	25[c]	>25[c]
1905	3	3	3	12[c]
Cryptococcus neoformans				
222	1.6	0.8[c]	3	25[c]
843	0.8	12[c]	12[c]	>25[c]

[a] L–AmpB–C, cholesterol-containing L–AmpB.
[b] L–AmpB–E, ergosterol-containing L–AmpB.
[c] Indicates MFC with a $\geq$ fourfold difference compared with free AmpB.

Adapted from Mehta RT, et al. Infect Immun 47:429–433, 1985.

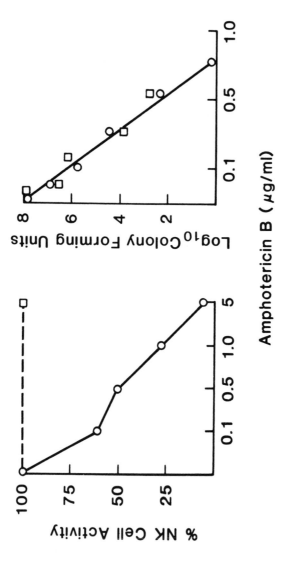

FIGURE 1. In vitro toxicity and antifungal efficacy of L-AmpB. (-o-) Free AmpB; (-□-) L-AmpB.

TOXICITY AND ANTIFUNGAL EFFICACY OF LIPOSOMAL - AMPHOTERICIN B

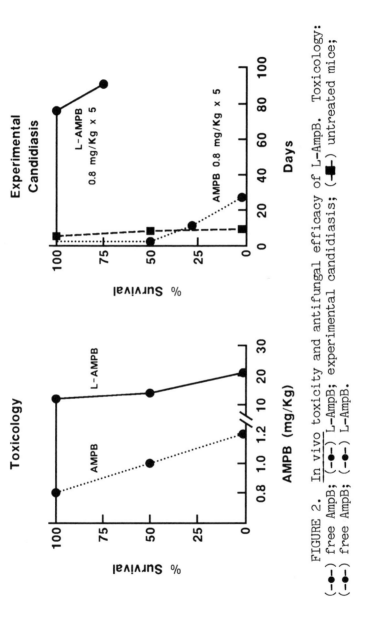

FIGURE 2. In vivo toxicity and antifungal efficacy of L-AmpB. Toxicology: (—●—) free AmpB; (—●—) L-AmpB; experimental candidiasis; (—■—) untreated mice; (—●—) free AmpB; (—●—) L-AmpB.

1.0 mg/kg (updated from ref. 9). Following daily doses of
L-AmpB at 5 mg/kg, we did not observe any renal or liver
toxicity 90 days after the drug administration. The
efficacy of free versus L-AmpB was tested in a model of
experimental candidiasis developed in our laboratory
(10-12). All treatments were administered i.v. and started
two days following the Candida albicans inoculum to ascertain that a well-established fungal infection was present.
All untreated animals were dead by day 10. Infected mice
treated with free AmpB at its MTD dose (0.8 mg/kg) daily
for 5 days showed significant increase in survival; however, all mice were dead by day 20. Death was not related
directly to AmpB toxicity since in previous experiments we
had shown that mice tolerated this regimen well. However,
100% of the mice treated with L-AmpB using the same protocol were alive by day 60. By day 90, all mice were
sacrificed with 50% of the survivors being microbiologic-
ally free of infection. These studies demonstrated that
L-AmpB was by far less toxic and more active in experimental candidiasis than free AmpB. L-AmpB composed of
DMPC:DMPG in a 7:3 molar ratio was also shown to be
effective in the treatment of systemic leishmaniasis in
hamsters and monkeys (13).

Clinical Trials

In 1983, we started a clinical trial of L-AmpB in patients with documented fungal infections failing to respond
to the conventional form of the drug (Table 2). Sixteen
patients with hematologic malignancies developed systemic
fungal infections. Nine patients presented with hepatosplenic mycoses (14) and seven patients with (15) invasive
sinonasal aspergillosis. Of the nine patients with hepatosplenic mycoses, eight had biopsy- or culture-documented
Candida, and one had an unclassified fungus. Eight patients
had a complete remission, and one showed no improvement.
Eight of the nine patients studied had a history of severe
fever and chills secondary to the administration of AmpB.
Only three patients had fever and chills or both that
occurred within one to two hours after L-AmpB administration; the fever and chills were usually mild and lasted ten
to 15 minutes. When the symptoms persisted longer, they
were suppressed by the administration of diphenhydramine,
acetaminophen, or meperidine. No nephrotoxicity was
observed that could be associated with L-AmpB. Decreased
levels of serum K^+ requiring supplementation were observed

TABLE 2

CHARACTERISTIC OF THE TREATED PATIENTS

Age (yrs)	Underlying disease	Fungi	Site of fungal disease	Response to treatment[a]
2	Leukemia	Candida spp	Liver, spleen, skin	CR
2.5	Leukemia	Candida spp	Liver, spleen	CR
64	Leukemia	Candida spp	Liver	CR
2.5	Leukemia	Candida spp	Liver, spleen, kidney	CR
16	Leukemia	Candida spp	Liver	CR
26	Leukemia	Candida spp	Liver	CR
37	Leukemia	Candida spp	Liver	NR
22	Leukemia	Candida spp	Liver	CR
13	Lymphoma	Unclassified	Liver, spleen	CR
22	Leukemia	Aspergillus flavus	Sinus, orbit	CR
41	None	Aspergillus fumigatus	Sinus, extradural	NR
60	Leukemia	Aspergillus spp	Sinus	CR
22	Leukemia	A. flavus	Sinus, nose	CR
18	Aplastic anemia	A. flavus	Sinus, nose	CR
16	Leukemia	Aspergillus spp	Sinus, nose	NR
32	Leukemia	Aspergillus spp	Sinus, nose	CR

a CR – complete response, NR – no response

in the patients, particularly at doses of L-AmpB >3 mg/kg.
At onset of therapy, seven of the nine patients had a 20%
to 80% reduction of creatinine clearance (range, 22 cc/min
to 105 cc/min). In six patients, the creatinine clearance
remained stable and in two it improved by more than 20%.
The eight patients for whom a follow-up evaluation of more
than six months is available had no evidence of chronic
renal or liver toxicity as determined by liver enzyme
measurements and BUN and serum creatinine determinations.
No clinical evidence of central nervous system or hepato-
toxicity was observed on an acute or chronic basis. Four
of the patients with hepatosplenic candidiasis whom we have
followed for more than three years have had no recurrent
fungal infection nor evidence of chronic toxicities.

Seven patients with sinonasal aspergillosis who failed
to respond to conventional AmpB were treated with L-AmpB.
Five patients had underlying hematologic malignancies, one
patient had aplastic anemia, and one patient had no underlying disease. All patients had biopsy-proven invasive
Aspergillus sinusitis and had failed conventional antifungal therapy including AmpB. Five patients had a complete
response, and two did not respond to treatment. When they
occurred, fever and chills were infrequent and mild, and
responded well to conventional management. No severe renal
or central nervous system toxicity was observed.

Mechanisms of Action

Liposome incorporation leads to an enhanced uptake of
L-AmpB in tissues rich in cells of the mononuclear phagocyte system (6,7). We observed enhanced distribution of
L-AmpB to tissues infected with C. albicans. This latter
finding could be related to the inflammatory process and
brought up the possibility that capillary leakage or
secondary phagocyte transport may play a role. Furthermore, Christiansen et al (16) observed high concentrations
of AmpB far exceeding the drug's minimum inhibitory concentrations (MIC) in patients dying of invasive tissue
candidiasis. However, AmpB extracted from the infected
tissues had MICs corresponding to AmpB against isolates
from the same tissues. These results indicated that
microenvironmental conditions affected the in vivo activity
of AmpB and that tissue concentrations did not correlate
with in vivo antifungal activity.

To test whether phagocyte transport played a role in the enhanced therapeutic activity of L–AmpB, we determined AmpB concentrations in peritoneal exudate cells (PEC) and peritoneal lavage fluid following the intraperitoneal administration of thyoglycollate (a yeast extract). Subsequently PECs were recovered by peritoneal lavage 1, 3 and 6 hours following the iv administration of AmpB or L–AmpB (Table 3). We observed that when L–AmpB was injected iv 48 hours after the thyoglycollate challenge high levels of AmpB were detected in the cell extracts and not in the peritoneal fluid in the animals studied. These results support the concept that indeed L–AmpB is transported by phagocytes to inflammatory areas.

TABLE 3
UPTAKE OF L–AMPB BY MURINE PERITONEAL EXUDATE CELLS

	Time after L–AmpB injection[a]		
	1 hr	3 hr	6 hr
AmpB[b] concentration	2.79	3.05	10.5
Range	(1.6 – 4.17)	(1.3 – 3.6)	(7.2 – 12.9)

[a]L–AmpB was injected i.v. 48 hr after i.p. thyoglycollate administration
[b]Mean ng $\pm$ range AmpB/10^6 cells

Perspective

The successful development of a drug–drug carrier complex will be dependent on the right selection of drug, drug carrier, and disease target. L–AmpB development meets these criteria. The experimental and clinical data accumulated indicate that L–AmpB is far less toxic than the conventional form of the drug. In animal models L–AmpB is far less toxic and more active than the free drug. In our clinical experience, most of the patients treated had

received AmpB and failed to respond; the rest of the
patients had either severe side effects or allergic
reactions that precluded the administration of the free
drug. In general these patients were critically ill, with
severely deteriorated overall status at the onset of therapy
with L-AmpB. The reduced toxicity of L-AmpB allowed us in
most instances to resume better nutritional support and to
continue of antileukemic chemotherapy.

The observation of secondary phagocytic transport as a
possible mechanism involved in the enhanced therapeutic
index of L-AmpB has implications beyond the area of systemic
mycoses, and creates a potential avenue for delivering
antiinfective agents to intracellular sites. The true
impact of L-AmpB in the management of systemic mycoses and
parasitic diseases will be more apparent once clinical
trials are conducted in populations other than cancer
patients and immunocompromised hosts. In another chapter,
Dr. Dan Bonner reviews further pharmaceutical development of
the formulation used in our studies.

REFERENCES

1. Edwards JE, Lehrer RI, Stiehm ER, Fischer TJ, Young LS
    (1978). Severe candidal infections. Clinical
    perspective, immune defense mechanisms, and current
    concepts of therapy. Ann Intern Med 89:91-106.
2. Hermans PE, Keys TF (1983). Antifungal agents used for
    deep-seated mycotic infections. Mayo Clin Proc
    58:223-231.
3. Horn R, Wong B, Kiehn TE, Armstrong D (1985). Fungemia
    in a cancer hospital: Changing frequency, earlier onset,
    and results of therapy. Rev Infect Dis 7:646-655.
4. Mehta K, Juliano RL, Lopez-Berestein G (1984).
    Stimulation of macrophage protease secretion via
    liposomal delivery of muramyl dipeptide derivatives to
    intracellular sites. Immunology 51:517-527.
5. Mehta K, Lopez-Berestein G, Hersh EM, Juliano RL (1982).
    Uptake of liposomes and liposome-encapsulated muramyl
    dipeptide by human peripheral blood monocytes. J
    Reticuloendothel Soc 32:155-164.
6. Kasi LP, Lopez-Berestein G, Mehta K, Rosenblum M, Glenn
    HJ, Haynie TP, Mavligit G, Hersh EM (1984). Distribution
    and pharmacology of intravenous ^{99m}Tc-labeled
    multilamellar liposomes in rats and mice. Int J Nucl Med
    Biol 11:35-37.

7. Lopez-Berestein G, Kasi L, Rosenblum MG, Haynie T, Jahns M, Glenn H, Mehta R, Mavligit GM, Hersh EM (1984). Clinical pharmacology of ^{99m}Tc-labeled liposomes in patients with cancer. Cancer Res 44:375-378.

8. Mehta RT, Mehta K, Lopez-Berestein G, Juliano RL (1985). Effect of liposomal amphotericin B on murine macrophages and lymphocytes. Infect Immun 47(2):429-433.

9. Lopez-Berestein G, Mehta R, Hopfer RL, Mills K, Kasi L, Mehta K, Fainstein V, Luna M, Hersh EM, Juliano R (1983). Treatment and prophylaxis of disseminated infection due to Candida albicans in mice with liposome-encapsulated amphotericin B. J Infect Dis 147:939-944.

10. Lopez-Berestein G, Mehta R, Hopfer R, Mehta K, Hersh EM, Juliano R (1983). Effects of sterols on the therapeutic efficacy of liposomal amphotericin B in murine candidiasis. Cancer Drug Deliv 1:37-42.

11. Lopez-Berestein G, Hopfer RL, Mehta R, Mehta K, Hersh EM, Juliano RL (1984). Liposome-encapsulated amphotericin B for treatment of disseminated candidiasis in neutropenic mice. J Infect Dis 150:278-283.

12. Lopez-Berestein G, McQueen T, Mehta K (1985). Protective effect of liposomal-amphotericin B against C. albicans infection in mice. Cancer Drug Deliv 2:183-189.

13. Berman JD, Hanson WL, Chapman WL, Alving CR, Lopez-Berestein G (1986). Antileishmanial activity of liposome-encapsulated amphotericin B in hamsters and monkeys. Antimicrob Agents Chemother 30:847-851.

14. Lopez-Berestein G, Bodey GP, Frankel LS, Mehta K (1987). Treatment of hepatosplenic candidiasis with liposomal-amphotericin B. J Clin Oncol 5(2):310-317.

15. Weber RS, Lopez-Berestein G (1987). Treatment of invasive Aspergillus sinusitis with liposomal- amphotericin B. Laryngoscope 97:937-941.

16. Christiansen KJ, Bernard EM, Gold JWM, Armstrong D (1985). Distribution and activity of amphotericin B in humans. J Infect Dis 152:1037-1043.

Liposomes in the Therapy of Infectious Diseases and Cancer, pages 329–342

A PILOT PHASE I TRIAL OF LIPOSOMAL N-ACETYL-MURAMYL-L-ALANYL-D-ISOGLUTAMINYL-L-ALANYL-PHOSPHATIDYLETHANOLAMINE [MTP-PE (CGP 19835A)] IN CANCER PATIENTS

J. Lee Murray[1], Eugenie S. Kleinerman[2], Janet R. Tatom,[1] Joan E. Cunningham,[1] Jose Lepe-Zuniga,[1] Jordan U. Gutterman[1], Kathe Andrejcio,[3] Isaiah J. Fidler,[2] and Irwin H. Krakoff[4]

Departments of Clinical Immunology and Biological Therapy[1] and Cell Biology,[2] Division of Medicine,[4] M. D. Anderson Hospital and Tumor Institute, Houston, Texas 77030; and CIBA-GEIGY Corporation,[3] Summit, New Jersey 07901

ABSTRACT   Twenty-one patients with metastatic cancer refractory to standard therapy received escalating doses of MTP-PE (.05 mg/m^2 - 4 mg/m^2) in PS:PC liposomes (lipid: MTP-PE ratio 250:1). Liposomal MTP-PE was infused over 1 h twice weekly; doses were escalated within individual patients every three weeks as tolerated for a total treatment duration of 9 weeks. X-rays to evaluate responses, routine clinical laboratory parameters, acute phase reactants (fibrinogen, C-reactive protein, β_2-microglobulin, ceruloplasmin), and immunologic tests including lymphocyte surface markers, monocyte tumoricidal activity (MTA), and serum interferon and IL-1 levels were monitored at various time points. Three patients did not complete the full 9 weeks of therapy due to rapidly progressive disease, leaving 18 evaluable for cumulative toxicity and response. Toxicity was mild ($\leq$ grade II in 19 pts) with chief side effects being chills (78% of pts), fever (69%), malaise (49%) and nausea (42%). Toxicity was neither cumulative or dose related; there were no consistent changes in liver function or renal function tests. Significant increases in WBC, absolute granulocyte count, acute phase reactants and MTA occurred. IL-1 and alpha interferon were not detected in serum. No objective tumor responses were seen. Continuing studies are in progress to determine the maximal tolerated dose and optimal biologic dose of this agent.

INTRODUCTION

Muramyl tripeptide phosphatidyl ethanolamine [N-acetyl muramyl-L-alanyl-D-isoglutaminyl-L-alanyl-phosphatidyletha-nolamine (MTP-PE)] is a synthetic muramyl dipeptide (MDP) analog which can be incorporated into multilamellar lipid vesicles (MLV), liposomes, with high efficiency. The encapsulation of MTP-PE in liposomes has been shown to enhance the activation of murine macrophages (1) and human monocytes (2) to a 100 fold greater extent than free MDP. In addition, systemic administration of liposomes containing either MDP or MTP-PE has been shown to eradicate spontaneous metastases in animal tumor models (3-6). Recent preclinical studies have demonstrated antitumor activity and immunomodu-lating properties for MTP-PE given orally (7) or by the intranasal route (8).

A stable, reproducible preparation of liposomal MTP-PE (ℓMTP-PE) has recently been produced by CIBA-GEIGY Corpora-tion for clinical use in man. In light of its enhanced stability, anti-cancer properties, and a 10-fold reduction of toxicity in animals when incorporated into liposomes (CIBA-GEIGY, unpublished), we elected to perform a phase I trial in cancer patients. The main objectives of prelimi-nary studies reported below were to determine the toxicity and the maximum tolerated dose of ℓMTP-PE and to examine the immunomodulating activity of the preparation.

METHODS

Preparation of ℓMTP-PE

Freeze dried liposomes containing MTP-PE were produced at CIBA-GEIGY Corporation by mixing MTP-PE with phospholipid in a 7:3 ratio of phosphatidylcholine to phosphotidylserine followed by lyophylization. Prior to administration, 2.5 ml of CA^{++} and Mg^{++} free phosphate buffered saline (PBS) was added to vials containing lipids in the above ratio along with 1 mg of MTP-PE (7). The lipid to MTP-PE ratio in the final preparation was constant at 250:1. After mixing, the vials were agitated for 5 minutes at high speed. The resul-ting suspension was stable and could be stored at 4° from 4 to 6 weeks without loss of biologic activity. Prior to admin-istration, the preparation was added to 50 ml of normal saline.

Patients

Patients eligible for study included adults greater than 18 years of age with histologic proof of metastatic cancer who had failed previous therapy. Patients had to have an estimated performance status of 0-2 using Zubrod's criteria (9) and an estimated life span of $\geq$ 12 weeks. All patients gave written informed consent to participate in the study in accordance with established guidelines from the Surveillance Committee at M. D. Anderson Hospital and Tumor Institute. All anti-cancer therapy had been discontinued a minimum of three weeks prior to study. To be eligible for study, patients had to have a Hgb of $\geq$ 9 mg%, a white blood cell count (WBC) of $\geq$ 4,000/mm^3, granulocyte count of $\geq$ 2000/mm^3, and platelets of $\geq$ 100,000/mm^3. Patients had to have a bilirubin $<$ 1.5 mg%, serum glutamyl pyruvate transaminase (SGPT) of $\leq$ 75 mg%, BUN of $\leq$ 30 mg% and creatinine $\leq$ 1.5 mg%. In view of the propensity for free MTP-PE to cause vasculitis in animals (CIBA-GEIGY, unpublished) patients had to have no previous history of autoimmune disease or vasculitis. Prior to study all patients had physical exam, x-rays, CT scans, and other tests performed to evaluate extent of disease.

Study Design

Liposomal MTP-PE was administered intravenously over one hour twice weekly for a total duration of nine weeks. The initial three patients entered received ℓMTP-PE at a dose of .05 mg/m^2 MTP-PE:12.5 mg/m^2 lipid. After three weeks of therapy, they were then escalated to the next dose level (0.1 mg/m^2), and subsequently to 0.25 mg/m^2 ℓMTP-PE for the final three weeks of therapy. If no major toxicity was observed, additional patients were entered at the next highest level. The dose levels administered were 0.05, 0.10, 0.25, 0.50, 1.0, 1.5, 2.0, 3.0 and 4.0 mg/m^2. Because doses were escalated within patients, the total number of treatment courses administered at each dose level varied. Patients could continue to receive ℓMTP-PE at the ending dose provided their tumors were stable or responding to treatment after nine weeks.

During study, patients had physical exam, routine chest x-rays, electrocardiogram, and blood for immunologic parameters drawn every three weeks. Complete blood counts (CBC) with differential, platelet counts and serum chemistries were monitored weekly. Serum cholesterol, triglycerides,

anti-nuclear antibodies (ANA) and rheumatoid factor assays
(RhF) were also performed weekly. At the end of nine weeks,
x-rays, CT scans, etc., were repeated to evaluate tumor
status.
     During study the following immunologic parameters were
examined: lymphocyte subpopulations, in vitro monocyte
tumoricidal activity, serum IL-1, alpha interferon levels,
and acute phase reactants including fibrinogen, ceruloplasmin, β_2-microglobulin, and C-reactive protein were
performed prior to study and at three week intervals. Skin
tests to seven recall antigens were performed prior to study
and at eight weeks.

Immunologic Tests

     Peripheral blood lymphocytes were analyzed for the
presence of the surface antigens, T_3 (Pan-T cell antigen),
T_4 (T helper cells), T_8 (T suppressor cells), T_{11} (E-rosette
forming cells), T_{10} (pre-T cells), Ia (class II, MHC), and
SIg (surface immunoglobulin-B cells) using previously published techniques (10). In brief, immunofluorescent staining
was performed by incubating 100 µl whole blood with 10 µl of
fluorescein isothiocyanate-conjugated monoclonal antibodies
against the above antigens (Ortho-Diagnostics, Raritan, NJ)
or in the case of SIg with IgG specific for Fab fragments of
human IgM and IgD (Kallstadt Laboratories, Dallas, TX) in 12
x 75 cm^2 test tubes on ice for 30 minutes. Two ml of erythrocyte lysing reagent were then added and cells were incubated for an additional 10 minutes at room temperature.
Samples were then washed x3 in PBS (Gibco, Grand Island,
NY), resuspended in PBS and analyzed for surface fluoresence
using an Ortho Spectrum III flow cytometer.
     Monocyte tumoricidal activity (MTA) against A375 mela-
noma cells was assayed using a previously published technique (2). In essence, peripheral blood mononuclear cells
were harvested by Ficoll-Hypaque gradients and 2 x 10^5 cells
were added to each well of 96 well flat-bottomed microtiter
plates. Monocytes were allowed to adhere for 1 h, washed
with media and allowed to adhere for an additional 24 hours.
[^{125}IUdr]-labeled tumor cells were then added to the
monolayers such that the ratio of monocytes to tumor cells
was 10:1. After 72 hour incubation, plates were washed to
remove non-adherent cells and adherent viable cells were
lysed with 0.1 ml 0.5 n NaOH. Radioactivity of lysate was
measured in a gamma counter. Percent cytotoxicity was
calculated as:

$$= \frac{\text{cpm of target cells added} - \text{cpm in lysate}}{\text{total cpm target cells added}} \quad \text{x100}$$

Serum interleukin-1 (IL-1) levels and IL-1 activity in monocyte supernatants was measured using a radioimmunoasssay developed by Cistron Biotechnology (Pine Brook, NJ). Serum alpha interferon levels were measured by a standard bioassay (11). Acute phase reactants were measured using standard radiometric and ELISA techniques in the Department of Laboratory Medicine at M.D. Anderson Hospital and Tumor Institute.

Skin tests to seven recall antigens along with a saline control were applied using a multitest-CMI device (Miriaux Institute, Miami, FL). Details of application and evaluation have been described elsewhere (12).

Statistical Analysis

Comparisons between baseline values and several immune tests obtained at different dose levels were analyzed using one-way analysis of variance (ANOVA) and TUKEY test. To immunize wide fluctuations noted in individual patients between baseline values and serial samples, and to assure that equal percentage changes were counted equally, data were analyzed by dividing the natural logarithm (ln) of the value obtained while receiving ℓMTP-PE by the ln of the baseline observation. The value obtained - either a positive or negative number representing the average change between pre- and post-tests - was also tested by paired t test to see whether it differed significantly from 0 (i.e., ln 1) (10).

RESULTS

Patient Characteristics

Table 1 demonstrates the characteristics of patients in the trial. Twenty-one patients were entered, 13 males and 8 females, with a median age of 50. Three patients were considered unevaluable due to early discontinuance of therapy, leaving 18 patients evaluable for toxicity and therapeutic efficacy. The majority of patients entering had metastatic adenocarcinoma of the gastrointestinal tract with a scattering of other tumor types present. Eighteen patients had received previous chemotherapy, 15 previous radiotherapy and 7 previous immunotherapy.

TABLE 1
PATIENT CHARACTERISTICS

NO. PATIENTS ENTERED		21
NO. PATIENTS INEVALUABLE		3
TOO EARLY	0	
DID NOT COMPLETE FULL COURSE	3	
TOTAL NO. EVALUABLE (i.e.,		18
Completed 9 Weeks of Treatment)		
SEX: M/F		13/8
AGE: Median		50
Range		18-71
MEDIAN P.S.		1
TUMOR HISTOLOGY:		
Colorectal		8
Melanoma		1
Renal Cell		2
Lung		1
Breast		1
Stomach		2
H & N		1
Sarcoma		3
Salivary Gland		1
Undifferentiated		1
PREVIOUS TREATMENT:		
Chemotherapy		18
Radiotherapy		13
Immunotherapy		7

Toxicity

Table 2 details the percentage of patients experiencing side effects at a range of dose levels shown. In general, ℓMTP-PE was well tolerated at all doses. All patients except two experienced side effects which were $\leq$ grade II by NCI toxicity grading criteria. The major side effects noted were chills, fever, malaise, and nausea. Mild headaches were also a fairly frequent occurrence. Although there was a trend towards a greater percentage of patients experiencing side effects at higher dose levels, there was no evidence of cumulative toxicity noted. Of interest was the observation that the majority of patients experienced side

effects with the initial dose of MTP-PE and developed a
tolerance to subsequent doses administered. Two patients
developed grade III-IV toxicity and had the dose of ₤MTP-PE
decreased one level without further sequelae (Table 2). One
patient experienced grade III fever with hypotension at a
dose of 3 mg/m^2 ₤MTP-PE; his blood pressure eventually rose
after 2-3 hours of i.v. fluids. Patient 2 experienced grade
III dyspnea which responded to antihistamines and cortico-
steroids. There were no significant changes in ANA, RhF,
cholesterol, triglycerides, or serum chemistries over time;
specifically, there were no consistent changes in hepatic or
renal function secondary to ₤MTP-PE.

TABLE 2
PERCENT PATIENTS EXPERIENCING TOXICITIES
TO MTP-PE

PARAMETER	DOSAGE GROUPS (mg/m^2)		
	0.05-0.25	0.50-1.50	2.00-4.00
Chills	72	76	87
Fever	61	60	87
Malaise	41	40	67
Nausea/Vomiting	37	48	42
Anorexia	0	8	18
Tachycardia	4	12	18
Diaphoresis	0	8	13
Diarrhea	11	4	6
Dry Skin	0	0	9
Dyspnea/Tachypnea	4	4	7*
Headache	13	25	24
Hypertension	4	21	20
Hypotension	10	16	7**
Myalgia	10	0	0

* Includes 4% as Grade 3
** Includes 4% as Grade 4

Cell Counts and Immunologic Parameters

An increase in mean absolute granulocyte count was
observed with significant (p<.05) increases over baseline
occurring at the 3 and 4 mg/m^2 doses (Figure 1). In

contrast there were no consistent changes noted in mean
absolute lymphocyte count, lymphocyte subpopulations, or
absolute monocyte count as assessed by Wright's stain and
non-specific esterase stain (data not shown).

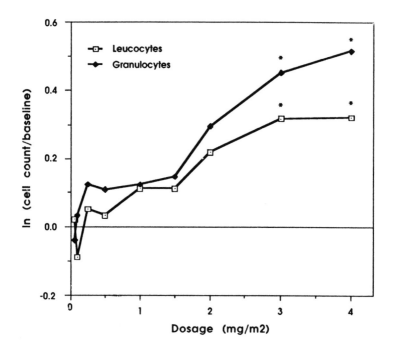

FIGURE 1.   Changes in ln mean WBC and ln mean granulocyte count from baseline (solid horizontal line) were
compared (see Methods).   There were significant (*)
increases in each parameter with respect to baseline in
patients receiving 3 and 4 mg/m^2 ℓMTP-PE (p<.05).

Along with increases in WBC and granulocyte count,
there were significant increases in acute phase reactants
noted, particularly C-reactive protein β_2-microglobulin and
ceruloplasmin (Figure 2).

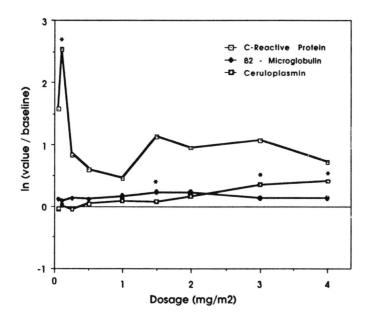

FIGURE 2. Changes in acute phase reactants data plotted as in Figure 1. Significant (*) increases in C-reactive protein, β2 microglobulin, and ceruloplasmin were noted at various dose levels.

Preliminary studies had shown that the optimal MTA for individual patients was observed at either 1 h or 24 h post ℓMTP-PE, hence, cytotoxicity was measured at 1 h, 24 h and 72 h after each dose escalation. Values plotted in Figure 3 represent the mean percent cytotoxicity for patients studied at each dose level. Because of inherent variability in MTA among patients, percentage cytotoxicity values represent the highest value obtained per individual (i.e., at either 1, 24 or 72 h). The majority of patients had increases in cytotoxicity above 15% (the upper range for normal controls). When grouped with respect to dose, higher cytotoxicity values were evident at doses above .25 mg/m^2, however, a significant fall-off in MTA occurred at the highest doses. Of interest was the observation that several patients had elevated spontaneous cytotoxicity which either decreased or remained stable following ℓMTP-PE treatment (not shown).

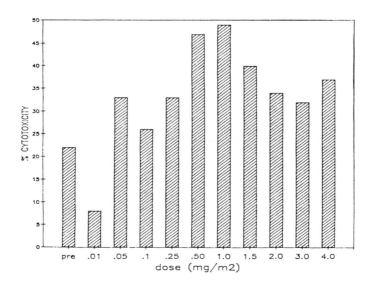

FIGURE 3.   Effect of ℓMTP-PE on in vivo MTA.   The
majority of patients studied on an individual basis had
increases in MTA over baseline.   There was no consistent
time point at which MTA was maximum for each patient
studied.

There was no measurable IL-1 or alpha interferon
detected in serum at either 1 h or 24 h post ℓMTP-PE
treatment.   Likewise, there was no measurable IL-1   in
monocyte supernatants obtained after 24 h incubation of
patient monocytes in vitro.   Interestingly, IL-1   was
detected in monocyte supernatants following stimulation
with lipopolysaccharides (range 1.4 - 29.4 ng/ml).
    Skin tests were analyzed by comparing the number of
skin tests converting from negative to positive divided by
the number of tests which were originally positive that
turned negative.   Numbers greater than one would indicate a
positive response.   There were no consistent changes
observed in skin tests when analyzed in this fashion.

Efficacy of lMTP-PE

There were no complete or partial tumor responses observed. Three patients (1 colorectal cancer, 1 lung cancer, 1 sarcoma) had long term stabilization of disease ranging from 14 to 21 weeks.

DISCUSSION

The most important findings in this preliminary study were 1) lMTP-PE administered at this dose and schedule was safe; the maximum tolerated dose has not been reached and 2) significant increases in absolute WBC, granulocyte count, acute phase reactants and in vivo monocyte tumoricidal activity were seen.

lMTP-PE was well-tolerated. The most consistent side effects noted in the majority of patients on study were fever, chills, malaise and nausea. Side effects were self-limited and occurred on the day of treatment. If the number of toxic events per treatment at each dose level was examined there was a tendency for the frequency of toxic events to increase at doses of lMTP-PE above 1 mg/m^2. In several patients studied at these higher doses, fever and chills occurred over a longer interval with malaise lasting as long as 24 hours. However, these observations were the exception rather than the rule. In the majority of patients, side effects were inconsistent, not dose related, and not cumulative. Additional patients are currently being entered at doses greater than 4 mg/m^2 in an attempt to determine the maximal tolerated dose.

A consistent increase in absolute WBC and granulocyte count was observed particularly at dose levels of 3 and 4 mg/m^2. The explanation for this finding is unknown, but might relate to the production of colony stimulating factor(s) by activated monocytes particularly G-CSF along with IL-1 (13,14). Another cytokine, IL-6 (BSF$_2$ or β_2 interferon) also produced by monocytes (15) can act as a hepatocyte stimulating factor (16). For this reason, it was interesting to note an increase in acute phase reactants with treatment.

Monocyte tumoricidal activity was enhanced over baseline in the majority of patients on an individual basis. However, the time course of maximal monocyte activity was variable from patient to patient and there did not appear to be an optimal dose of lMTP-PE at which cytotoxicity was

maximal for all patients. More studies are ongoing to
determine whether there are any correlations with monocyte
tumoricidal activity and other clinical parameters.

The clinical side effects observed, especially fever
and chills, could be secondary to the production of various
cytokines (i.e., IL-1, tumor necrosis factor α, IL-6) by
activated monocytes. Unfortunately, we were unable to
detect measurable levels of IL-1 in patient serum obtained
either 1 h or 24 h post treatment. Neither was IL-1 detected in monocyte supernatants in vitro. The reasons for this
finding are unclear; however, it is possible that IL-1 is
either cleared too rapidly from serum to be measurable or
that various inhibitory factors present in serum affect
accurate measurement. Another possibility is that IL-1
remains intracellular and is not secreted into the media.
Bakouche et al. (18) noted an increase in intracellular IL-1
in human monocytes stimulated with LPS encapsulated in
liposomes, however, there was no extracellular IL-1
detected. In contrast, preliminary experiments have shown
that patient monocytes were capable of secreting from 1 to
29 n/ml of IL-1 when incubated with LPS alone. Further
studies into the mechanisms accounting for these
interesting observations are warranted.

In summary, the results of this Phase I trial suggest
that ℓMTP-PE is safe, and may have biological activity in
vivo. Studies are continuing to determine the optimal
administration schedule, maximal tolerated dose, and optimal
biologic dose of this agent.

REFERENCES

1. Key ME, Talmadge JE, Fogler WE, Bucana C, Fidler IJ
    (1982) Activation of tumoricidal macrophages from lung
    melanoma metastases of mice treated systemically with
    liposomes containing a lipophilic derivative of muramyl
    dipeptide. J Natl Cancer Inst 69:1189-1195.
2. Kleinerman ES, Erickson KL, Schroit AJ, Fogler WE,
    Fidler IJ (1983) Activation of tumoricidal properties
    in human blood monocytes by liposomes containing lipo-
    philic muramyl tripeptide. Cancer Res 43:2010-2014.
3. Fidler IJ, Sone S, Fogler WE, Barnes ZL (1981)
    Eradication of spontaneous metastases and activation of
    alveolar macrophages by intravenous injections of
    liposomes containing muramyl dipeptide. Proc Natl Acad
    Sci USA 78:1680.

4. Lopez-Berestein G, Milas L, Hunter N, Mehta K, Eppstein D, Vander Pas MA, Mathews TR, Hersh EM (1986) Prophylaxis and treatment of experimental lung metastases in mice after treatment with liposome encapsulated 6-0-steroyl-N-acetyl-muramyl-L-ammohtyryl-D-isoglutamine. Clin Exp Metastasis 2:336.

5. Phillips NC, Mora ML, Cheslid L, Lefranirer P, Bernard JM (1985) Activation of tumoricidal activity and eradication of experimental metastases by freeze-dried liposomes containing a new lipophilic muramyl dipeptide derivative. Cancer Res 45:128.

6. Talmadge JE, Lenz BF, Klalansky R, Simon R, Riggs C, Guo S, Olkham RK, Fidler IJ (1986) Therapy of autochthonous skin cancers in mice with intravenously injected liposome containing muramyl tripeptide. Cancer Res 46:1160.

7. Fidler IJ, Fogler WE, Brownbill AF, Shumann G (1987) Systemic activation of tumoricidal properties in mouse macrophages and inhibition of melanoma metastases by the oral administration of MTP-PE, a lipophilic muramyl dipeptide. J Immunol 138:4509-4514.

8. Brownbill AF, Braun DG, Dukor P, Shumann G (1985) Induction of tumoricidal leukocytes by the intranasal application of MTP-PE, a lipophilic muramyl peptide. Cancer Immunol Immunother 20:11.

9. Zubrod CG, Schneiderman M, Frei E, et al. (1960) Appraisal of methods for the study of chemotherapy of cancer in man: Comparative therapeutic trial of nitrogen mustard and triethylene thiophos-phoramide. J Chron Dis 11:7-33.

10. Murray JL, Reuben JM, Smith TL, Gehan EA, Koretz SM, Hersh EM (1987) A pilot clinical trial of the toxicity and immunorestorative effects of T cell reconstituting factor (SR270258) in cancer patients. J Biol Resp Modif 6:56-58.

11. Rubinstein S, Familletti PC, Pestka S (1981) Convenient assay for interferons. J Virol 37:755-758.

12. Reuben JM, Hersh EM (1984) Delayed hypersensitivity responses of cancer patients to recall antigens using a new "multitest" applicator. Ann Allergy 53:390-394.

13. Shah RG, Caporale LH, Moore MAS (2977) Characterization of colony-stimulating activity produced by human monocytes and phytohemagglutamin-stimulated lymphocytes. Blood 50:811, 1977.

14. Moore MAS, Warren DJ (1987) Interleukin-1 and G-GSF
     synergism: In vivo stimulation of stem cell recovery
     and hemalopoietic regeneration following 5-fluorouracil
     treatment of mice. Proc Natl Acad Sci USA 84:7134.
15. Vaquero C, Sanceari J, Weissenbach J, Beranger F,
     Falcoff R (1986) Regulation of human gamma-interferon
     and beta-interferon gene expression in PHA-activated
     lymphocytes. J Interferon Res 6:161-170.
16. Gauldie J, Richards C, Hamish D, Lansdorp P, Baumann H
     (1987) Interferon beta 2/β-cell stimulatory factory
     type 2 shares identity with monocyte-derived
     hepatocyte-stimulating factor and regulates the major
     acute phase protein response in liver cells. Proc Natl
     Acad Sci USA 20:7251-7255.
17. Bakouche D, Koff WC, Brown DC, Lachman LP (1987)
     Interleukin-1 release by human monocytes treated with
     liposome-encapsulated lipopolysaccharide. J Immunol
     139:1120-1126.

Liposomes in the Therapy of Infectious Diseases and Cancer, pages 343–352
© 1989 Alan R. Liss, Inc.

WATER-INSOLUBLE DRUGS ENTRAPPED INTO SONICATED LIPOSOMES:
INTRAVENOUS ADMINISTRATION OF LARGE VOLUMES
IN CANCER PATIENTS. PHASE-I STUDIES[1]

Jean-Paul Sculier, André Coune, C. Brassinne,
C. Laduron, C. Hollaert, G. Atassi

Service de Médecine Interne et Laboratoire
d'Investigation Clinique H.J. Tagnon, Institut J. Bordet,
Centre des Tumeurs de l'Université Libre de Bruxelles,
1 rue Héger-Bordet, 1000 Brussels, Belgium

ABSTRACT During our 6-year clinical experience on the
use of liposomes made of egg phosphatidylcholine,
cholesterol and stearylamine (molar ratio 4:3:1), 2
lipophilic antimitotic agents - NSC-251635, a quinazolone derivative, and 6-aminochrysene - and 1 amphiphilic antifungal agent - amphotericin B - have been
given intravenously to cancer patients. Twenty-two
liters of liposomes containing NSC-251635 were given
to 14 patients (40 infusions). Thirty-two liters and a
half of liposomes containing 6-aminochrysene (30 to
200 mg/m^2/infusion) were given to 13 patients (47
infusions). Tolerance was excellent. One objective
response was observed. Amphotericin B entrapped in
liposomes was given to 27 cancer patients with severe
fungal infections. A total of 70.4 liters of liposomes
was given in 206 courses (1 to 20/patient; daily dose
0.4 to 4 mg/kg). Limiting toxicity was distal tubular
acidosis with hypokalemia. Tolerance was better than
with Fungizone^R and much higher serum amphotericin B
levels were obtained as well as increased antifungal
activity as suggested by the cure of 2 neutropenic
patients with candidemia resistant to Fungizone^R. Our
data indicate that the liposomes we tested might be
used safely as carriers to administer by the intravenous route water-insoluble drugs.

---

[1]This work was supported by the Fondation Lefèbvre
(Belgium)

Among the potential applications of liposomes in therapeutics, entrapment of water-insoluble drugs for intravenous (iv) administration is one of the most promising. Sonicated liposomes made of dipalmitoyl phosphatidylcholine, cholesterol and stearylamine (molar ratio 4:3:1) containing a lipophilic antimitotic agent, Nocodazole[R] (NSC-238159), were shown to interact in vitro with L1210 leukemia cells and to have enhanced therapeutic activity against L1210 murine leukemia (1,2). Another lipophilic compound, a quinazolone derivative, NSC-251635, could be entrapped in liposomes of the same type, where phosphatidylcholine was the phospholipid. These liposomes were active in CDF1 mice against L1210 leukemia, after intraperitoneal (ip) or iv injections, while suspensions of NSC-251635 were not (3). These experimental data prompted us in 1981 to start a phase I study with liposome-entrapped NSC-251635 in patients with advanced cancer. Because of the good tolerance of the preparation, another lipophilic cytostatic agent, 6-aminochrysene (6AC), and an amphiphilic polyene antibiotic, amphotericin B (AmB), entrapped in liposomes of the same type and composition, were investigated in cancer patients (4). We will give here an overview of our 6-year clinical experience in the intravenous administration of water-insoluble drugs entrapped in sonicated liposomes.

LIPOSOMES PREPARATION AND CHARACTERISTICS

Sterile and pyrogen-free liposomes were freshly prepared as previously described (3). Briefly, egg phosphatidylcholine, cholesterol and stearylamine at molar ratio of 4:3:1 were dissolved in chloroform: methanol at 2:1 (vol: vol). After mixing 2.25 mM of NSC-251635 or 2.05 mM of 6AC dissolved in methanol, the lipids were dried by evaporation under vacuum. One ml of 50 mM Tris saline buffer (pH 7.4) was added for each 20 (NSC-251635) or 10 (6AC) mg of dried lipids. The mixture was shaken vigorously until suspension of the lipid film was complete. The suspension was sonicated for 15 min at 140 W, under an N_2 atmosphere, using a model B-30 Branson sonifier. After centrifugation at 2,000 g for 30 min, liposomes were recovered in the supernatant.

For AmB, empty liposomes of the same lipid composition (20 mg of lipids per ml of buffer) were sonicated on the powdered drug (0.52 mM per ml of liposomal preparation) during 30 min at 140 W, under an N_2 atmosphere.

Characteristics of the liposomes infused are shown in table 1.

TABLE 1
LIPOSOMES CHARACTERISTICS

| DRUG | NSC-251635 | 6AC | AmB | |
			Study 1	Study 2
Lipid concentration (mg/ml)	20	10	20	
Mean drug concentration (mcg/ml)	641	294	297	440
Mean drug entrapment yield (%)	64	59	59	88
Predominant vesicle size (nm)	33	20	60	

Hydrodynamic diameters of the liposomes were measured by dynamic laser light scattering (Nicomp Model 370). Concentrations of the drug were measured by optical density (liposomes) or by HPLC (liposomes, serum) as a methanol extraction of the liposomes or of the serum.

PHASE I STUDIES WITH LIPOPHILIC CYTOSTATIC AGENTS

NSC-251635 and 6AC were investigated in patients with advanced cancer resistant to conventional antitumoral therapy. In the first phase I trial (5,6), a total of 40 infusions of liposomes containing NSC-251635 was given to 14 patients in 38 courses. The volume of liposomes iv administered was progressively escalated from 210 ml to 1,000 ml. The infusion rate ranged from 100 to 500 ml/hour (h), with a mean value of 400 ml/h. The maximum dose of lipids administered per infusion was 20 g. The NSC-251635 doses ranged from 82 to 456 mg/m^2 of body surface, with a mean value of 236 mg/m^2. Three patients received repeated single courses, each of a high liposomes volume (500 to 1,000 ml). The interval between the courses varied from 7 to 50 days. Whatever their volume, duration and administration frequency, infusions were well tolerated. Acute lumbar pain occurring a few minutes after the start of infusion in 3 patients whose initial infusion rate was rapid, was rapidly controlled by slowing down. Mild and transient drowsiness during the infusion was the most common side-effect and occurred in 5 patients. Fever and chills subsiding rapidly were observed in 3 patients during the initial part of the infusion; no causal pathogen was demonstrated. An urticarial rash developed in 1 patient at the start of his 6th infusion and recurred during each of the 3 following infusions. It is possible that this side-effect be related to the activation of the complement system, as shown by the strong decrease in CH'50 (total hemolytic complement activity) and the increase in C_{3d}/C_3 ratio reaching a peak value 2 to 4 h after the start of the infusion. No cardiovascular, pulmonary (fat embolism), hematologic or chronic toxicity was observed. No objective regression of tumor was demonstrated.

In the 6AC phase I trial, the dose of the drug was progressively escalated, starting at 30 mg/m^2 and increasing it by steps of 10 mg/m^2. Two patients were treated at each step. Interval between 2 courses was 2 weeks, except for one patient who received the drug twice a week for 3 weeks. Iv infusion of the liposomal preparation was performed over 2 h. A total of 47 infusions of liposomes containing 6AC was given in 13 patients. Number of infusions per patient ranged from 1 to 10 with a mean of 4. Two patients received 9 and 10 courses. A maximal dose of 200 mg/m^2 of 6AC was reached. The maximum volume of liposomes infused was 1,196 ml, corresponding to a total of 12 g of lipids. Few side-effects were observed: sedation (11 episodes in 4 patients), nausea and/or vomiting (6 episodes in 3 patients), venous irritation (2 episodes in 2 patients) and lumbar pain (1 episode). They did not appear to be dose-related. An activation of the complement system was also demonstrated by the increase in C_{3d}/C_3 ratio with a peak value 2 to 4 h after the start of the infusion. No other acute or chronic side-effects were observed. One patient with brain and adrenal metastases of a relapsing lung adenocarcinoma had an objective regression of both lesions after 4 courses of 6AC.

TABLE 2
PHASE I STUDIES WITH ANTIMITOTIC AGENTS

Drug	NSC-251635	6AC
Number of treated patients	14	13
Total number of infusions	40	47
Total volume of liposomes	22 1	32.5 1
Maximum volume of liposomes per course	1,000 ml	1,196 ml
Mean number of infusions per patient (range)	3 (1-10)	4 (1-10)
Side-effects	sedation chills, fever lumbar pain urticarial rash	sedation lumbar pain nausea, vomiting phlebitis
Objective response	0	1
Limiting factor	liposomes volume	liposomes volume

Table 2 summarizes the results of the two phase I trials. In both studies the limiting factor was not the toxicity of the liposomal preparation but the volumes of liposomes that could be prepared in the hours preceding the infusions. We avoided the use of stored liposomes to prevent side-effects that could be related to possible alterations occurring during the storage period.

In the NSC-251635 trial, biodistribution of the liposomes was also investigated. After iv infusion of ^{111}In-oxinate radiolabelled liposomes uptake was mainly observed in the liver and the spleen (7). There was no difference of distribution between drug-free and drug-containing liposomes. Three patients received ^{14}C-phosphatidylcholine labelled liposomes containing NSC-251635 with traces of ^{3}H labelled drug. Radioactivity was measured in tissue specimens of various organs obtained from these patients at post-mortem examination. Phospholipid and drug radioactivities were mainly found in liver, spleen, lung, kidney and adrenals. There was no preferential uptake by cancer tissue.

Pharmacokinetic analysis showed that maximal serum phospholipid and NSC-251635 concentrations were obtained at the end of the liposome infusion (6). The drug peak was followed by an exponential decrease phase leading to a plateau-like phase characterized by a prolonged presence of the drug in the blood up to 120 h after its administration. For the 6AC trial, a pharmacokinetic modelisation was performed. Serum drug concentration profiles were best fitted by a linear bicompartmental model. Total mean transit time varied from 8.15 to 14.76 h. Volumes of both compartments were large but the storage compartment was much more important that the central one. Metabolic clearance ranged between 14.5 and 21.4 l/h.

PHASE I STUDIES WITH AMPHOTERICIN B

AmB is a poorly water-soluble drug supplied for iv administration as a colloidal suspension with sodium deoxycholate as a dispersing agent (Fungizone^R). This preparation induces many serious side-effects such as high fever, chills, bronchospastic attacks or nephrotoxicity. We performed in cancer patients with suspected or proven invasive fungal infections 2 phase I studies with AmB entrapped in sonicated liposomes (ampholiposomes). A total of 70.4 liters was given to 27 patients in 206 courses.

In the first trial (8), AmB was given as ampholiposomes at usual doses (0.4 to 1.8 mg/kg/course). The initial dose of AmB infusions to the first patient was 0.4 mg/kg. The subsequent daily doses and the intervals between 2 infusions of ampholiposomes were decided according to the level of AmB measured in the serum of the patient. Infusion rate was 420 ml/h. Fifteen patients received a total of 117 iv infusions of ampholiposomes. The total dose of AmB administered per patient ranged from 20 to 1,004 mg (mean 472 mg), the number of infusions from 1 to 20 (mean 8) and the duration of treatment from 1 to 29 days (mean 10 days). None of the common side-effects of Fungizone^R occurred; especially, no renal function impairment was observed. The most common side-effects were slight somnolence (6 patients), nausea and vomiting (3), arthralgia (1) and lumbar pain (1). In this last case, a concomitant elevation of the serum amylase and lipase levels was measured, suggesting that the acute lumbar pain might be related to an acute pancreatitis attack.

In the second trial, an interpatient escalation of the dose of AmB entrapped into liposomes was performed, starting at a 2 mg/kg/day (d), dose that was increased by steps of 1 mg/kg. Total dose was limited to 30 mg/kg and 2 patients had to be completely treated in a same step before a new patient could be entered in the next step. Infusion rate was 400 ml/h. Eleven patients received a total of 88 infusions of ampholiposomes; 2 received a complete treatment at 2 mg/kg/d, 6 were treated at 3 mg/kg/d and 3 at 4 mg/kg/d but only 3 and 1 respectively received the full treatment. Various side-effects were observed: severe nausea and vomiting (5 patients), transient acute lumbar pain (1), mild chills and fever during the 2 or 3 first infusions (7), somnolence (3) and cardiac arrhythmias related to hypokalemia (2). Limiting but manageable toxicity related to a high cumulative dose was severe distal tubular acidosis with hypokalemia and hypomagnesemia. Notwithstanding this well-known side-effect of AmB, no case of renal failure was observed.

As phase I studies are not designed to evaluate the therapeutic response, the effectiveness of ampholiposomes was rather difficult to assess. Five patients on 11 with a lung aspergillosis were improved and 5 on 9 with a fungemia were cured. Two fungemic patients whose clinical condition was still deteriorating during Fungizone[R] therapy were cured with ampholiposomes in spite of a persisting neutropenic state (table 3). These 2 cases clearly suggest an advantage for the treatment of fungemia with ampholiposomes. This observation indicates how desirable it would be to initiate controlled clinical studies in this field.

One possible mechanism by which ampholiposomes could be more effective than Fungizone[R] may be the much higher serum levels reached by the use of lipid vesicles (8). With a daily standard treatment schedule, peak and trough serum AmB concentrations, as measured by HPLC, were always ≥10 mcg/ml and ≥5 mcg/ml respectively, while they did not exceed 2.5 mcg/ml and 1 mcg/ml with Fungizone[R] (figure 1). These high serum concentrations were significantly associated with increased serum fungistatic activities and were obtained without inducing the usual Fungizone[R] side-effects. Pharmacokinetic modeling showed that AmB distribution followed a non-linear bicompartmental model incorporating a liposome-free drug subsystem.

TABLE 3
TREATMENT OF FUNGEMIA BY HIGH DOSES OF AMPHOLIPOSOMES
IN TWO NEUTROPENIC PATIENTS

Patients number	1	2
Pathogen	Candida	Candida
	albicans	tropicalis
1st treatment: Fungizone[R] (mg/kg)	3.6	1.2
2nd treatment: ampholiposomes		
- AmB (mg/kg)	30	18
- courses (number)	10	6
- duration (days)	11	6
Granulocytes counts:		
- start of treatment	<100	<100
- end of treatment	<100	<100
AmB serum concentration:		
- highest peak (mcg/ml)	36.65	28.65
- highest trough (mcg/ml)	15.02	12.11

CONCLUSIONS

Data collected by our group during a 6-year clinical experience have shown that sonicated liposomes made of egg phosphatidylcholine, cholesterol and stearylamine (molar ratio 4:3:1) can be considered as a safe carrier for administering iv water-insoluble drugs to human beings. Two unrelated lipophilic antimitotic compounds could be given without major toxic side-effects, suggesting that lipophilic compounds should no longer be rejected from therapeutics. Amphotericin B, an amphiphilic antibiotic, entrapped in liposomes had its toxicity markedly reduced although its administration resulted in high serum concentrations. A higher clinical efficacy as compared to Fungizone[R] was suggested in some cases. This should prompt the initiation of controlled clinical studies.

It is probable that in the next years the scope of clinical applications of liposomes as a drug delivery system will be broadened.

ACKNOWLEDGEMENTS

We thank Drs Frühling, Meunier, Delcroix & Duchâteau for their respective help in isotopic, microbiological, pharmacokinetics and complement studies and also the nursing team of the intensive care unit of the Department of Medicine (Institut J. Bordet) for its excellent help in the management of the patients.

FIGURE

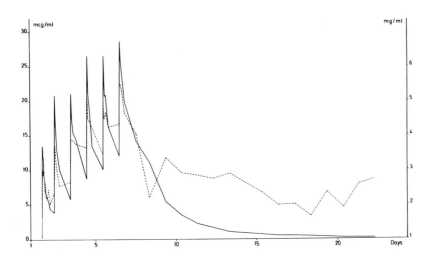

FIGURE 1. Serum profiles of AmB (——) and phospholipids (---) concentrations measured in patient 2 of table 3.

REFERENCES

1. Frühling J, Penasse W, Laurent G, Brassinne C, Hildebrand J, Vanhaelen M, Vanhaelen-Fastre R, Deleers M, Ruysschaert JM (1980). Intracellular penetration of liposomes containing a water-insoluble antimitotic drug in L1210 cells. Eur J Cancer 16:1409.

2. Laduron C, Coune A, Atassi G, Hildebrand J, Ruysschaert JM, Stryckmans P, Brassinne C (1983). Chemotherapeutic efficacy of Nocodazole^R encapsulated in liposomes on L1210 murine leukemia. Res Commun Chem Pathol Pharmacol 39:419.

3. Brassinne C, Atassi G, Frühling J, Penasse W, Coune A, Hildebrand J, Ruysschaert JM, Laduron C (1983). Antitumor activity of a water-insoluble compound entrapped in liposomes on L1210 leukemia in mice. J Ntl Cancer Inst 70:1081.

4. Sculier JP, Coune A, Brassinne C, Laduron C, Hollaert C (1987). Premiers essais d'utilisation intraveineuse du liposome ultrasoniqué en thérapeutique humaine. Médecine/Sciences 3:41.

5. Coune A, Sculier JP, Frühling J, Stryckmans P, Brassinne C, Ghanem G, Laduron C, Atassi G, Ruysschaert JM, Hildebrand J (1983). Iv administration of a water-insoluble antimitotic compound entrapped in liposomes. Preliminary report on infusion of large volumes of liposomes to man. Cancer Treat Rep 67:1031.

6. Sculier JP, Coune A, Brassinne C, Laduron C, Atassi G, Ruysschaert JM, Frühling J (1986). Intravenous infusion of high doses of liposomes containing NSC 251635, a water-insoluble cytostatic agent. A pilot study with pharmacokinetic data. J Clin Oncol 4:789.

7. Frühling J, Coune A, Ghanem G, Sculier JP, Verbist A, Brassinne C, Laduron C, Hildebrand J (1984). Distribution in man of ^{111}In-labelled liposomes containing a water-insoluble antimitotic agent. Nucl Med Comm 5:205.

8. Sculier JP, Coune A, Meunier F, Brassinne C, Laduron C, Hollaert C, Collette N, Heymans C, Klastersky J (1988). Pilot study of Amphotericin B entrapped in sonicated liposomes in cancer patients with fungal infections. Eur J Cancer Clin Oncol 34:527.

Liposomes in the Therapy of Infectious Diseases and Cancer, pages 353–365
© 1989 Alan R. Liss, Inc.

LIPOSOME ENCAPSULATED DOXORUBICIN
PRELIMINARY RESULTS OF PHASE I AND PHASE II TRIALS

Joseph Treat, M.D.
Andrew R. Greenspan, M.D.
Aquilur Rahman, Ph.D.

Division of Medical Oncology
Lombardi Cancer Research Center
3800 Reservoir Road, N.W.
Georgetown University Hospital
Washington, D.C. 20007

ABSTRACT Liposome encapsulated doxorubicin
(LED) represents an innovative approach in antineoplastic therapy. Our Phase I trial using
doxorubicin liposomes prepared from cardiolipin,
phosphatidyl choline, cholesterol and stearylamine involved 14 patients. This study defined
the maximum tolerated dose (myelosuppression
was the limiting toxicity). The Phase II trial
in recurrent breast cancer patients who have
failed one prior regimen is ongoing. To date 5
of 8 evaluable patients have responded. Two
patients have exceeded 900 mg/m^2 of doxorubicin
without any change in cardiac function. Preliminary results in the Phase II recurrent breast
cancer trials indicate LED has significant
activity in recurrent breast cancer.

INTRODUCTION

Doxorubicin (an anthracycline) is an important
antineoplastic agent with a wide range of antitumor
activity. It has significant clinical activity in lymphomas and leukemias (1,2,3) as well as solid tumors such as
breast and stomach carcinomas (4,5). However its clinical
usefulness is limited by its toxicities of which the most
notable is cardiotoxicity.

Clinically significant cardiotoxicity may develop as cumulative dosages exceed 450 mg/m^2 (6,7). Generally therapy is discontinued in the 450 to 550 mg/m^2 range to avoid cardiotoxicity.

The antitumor activity of LED has been evaluated in P388 ascitic leukemia, disseminated gross leukemia and advanced mammary carcinoma (8). All these studies demonstrated either equivalent anticancer activity compared to free drug or have demonstrated enhanced therapeutic response accompanied by higher doses of LED in the three murine tumor types evaluated.

Animal studies conducted at our laboratories also have shown that the delivery of doxorubicin with cardiolipin can significantly reduce cardiotoxicity in mice and dogs as compared to free drug (9,10).

Thus based upon preclinical data demonstrating no loss of antineoplastic effect and protection against cardiac toxicities, we embarked upon clinical trials in our patients under an FDA approved IND.

MATERIAL AND METHODS

Lipids and Drugs: Chromatographically pure cardiolipin, phosphatidyl choline, cholesterol, and stearylamine were purchased from Sigma Food and drugs (St. Louis, Mo.). Doxorubicin (Adriamycin HCL) for injection was obtained from Adria Labs (Columbus, Ohio). All other chemicals were high quality analytical grades.

Preparation of Liposomes

For the preparation of liposomes, endotoxin and pathogen free glass wares were used during the whole process and all the subsequent processes were done in a laminar flow hood. Doxorubicin was encapsulated in liposomes as described previously (8). Doxorubicin was dissolved in methanol (2 mg/ml) and was mixed thoroughly with cardiolipin solution in ethanol. For a typical batch of liposomes preparation, 280 mg of doxorubicin was complexed with 420 mg of cardiolipin and evaporated to dryness with a flash evaporator. To this dried film were then added 1050 mg of phosphatidylcholine, 350 mg of

cholesterol and 140 mg of stearylamine. These mixtures
were thoroughly mixed in the same flash until a clear
solution was obtained. This mixture of lipids and drug
was then evaporated to dryness with a flask evaporator,
under vacuum. Following this evaporation period, 140 ml
of USP saline was added to the flask and was wrapped in
an aluminum foil and kept in the dark for half-hour to
hydrate. The liposomes were then sonicated in a cup-horn
type sonicator (Heat System Model W-220F) in a fixed temperature bath at 37°C for 90 minutes. The non-entrapped
doxorubicin was separated from liposome-encapsulated drug
by extensive dialysis against USP saline at 4°C over a
period of 20 hours with at least two changes of saline
solution. The percentage of entrapment of doxorubicin in
cardiolipin was determined by fluorescence after completion of dialysis and was found to be 45-55% of the total
input dose. Thus for each milligram of doxorubicin
administered in liposomes 14 mg of lipid needs to be
administered. The doxorubicin liposomes were then transferred to a sterile plastic bag (Viaflex, Travenol) for
storage and transport to the pharmacy for patient administration.

Liposomes Testing for Endotoxin and Sterility

Liposomes thus prepared using aseptic techniques
were tested for endotoxin by limulus Amebocyte lysate
assay using Sigma Chemical Kit #210-2, 210-10. The sensitivity of the tests ranged from 0.05 ng to 1.0 ng/ml. In
addition the liposome samples did not inhibit endotoxin-
induced coagulation of the lysate at a concentration of
endotoxin of approximately 1 ug/ml. Sterility of the
liposome preparations was determined both radiometrically
(Bactec Model #460, Johnston Laboratories, Cockeysville,
Maryland) and by direct inoculation onto blood and chocolate agar plates. All cultures were incubated for one
week before being considered negative for growth. However,
the liposome batches were found completely sterile by both
methods of evaluation. Liposome size distribution was
assessed by Ortho Cytofluorograph 50 H using standard
fluorescence beads. The liposomes gave a 90% size distribution of 0.9 to 1.2 um. After all these quality controls
and testings, the liposomes were then released to be
infused in patients.

Phase I Study Summary

        Patients were eligible for LED Phase I trial if
there was a biopsy proven diagnosis of malignancy for which
either no standard therapy exist or standard therapy had
failed. Fourteen patients were entered in this trial.
Ages ranged from 39 to 72 with a median age of 56. A wide
range of tumor types were treated in this Phase I trial.
These included adenocarcinoma of unknown primary (3),
adenocarcinoma of lung (3), adenocarcinoma of pancreas (1),
breast (1), colon (1), melanoma (1), small cell (1), sarcoma (1) cystosarcoma phylloides (1) and multiple myeloma
(1). All patients had an ECOG performance status of 0 to 2.
        LED was administered in either a 30 or 45 minute
intravenous infusion every 21 days. Four dose levels were
ultimately used. Three patients were entered at each dose
level without dose escalation for an individual patient.
If toxicities were acceptable at a given level then the
dose was escalated for the next group of 3 patients.
Patient eligibility also required no prior therapy with
anthracyclines. Serum creatinine of less than 1.5 mg/dl
and normal hepatic function were required. An initial
total white blood cell count of greater than $3500/mm^3$
and a platelet count of greater than $100,000/mm^3$ were
necessary. Cardiac function was assessed by a resting
radionucleotide ventriculogram (RVG). A greater than
50% ejection fraction was required for entrance to study.
The RVG was repeated at approximately 100 mg/m^2 increments
and more frequently when total cumulative dose exceeded
500 mg/m^2. Patients were removed from study for either
disease progression or unacceptable toxicity. Potential
toxicities which were monitored included myelosuppression
(weekly complete blood and platelet count), nausea/
vomiting, alopecia, liver function abnormalities (measured by serum liver function tests) and cardiotoxicity.

                            RESULTS

        A total of 48 treatment cycles were administered.
Patients received a range of 1 to 19 cycles summarized
according to dosage level. Three patients were entered at
the 30,45,60 mg/m^2 levels. Five were entered at the 90
mg/m^2 level. The toxicity profile of each dose level is
presented below as a short summary.

$30mg/m^2$: myelosuppression (thrombocytopenia 3200 mm^3) occurred in one patient who had been heavily pretreated for multiple myeloma. No other patients exhibited any sign of myelosuppression. No nausea/vomiting, alopecia, mucositis, phlebitis were seen. No alterations in liver function tests were noted. A total of 7 cycles were administered at this dose level.

$45mg/m^2$: no myelosuppression was seen at this dose. Mild nausea/vomiting was seen in one patient. There were no mucositis, phlebitis or alopecia seen in any patient. No alteration in liver function tests were noted. One patient (adenocarcinoma of lung) received 19 cycles of therapy for a cumulative dose of 885 mg/m^2 (17 cycles at 45 mg/m^2, 2 at 60 mg/m^2). Cardiac function as measured by RVG remained unchanged compared to pre entry testing. The patient was removed from study for disease progression. A total of 23 cycles were administered at this dose level.

$60mg/m^2$: Again at this level no myelosuppression was noted. One patient developed total alopecia. Neither mucositis nor phlebitis was noted. No liver function abnormalities were noted. A total of 7 cycles were administered at this dose level.

$90mg/m^2$: Of the 5 patients entered at this dose level, 3 patients developed significant myelosuppression (total WBC less than $1000/mm^3$ in one, two less than $1500/mm^3$, two with platelets less than $100,000/mm^3$). All patients developed alopecia. No abnormalities in liver function tests, mucositis, phelebitis were seen. A total of 11 cycles were administered at this dose level.

In 48 total cycles of therapy only 4 treatment related reactions occurred during infusion. One patient experienced chills without fever or change in vital signs which lasted 30 minutes during this patient's first and second cycle. The chills subsided with benadryl. The addition of solumedrol before the third cycle prevented this reaction. In another patient the third and fourth reactions were the development of moderate lower back pain of one hour duration with the patient's first cycle and the development of severe lower back and chest pain with the second cycle. The infusion was stopped. No change in EKG was seen. The level of LDH serum enzyme performed immediately post infusion was 287 (baseline 167). Twenty-four hours later this returned to baseline.

In all instances, other patients received LED
from the same preparation without event.

Conclusions from this Phase I study are that
significant myelosuppression occurred at 90 mg/m^2 dose
level. Myelosuppression was not evident at doses of 30,
45 or 60 mg/m^2. No hepatic, renal or pulmonary toxicity
was seen. No phlebitic reactions were noted. No objective responses were seen. Only occasional mild nausea
and vomiting occurred. No mucositis was seen. In regard
to cardiac toxicity, none was seen. However, sufficient
data was not generated. Only 3 patients received more
than 240 mg/m^2. One of whom received 885 mg/m^2 showed
no change in repeated RVG testing.

Phase II Study: Preliminary Summary of LED in Treatment
of Recurrent Breast Carcinoma

Patients with recurrent measurable breast
carcinoma are eligible for the Phase II study. Patients
must have failed one standard non-anthracycline containing regimen for recurrent disease. Patients may have
received an anthracycline (doxorubicin) as adjuvant
therapy if at the time of entry into the study at least
one year has elapsed since adjuvant therapy was completed. All patients must have a pre-study RVG. A minimum
of 2 cycles is given before evaluation for response.
Patients begin therapy at 75 mg/m^2 or less (60 or 45
mg/m^2) depending upon extent of prior chemotherapy and
radiation therapy and the severity of myelosuppression
seen with these prior therapies.

Patients are discontinued from therapy if there
is disease progression.

Patients are treated every 21 days by an intravenous 45 minute infusion in an outpatient setting. Dose
reductions are scheduled for patients who develop significant myleosuppression (WBC less than 1000/mm^3 or platelet
counts less than 100,000/mm^3).

RESULTS

To date (study is ongoing) 12 patients have been
entered. Table II summarizes the clinical data currently
available.

TABLE 1

SEX/AGE	PRIMARY	PRIOR THERAPY	PERFORMANCE STATUS	LED DOSE mg/m^2	NUMBER OF CYCLES
M/52	Multiple Myeloma	Melphalan Prednisone	I	30	I
M/41	Colon	5-Fluorouracil	0	30	3
M/65	Melanoma	None	0	30	3
M/64	Adenocarcinoma Unknown Primary	None	0	45	2
F/49	Adenocarcinoma Unknown Primary	None	0	45	2
	Adenocarcinoma Lung	None	0	45 × 17 60 × 2	19
F/45	Adenocarcinoma Pancreas	Intraperitoneal 5-Fluorouracil	0	60	5
F/46	Adenocarcinoma Breast	CMF	I	60	2
F/68	Adenocarcinoma Lung	Platinum dichloro- methotrexate	0	60	5
M/55	Small Cell Large Bowel	CMV VP-16 Platinum	0	90 × I 60 × I	2
F/43	Cytosarcoma Phylloides	Radiation	0	90	2
M/73	Adenocarcinoma Unknown Primary	None	0	90	I
M/39	Hemangiosarcoma of extremity	None	0	90	3
M/71	Adenocarcinoma Lung	None	I	90 × I 60 × 2	3

TABLE II

Preliminary Results of Phase II Trials: LED for Recurrent
Measurable Breast Carcinoma

Age	Measurable Lesion	Other Lesion Sites	Prior Therapy	Dose/m^2 LED	Response By Site
72	Skin lesions pleural effusion	Bone	CMFVP (Adj)x24 cycles 5-FU for recurrence	75 (1) 45 (4)	Skin: Complete resolution
					Pleural Effusion: Resolved
					Bone: Unchanged
					Response Duration: 5 months+
56	Supraclavicular Node	Bone	CMF (50 cycles) For Recurrence, mitomycin-velban (2) for Recurrence	75 (6)	Node: Complete Resolution
					Bone: Stable Response Duration: 6 months+

(continued on facing page)

39	Pleural effusion (biopsy proven);	None	CAF(Adj) ellip- tinium for recur- rence	75 (8) 60 (1)	Pleural Effusion: complete resolu- tion Response Duration: 6 months+
39	Lung nodules	Bone	CMF (24) for recur- rence radi- ation for bone recur- rences	60 (4)	Lung:Com- pletely resolved Bone: Unchanged Response Duration: 3 months+
80	Lung nodules	Bone	LPAM-5-FU (Adj) CMF (6) for recur- rence	45 (3)	Disease progres- sion
51	Lung nodules	Bone	CMF (6) for recur- rence	75 (4)	Stable
54	Lung nodules	Bone	CAF (8) (Adj) CMF (3) recurrence	75 (6)	Lung: Stable Bone: Improved Stable: 3 months+
33	Liver nodules Skin lesions	Bone	CMF (6) (Adj) refused standard first line	60 (4)	Skin: Partial resolu- tion Liver: Stable at 3 months

Of the 12 patients who have entered study, 8 are evaluable presently. Six of the 8 patients have obtained responses. Responses seen include areas of soft tissue (lymph nodes, skin) as well as visceral areas (lung). Response duration of 5,6,6,3,3 are seen in patients 1,2,3,4,7 respectively. In all patients at this time response is continuing with patients remaining on therapy.

In 4 of 5 of the responders, the measurable lesion has completely resolved. Four of these five patients also had disease in non-measurable areas (bone). This boney metastatic disease is followed by radionucleotide bone scans. Bone scans are not amenable to strict measurements of response and are considered not measurable sites of disease. In all four patients the scans remained stable. Although the measurable lesions has completely resolved, due to the fact that the bone disease is unchanged, these patients are considered partial responders. In patient 7 the bone scan has improved. Patient 1,4,8 also had notable improvement in their performance status to correlate with their objective tumor response. Additionally responding patients 1 and 4 also had subjective elimination of bone pain correlating with their objective tumor regression.

Toxicities

Toxicities which were evaluated included alopecia, nausea and vomiting, phelebitis, and myelosuppression. Cardiac function as measured by RVG was also monitored. Table II summarizes these results.

In general LED is well tolerated. No treatment related reaction during administration of liposomes have been noted in this on-going Phase II trial. Nausea and vomiting has been occasional. Alopecia has occurred in 7 of 8 patients. Despite multiple cycles of therapy in individual patients, no sign of chemotherapy related phlebitis has occurred. Significant myelosuppression (WBC less than 1500/mm^3 or platelets less than 100,000/mm^3) has occurred in only 2 treatment cycles. Dose reductions were employed in these two patients without additional occurrence of significant myelosuppression. No alterations in liver function tests were seen secondary to therapy.

Cardiac function has been monitored by radionucleotide ventriculograms (RVG). Pre-study RVG are obtained. Additional RVG are performed when cumulative doses exceed 300 mg/m^2. At that point RVG are repeated approximately at every additional 100 mg/m^2 increment. Four patients have received over 300 mg/m^2 total dose (300,450, 450,660 respectively) of LED.

Of note the patient who received 660 mg/m^2 of LED had also received 300 mg/m^2 of free doxorubicin as prior adjuvant therapy. One of the patients who received 450 mg/m^2 of LED had also received 400 mg/m^2 of free doxorubicin as prior adjuvant therapy. Thus these two patients have received 960 and 850 mg/m^2 total of doxorubicin in either the free or liposomal form. RVG computed ejection fractions remain unchanged from pre-study evaluation.

SUMMARY

LED represents an innovative approach in cancer therapy. Our Phase I study defined a maximum tolerated dose. No new toxicities were noted. Myelsuppression was not seen at dose levels less than 90 mg/m^2.

The preliminary results of the Phase II study are very encouraging. LED has shown to have significant activity in recurrent breast cancer. Tumor regressions have been documented in soft tissue and visceral areas of disease as presented in Table 2. These responses have been seen in patients after 2 or 3 cycles of LED administration. Patients who have responded objectively to LED also have demonstrated subjective improvement in symptoms.

Toxicities have not proven unusual. Myelosuppression remains the most important toxicity. Although a randomized trial has not been performed, the results of free doxorubicin Phase II trials (11,12) demonstrate a greater degree of myelosuppression. Only 2 episodes of significant myelosuppression have occurred in 41 treatment cycles. In this light the minimal degree of myelosuppression seen in the LED study is encouraging. Only occasional mild nausea and vomiting has been present with this agent. This minimal degree of gastrointestinal toxicity is remarkable considering the dosage of LED administered. Phlebitic reactions even after repeated doses are absent. Cardiac toxicity has not been observed in these preliminary data. Two patients in the Phase II Trial have now received cumulative doses far exceeding the point at which free doxorubicin is generally discontinued. Their cardiac function remains unchanged. More patients in future Phase III studies will be acquired to make a statistically significant statement regarding the preventive effect of LED upon cardiac toxicity.

This Phase II study has demonstrated the significant efficacy of LED in recurrent breast carcinoma. Toxicities have been acceptable and in some categories have been substantially reduced. Altogether this modality of treatment provides a much better quality of life for cancer patients and a detailed evaluation of efficacy in various human neoplasm is extremely desired with liposomal encapsulated doxorubicin.

Acknowledgment: The authors acknowledge the support of LyphoMed Inc., Rosemont, Illinois and Vestar Inc., Pasadena, California for these studies. The authors thank Ms. Karen O. Bivins for typing the manuscript.

REFERENCES

1.   Bonadonna G, Monfardini S, DeLena MD, Fossati-Bellani F, Beretter G (1970) Phase I and Preliminary Phase II Evaluation of Adriamycin (NSC-123127) Cancer Res 30:2572-2582.

2.   Bonadonna G, Delenar MD, Monfardini S, Milani F (1975) Combination Chemotherapy with Adriamycin in Malignant Lymphoma. In: Adriamycin Review. European Press Medicon, Ghent, pp 200-215.

3.   Haanen C, Hillen G (1975) Combination Chemotherapy with Doxorubicin in "Bad Risk" Leukemia Patients. In: Adriamycin Review. European Press Medicon. Ghent, pp 193-199.

4.   Wang JJ, Cortes E, Sinks LF, Holland JF (1971) Therapeutic Effect and Toxicity of Adriamycin in Patients with Neoplastic Disease. Cancer 28:837-843.

5.   Middleman E, Luce J, Frei E (1971) Clinical Trials with Adriamycin. Cancer 28:844-850.

6. Rinehart JJ, Louis RP, Baleerzak SP (1974) Adria-
    mycin Cardiotoxicity in Man. Ann Intern Med 81:475-
    478.

7. Chabner BA, Myers CE (1982) Clinical Pharmacology
    of Cancer Chemotherapy. In: DeVita VT Jr, Hellman
    S, Rosenberg SA (eds) Cancer: Principles and Prac-
    tice of Oncology. J.B. Lippincott Company,
    Philadelphia, p. 182.

8. Rahman A, Fumagalli A, Barbieri B, Schein, P,
    Casazza A (1986) Antitumor and Toxicity Evaluation
    of Free Doxorubicin and Doxorubicin Entrapped in
    Cardiolipin Liposomes. Cancer Chemother Pharmacol
    16:22-27.

9. Rahman A, White G, More N, Schein P (1985) Pharma-
    cological, Toxicological and Therapeutic Evaluation
    in Mice of Doxorubicin Entrapped in Cardiolipin
    Liposomes. Cancer Research 45:796-803.

10. Herman E, Rahman A, Ferrans V, Vick J, Schein P
    (1983) Prevention of Chronic Doxorubicin Cardio-
    toxicity in Beagles by Liposomal Encapsulation.
    Cancer Research 43:5427-5432.

11. Knight E, Horton J, Cunningham T, Rhie F, Lagakos S,
    Rosenbaum C, Taylor S, Tennant J (1979) Adriamycin:
    Comparison of a 5 Week Schedule with a 3 Week
    Schedule in Treatment of Breast Cancer. Cancer
    Treat Rep 63:121.

12. Frederickson D, Joergensen S, Roesdahl K, Thomsen J,
    Mouridison A (1978) Activity of Adriamycin in Meta-
    static Breast Cancer Resistant to a Combination
    Regimen with Cyclophosphamide, Methotrexate,
    5-Fluorouracil, Vincristine and Prednisone. Canc
    Treat 62:449

Liposomes in the Therapy of Infectious Diseases and Cancer, pages 367–389
© **1989 Alan R. Liss, Inc.**

PRECLINICAL AND CLINICAL PHARMACOLOGY OF DOXORUBICIN
ENTRAPPED IN CARDIOLIPIN LIPOSOMES

Aquilur Rahman, Jae-Kyung Roh, Joseph Treat

Division of Medical Oncology, Georgetown University,
3800 Reservoir Road, N.W., Washington, D.C. 20007

INTRODUCTION

The anthracycline antibiotics play an important
role in the treatment of leukemia and solid tumors in
humans (1,2). Doxorubicin (Adriamycin) is the prototype
of this family of compounds and has demonstrated
activity against a wide range of human cancers including
lymphomas, leukemia and solid tumors (3,4,5). Doxorubicin produces acute toxicity in the form of bone-
marrow depression, alopecia, and oral ulceration (6-8).
However, effective clinical use of these compounds has
been compromised by a serious dose-related cardiotoxicity (9,10). Juliano et al (11,12,13) and
Gregoriadis et al (14,15) have demonstrated that
liposomes can serve as effective carriers of anticancer
drugs by altering the pharmacokinetics and localization
of these agents in vivo. Subsequently, the use of
liposomes as carriers of doxorubicin has been demonstrated to offer important advantages with regard to the
attenuation of the dose-dependent cardiotoxicity. This
effect has been shown in rodents (16,18) and is
apparently at least partly attributable to the reduced
uptake of doxorubicin in cardiac tissue when it is
administered entrapped in liposomes. We have further
demonstrated that chronically administered doxorubicin
entrapped in cardiolipin liposomes completely protects
from drug-induced cardiotoxicity in beagle dogs (17).
Concurrent studies of the antitumor activity of this
liposome preparation in P388 ascitic leukemia,

disseminated Gross leukemia, and advanced mammary carcinoma demonstrated either antitumor activity equivalent to that of the free drug or an increase in therapeutic response accompanied by higher allowable doses of doxorubicin (18). In addition, the immuno-toxicity of liposomal doxorubicin administered on either acute or chronic schedules was less prefound than that of free drug, despite the fact that it was preferen-tially sequestered in the spleen (19,20).

In this report, we present the pharmacology of liposomal encapsulated doxorubicin in rats as well as clinical pharmacology in humans as a follow up of our Phase I trials in cancer patients with this modality of treatment.

MATERIALS AND METHODS

Preparation of Liposomes for Animal Use

Doxorubicin was kindly supplied by the Develop-mental Therapeutic Program, Division of Cancer Treat-ment, National Cancer Institute. Phosphatidylcholine, cardiolipin, cholesterol and stearyl amine were pur-chased from Sigma Chemicals Co. (St. Louis, Mo.). The lipids were tested for purity by thin-layer chromato-graphy on silica gel with a solvent system of chloro-form/methanol/water (70/30/5) and phosphatidyl choline, cardiolipin, cholesterol and stearylamine were found to be 99,98,99 and 90% pure respectively. Doxorubicin was encapsulated into liposomes using these lipids as described elsewhere (16).

In Vivo Studies

Male Sprague-Dawley rats (300-350g) were housed under laboratory conditions for 2 wk and kept on a purina chow diet and water ad libitum. Each rat was anesthetized with Ketaset, 45 mg/kg i.m., with Metofane. When necessary supplemental anesthesia by Metofane was provided. For biliary excretion studies, a midline abdominal incision was made in rats and the bile duct was isolated and cannulated with polyethylene tubing (PE 10). The right femoral vein and artery were isolated and polyethylene (PE 10) cannulas of constant length were inserted. The cannulas were filled with 100 units of heparin in 0.9% sodium chloride. Prior to injection, bile was collected from each rat and was used as the control. All incisions were sutured and the rats were placed in a restraining cage and allowed to recover from the anesthesia. Free doxorubicin or doxorubicin entrapped in cardiolipin liposomes were administered at a dose of 6 mg/kg over 2 min via the femoral vein in volumes corresponding to 1% body weight (0.01 ml/g). The cannula was flushed with heparinized saline. Blood was collected from the femoral artery before injection (t = 0) and at 5,15,30,60,120 and 240 min after drug administration. Plasma was separated by centrifugation at 2500 rpm for 20 min and the plasma was collected and frozen at $-20^{\circ}C$ until assayed.

Bile was collected into iced preweighed tubes at specified time intervals. Four h after being given injections, rats were sacrificed by administration of a large dose of Ketaset and selected tissues were rapidly excised, rinsed in 0.9% saline, and stored at $-20^{\circ}C$. Tissue distribution studies of free doxorubicin and doxorubicin entrapped in liposomes were performed in rats following a dose of 6 mg/kg i.v. Rats were sacrificed at specific times and selected tissues were excised.

For urinary excretion studies, free doxorubicin or doxorubicin entrapped in cardiolipin liposomes, at a dose of 6 mg/kg, was administered via a lateral tail vein of 4 rats in each group. Rats were housed separately in metabolic cages. Food and water were supplied ad libitum. At 4,8,12, and 24 h postdrug injection urine was collected, centrifuged at 5000 rpm for 20 min and the clear supernatant was separated and stored $-20^{\circ}C$. Urine samples collected from rats which were administered 0.9% NaCl or blank liposomes were processed similarly. Twenty-four h postdrug administration, rats were sacrificed and selected tissues were excised rapidly and stored at $-20^{\circ}C$.

Plasma, tissues, bile, and urine were analyzed for doxorubicin equivalents by the method of Formelli et al (21) as modified in our laboratories. Plasma (0.25 ml),

bile (50 ul), and urine (0.1 ml) were diluted to 1 ml
with distilled water, followed by addition of 0.20 ml of
AgNO₃ (33% wt/vol). Tissues were homogenized in 1 ml of
water in a Polytron homogenizer followed by addition of
0.2 ml of AgNO₃. The tubes were vortexed vigorously and
3 ml n-butyl alcohol saturated with water was added.
Each tube was vortexed for 1 min and then centrifuged at
5000 rpm for 10 min. The organic layer was removed
followed by further extracting of residue with 2 ml of
n-butyl alcohol. The tubes were vortexed for 30 s and
then centrifuged for 10 min again at 5000 rpm. The
second organic layer was removed and pooled with the
first. The butanol extract was read in a spectrofluorometer at 470 nm excitation and 585 nm emission.
Control plasma, bile, urine, and tissues obtained from
rats treated with 0.9 NaCl or blank liposomes were
processed the same way and read in the fluorometer to
correct for any endogenous fluorescence. Fresh
doxorubicin samples were prepared in n-butyl alcohol
each day for calculation of the concentration of
doxorubicin in the samples.

Pharmacokinetics Analysis. Plasma values of doxorubicin equivalents administered to rats at doses of 6
mg/kg i.v. of free drug and drug entrapped in liposomes
were utilized in obtaining the pharmacokinetic parameters. Visual inspection of the plasma level profile
of doxorubicin shows that a triexponential curve
adequately describes the pattern of plasma level
decreases according to the equation

$$P_d(t) = Ae^{-\alpha t} + Be^{-\beta t} + Ce^{-\gamma t} \qquad (A)$$

where $P_d(t)$ is the plasma doxorubicin concentration at
time t after i.v. administration of the drug; A, B, and
C are constants representing intercepts on the ordinate
at time zero; and α, β, and γ are the first-order
disposition constants with $\alpha > \beta > \gamma > 0$. The values of
the parameters of the triexponential function were
determined by submitting the individual plasma level
curves of doxorubicin to the Prophet Computer Program of
Drug Modeling (22) integrated with M-Lab of NIH (23).

RESULTS

The plasma pharmacokinetics of free and liposomal-
entrapped doxorubicin in rats at a dose of 6 mg/kg is
presented in Fig. I. Following i.v. administration of
free doxorubicin, the peak plasma concentration achieved
immediately following injection was 1.7 ug/ml. This was
reduced to 0.3 ug/ml by 1 h. Free drug cleared from
plasma very rapidly, with an apparent large volume of
distribution. With cardiolipin liposomes, the peak
plasma concentration of doxorubicin acheived was 20.9
ug/ml. The plasma levels of doxorubicin decreased
gradually and by 1 h the drug concentration in plasma
was 10 ug/ml. Fig. I also shows the goodness of fit as
predicted by computer. The comparative pharmacokinetics
parameters obtained from a single i.v. bolus administration of free doxorubicin and doxorubicin entrapped in
liposomes are presented in Table I. Following free
doxorubicin administration, the initial half-life of
plasma drug decay ($t1/2\alpha$) was 5.3 min. The second half-
life in plasma was about 3.0 h and the third half-life
($t1/2\gamma$) was 17.3 h. In contrast, the drug encapsulated
in liposomes produced a $t1/2\alpha$ of 10.3 min, $t1/2\beta$ of 3.6
h, and $t1/2\gamma$ of 69.3 h. The terminal plasma half-life
of doxorubicin entrapped in liposomes was 4-fold higher
than free drug. The volume of distribution of the
central compartment with free doxorubicin was 0.58
liters, which is 8-fold higher than that acheived with
doxorubicin entrapped in liposomes. The steady state
volume of distribution with free drug was 3.87 liters
compared to 0.168 liters with liposomal drug, which is
about 23-fold less than free doxorubicin. The rate of
clearance of free doxorubicin was 0.863 liters/h
compared to 0.014 liters/h with liposomal doxorubicin.
The area under the plasma concentration curve with
liposomal doxorubicin was 81.4 ug.h.ml^{-1} compared to
1.95 ug.h.ml^{-1} observed with free doxorubicin, which is
about 40-fold less.

The tissue distribution of free and liposomal-
entrapped doxorubicin in rats is presented in Table 2.
The peak cardiac concentration with free doxorubicin was
15.1 ug/g at 30 min; with cardiolipin liposomes, the
peak cardiac concentration of drug was 8.8 ug/g, also
observed at 30 min. The cardiac concentration with
doxorubicin entrapped in liposomes was 1.5- to 2-fold

FIGURE I

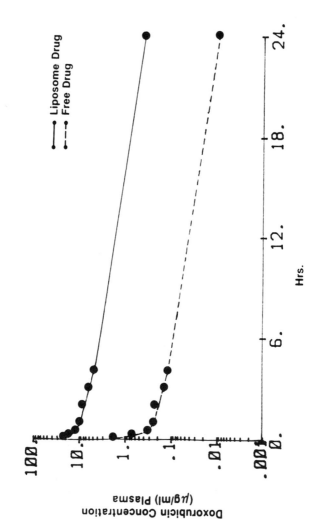

Plasma pharmacokinetic of doxorubicin in rats following a dose of 6 mg/kg i.v.,
● free doxorubicin, observed values, —— computer predicted doxorubicin
values, ● Doxorubicin entrapped in liposomes, observed values,
—— computer predicted doxorubicin values

Table I Plasma pharmacokinetics of free doxorubicin and doxorubicin entrapped in cardiolipin liposomes

	A(ug/ml)	α (h^{-1})	B(ug/ml)	β (h^{-1})	C(ug/ml)	γ (h^{-1})	t1/2 α (min)
Free doxorubicin	2.67	7.79	.296	0.229	0.083	0.040	5.3
Doxorubicin Lipo.	13.99	4.5	11.31	0.236	0.029	0.01	10.3

	t1/2 β (h)	t1/2 γ (h)	V_1 (liters)	V_2 (liters)	V_{ss} (liters)	Clearance (liters/h)	AUC (ug.h.ml^{-1})
Free doxorubicin	3.0	17.3	0.582	3.28	3.87	0.863	1.95
Doxorubicin Lipo.	3.6	69.3	0.068	0.100	0.168	0.014	81.38

Table 2 Pharmacologic disposition of free doxorubicin entrapped in cardiolipin liposomes following i.v. administration of 6 mg/kg to rats

Time	Heart FD[x]	Heart LD[xx]	Liver FD	Liver LD	Spleen FD	Spleen LD
30 min	15.1	8.8	26.4	54.3	26.4	71.9
2 h	11.5	8.7	6.5	36.1	21.8	60.7
4 h	9.8	5.8	15.2	33.9	16.4	46.0
24 h	4.7	2.3	4.1	31.8	11.5	42.5

Time	Lungs FD[x]	Lungs LD[xx]	Kidney FD	Kidney LD	S. Intestine FD	S. Intestine LD
30 min	16.31	12.9	37.2	23	12.1	8.0
2 h	14.5	10.1	20.6	21.6	11.3	7.2
4 h	12.2	11.7	18.1	18.6	7.9	3.7
24 h	5.01	6.48	5.18	5.28	5.94	3.59

[x]FD = Free Drug
[xx]LD = Liposomal Drug

less than free doxorubicin, and this relationship was maintained over 24 h. The pharmacokinetic parameters in tissues following administration of free doxorubicin and doxorubicin entrapped in liposomes are also evaluated. The terminal half-life with free drug in cardiac tissue was 17.9 h compared to 12.6 h with drug encapsulated in liposomes. The C X t values of cardiac tissue with free doxorubicin were 298.6 ug.h.g^{-1} compared to 147 ug.h.g^{-1} with liposomal drugs, an apparent 2-fold decrease. The levels of drug equivalents in liver following administration of liposomal doxorubicin were 2-fold higher than free doxorubicin. The levels of drug equivalents in spleen with doxorubicin entrapped in cardiolipin liposomes were increased 3-fold at all times of observation compared to free drug. Levels of drug in kidney and lungs in rats followed the same relationship as observed earlier (16,19). Drug equivalents in small intestine with liposomal doxorubicin showed a modest but very definite decrease in concentration compared to free drug (Table 2).

Since the anthracycline antibiotics, doxorubicin and daunorubicin are primarily excreted in the bile of rodents (24), biliary excretion studies of doxorubicin equivalents were evaluated in rats for 4 h following a dose of 6 mg/kg of free drug and drug entrapped in liposomes. The peak drug concentration in bile following administration of free doxorubicin was 166 ug/ml and occurred at 15 min; however, with liposomal doxorubicin, the peak biliary concentration of drug occurred at 30 min and was 175 ug/ml of bile. After this initial delay in biliary excretion, the levels of drug equivalents in bile were moderately higher in rats treated with liposomal doxorubicin compared to free drug. Over the 4-h period, about 17% of drug administered as free doxorubicin and 20% of drug administered as liposomal doxorubicin was recovered in rat bile (Fig. 2).

Urinary excretion of doxorubicin equivalents was monitored in rats administered comparable doses of free doxorubicin and liposomal doxorubicin. In both groups, equivalent drug levels occurred in urine. The total cumulative urinary excretion of drug was about 5% with free doxorubicin and 4% with doxorubicin entrapped in cardiolipin liposomes.

FIGURE 2

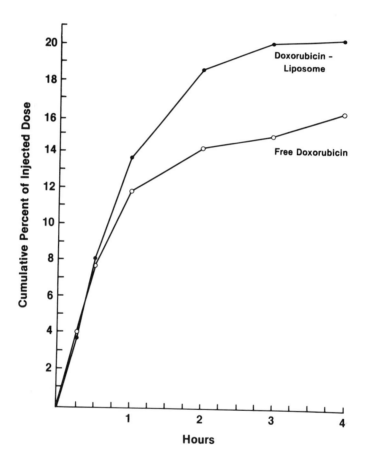

Percentage of cumulative biliary excretion of doxorubicin following administration of free drug and drug entrapped in liposomes.

CLINICAL PHARMACOLOGY STUDIES

Clinical pharmacology of liposomal encapsulated doxorubicin was evaluated in Phase I trials with cancer patients who had a biopsy-proven diagnosis of malignancy for which either no standard therapy exists or had failed standard therapy. The criteria of patients selection and dose escalation schedule is detailed in the accompanying chapter (Treat et al).

Lipids and Drugs: Chromatographically pure cardiolipin, phosphatidyl choline, cholesterol, and stearylamine were purchased from Sigma Food and Drugs (St. Louis, Mo.). Doxorubicin (Adriamycin HCL) for injection was obtained from Adria Labs (Columbus, Ohio). Doxorubicinol was kindly supplied by Farmitalia (Milan, Italy) and carminomycin was provided by Bristol Myers Co. (Wallingford, Connecticut). All other chemicals were of high quality analytical grades.

Preparation of Liposomes for Clinical Use

For the preparation of liposomes, endotoxin and pathogen free glass wares were used during the whole process and all the subsequent processes were done in a laminar flow hood. Doxorubicin was encapsulated in liposomes as described previously (16). Doxorubicin was dissolved in methanol (2 mg/ml) and was mixed thoroughly with cardiolipin solution in ethanol. For a typical batch of liposomes preparation, 280 mg of doxorubicin was complexed with 420 mg of cardiolipin and evaporated to dryness with a flash evaporator. To this dried film were then added 1050 mg of phosphatidylcholine, 350 mg of cholesterol and 140 mg of stearylamine all in chloroform solution. These mixtures were thoroughly mixed in the same flask until a clear solution was obtained. This mixture of lipids and drug was then evaporated to dryness with a flash evaporator, under vacuum. Following this evaporation period, 140 ml of USP saline was added to the flask and was wrapped in an aluminum foil and kept in the dark for half-hour to hydrate. The liposomes were then sonicated in a cuphorn type sonicator (Heat System Model W-220F) in a fixed temperature bath at 37°C for 90 minutes. The non-entrapped doxorubicin was separated from liposome-encapsulated drug by extensive dialysis against USP

saline at 4°C over a period of 20 hours with at least
two changes of saline solution. The percentage of
entrapment of doxorubicin in cardiolipin liposomes was
determined by fluorescence after completion of dialysis
and was found to be 45-55% of the total input dose.
Thus for each milligram of doxorubicin administered in
liposomes 14 mg of lipid needs to be administered. The
doxorubicin liposomes were then transferred to a sterile
plastic bag (Viaflex, Travenol) for storage and
transport to the pharmacy for patient administration.

Liposome Testing for Endotoxin and Sterility

Liposomes thus prepared using aseptic techniques
were tested for endotoxin and sterility. The samples
were tested for endotoxin by limulus Amebocyte lysate
assay using Sigma Chemical Kit #210-2, 210-10. The
sensitivity of the tests ranged from 0.05 ng to 1.0
ng/ml. In addition the liposome samples did not inhibit
endotoxin-induced coagulation of the lysate at a
concentration of endotoxin of approximately 1 ug/ml.
Sterility of the liposome preparations was determined
both radiometrically (Bactec Model #460, Johnston
Laboratories, Cockeysville, Maryland) and by direct
inoculation onto blood and chocolate agar plates. All
cultures were incubated for one week before being
considered negative for growth. However, the liposomes
batches were found completely sterile by both methods of
evaluation. Liposome size distribution was assessed by
Ortho Cytofluorograph 50 H using standard fluorescence
beads. The liposomes gave a 90% size distribution of
0.9 to 1.2 um. After all these quality controls and
testings, the liposomes were then released to be infused
in patients.

Pharmacokinetic Studies:

Pharmacokinetic studies were performed in patients
receiving liposomal encapsulated doxorubicin at a dose
of 60 mg/m^2 or 90 mg/m^2. Blood samples were drawn at
5,10,15,30 and 60 minutes and then at 2,4,8 and 24 hours
following (Liposomal entrapped doxorubicin) LED
infusion. Plasma was separated from these samples by
centrifugation immediately after being drawn and was
kept frozen until analysis. Urine samples were
collected in amber plastic bottles as voided. Urine

samples were pooled from five minutes to two hours, 2 to 4, 4 to 12 and 12 to 24 hours. Urine volumes were recorded and samples were immediately frozen.

For analysis of doxorubicin in plasma, an aliquot of 0.5 ml plasma was mixed with 6 ml of 0.4 N HCl -50% ETOH, vortexed vigorously and then centrifuged at 15,000 rpm for 15 minutes in a Sorvall Centrifuge and the supranatant collected. Control plasma was spiked with known concentration of doxorubicin and extracted similarly with 0.3 N HCl -50% ETOH. The supernatants were read in a Aminco Bowman spectrofluorometer Model J4-8960 set at 470 nm excitation and 580 nm emission. The concentration of drug in patients' plasma was calculated from the graph constructed with known concentrations of drug spiked with control plasma. Urine samples were treated similarly and drug concentration was determined as described above.

For analysis of doxorubicin metabolites in plasma of patients treated with LED, high pressure liquid chromatographic (HPLC) analysis was performed. For reverse phase HPLC, a Waters Associate Model ALC/244 liquid chromatograph fitted with a prepacked Waters C_{18}- uBondapak 30 cm x 3.9 mm ID column and U6K injector was used. Signal detection was by means of a McPherson FL-749 flow fluorescence detector, with the excitation wavelength at 475 nm and an emission wavelength at 585 nm. The optimal developing system was a programmed gradient of 0.05 M KH_2PO4 pH3.00 (solvent A) and acetonitrile: 0.05 M $KH PO_4$ (65:35) (Solvent B). A Waters Associate solvent programmer, Model 660 was set to run for 25 minutes at 1.5 ml/minute on profile #6 (linear gradient) with initial conditions set at 0% solvent B and final conditions 65% B. The programmer was put to reverse condition for five minutes to insure reequilibration for reproducible retention times. The retention times, under these conditions, for doxo-rubinol, doxorubicin and carminomycin were 16.5, 19.0, and 23 minutes respectively.

Plasma Sample Preparation for HPLC

Plasma samples (0.5 ml) were spiked with known concentration of carminomycin which was used as internal standard. Each tube was treated with 3 ml of n-butanol

saturated with water, and was agitated for one minute
and then centrifuged at 5,000 rpm for ten minutes at
4°C. The organic layer was removed followed by further
extraction of the residue with 2 ml of n-butanol, the
tubes were agitated and centrifuged again for ten
minutes at 5,000 rpm. The second organic layer was
removed and pooled with the first extract. The combined
organic layers were evaporated to dryness under vacuum
in a Haake Buchler vortex evaporator and redissolved in
400 ul of methanol. For HPLC analysis 25 to 50 ul
aliquots were injected.

Pharmacokinetic Analysis

Plasma values of doxorubicin administered to
patients at doses of 60 mg/m^2 and 90 mg/m^2 encapsulated
in liposomes were utilized in obtaining the pharmacokinetic parameters. Visual inspection of the plasma-
level profile of doxorubicin shows that a biexponential
curve adequately describes the pattern of plasma-level
decreases according to the equation.

$$Cp(t) = Ae^{-\alpha t} + Be^{-\beta t}$$

The values of the parameter of the biexponential
function were determined by subjecting the individual
plasma level curves of doxorubicin to Prophet Computer
Program of Drug Modeling (22) integrated with M-Lab of
NIH (23).

RESULTS

The time course of doxorubicin plasma levels after
i.v. infusion of LED at a dose of 60 mg/m^2 in three
patients is described in figure 3. The figure also shows
the computer fitted values of doxorubicin and the close-
ness of the two values is quite satisfactory. The
plasma concentration profile of doxorubicin appears to
be bifunctional with an initial rapid decrease and a
relatively slow terminal phase. The peak plasma level
of doxorubicin was 6.79 $\pm$ 1.04 ug/ml at 5 minutes which
is considerably higher than observed with free drug.
The plasma levels at 24 hours remained at 0.29 $\pm$ 0.15
ug/ml. These values are at least ten fold higher than
observed with free drug in previous studies (25).

FIGURE 3

PLASMA PHARMACOKINETICS OF DOXORUBICIN ENTRAPPED
IN LIPOSOMES FOLLOWING A 60mg/m2 DOSE

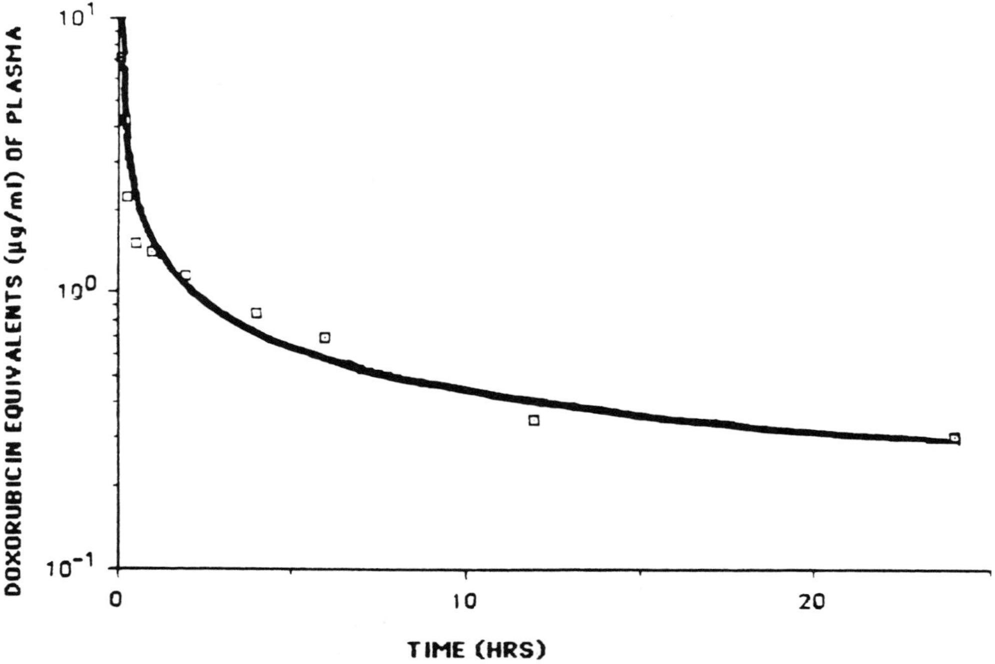

Table 3 presents the pharmacokinetic parameters of
doxorubicin in patients at doses of 60 mg/m^2 and 90
mg/m^2. The area under the plasma concentration curve
(AUC) is 26.72 and 29.47 ug.hr.ml^{-1} with 60 and 90 mg/m^2
dose respectively. These values are about 20 fold
higher than reported with free drug. The terminal half-
life is 22.0 hours whereas clearance is 3.65 and 5.84
liters/hr with doses of 60 and 90 mg/m^2. The volume of
distribution at steady state is 107.8 liters with 60
mg/m^2 dose and 176.3 liters with the dose of 90 mg/m^2.
All these parameters are significantly different when
doxorubicin is administered entrapped in liposomes
compared to free drug.

Another important feature of doxorubicin administered entrapped in liposomes is the relative lack of
metabolites in man. As evaluated by HPLC, the levels of
doxorubicinol, the predominant metabolite of doxorubicin as seen in studies with free drug, was essentially minimal after 12 hours of liposomal doxorubicin
administration. The lack of metabolism in plasma
demonstrates that liposomal encapsulation of doxorubicin
provides protection to the parent drug from metabolic
transformation.

Figure 4 represents the cumulative urinary
excretion of doxorubicin in patients following a dose of
60 mg/m^2 entrapped in liposomes. By four hours about 5%
drug is excreted which is increased to 10% by 24 hours.
These values are similar for drug excretion in urine
with either form of doxorubicin in patients.

DISCUSSION

Anthracycline antibiotics have been in clinical use
as antitumor agents for nearly 2 decades; however, their
usefulness in treating pediatric tumors, breast cancer,
leukemias, and lymphomas has been limited due to dose-
related cardiotoxicity. The anthracyclines, like most
other antineoplastic agents, fail to discriminate
efficiently between normal and target tissues: hence,
any approach enabling a chemotherapeutic agent to reach
its target in a selective and controlled fashion would
represent a major advantage in cancer chemotherapy.
Recently, liposomes have been shown to be effective as
carriers of drugs and other biologically active agents

TABLE 3

PLASMA PHARMACOKINETICS PARAMETERS OF DOXORUBICIN
ENTRAPPED IN LIPOSOMES

DOSE (MG/M^2)	AUC (UG.HR.MI^{-1})	TERMINAL HALF-LIFE (HRS)	CLEARANCE (LITERS/HR)	VDss (LITERS)
60	26.72 ± 5.2	22.0 ± 3.5	3.65 ± .21	107.83 ± 21.5
90	29.47 ± 6.1	21.6 ± 5.5	5.84 ± .41	176.34 ± 16.4

Three patients at each dose level of liposomal encapsulated doxorubicin were evaluated for pharmacokinetic
parameters. The individual plasma level were fitted
to a two-compartment open model of Prophet Drug Modeling
as described in the "Methods and Materials" section.

FIGURE 4

URINARY EXCRETION OF DOXORUBICIN ENTRAPPED IN LIPOSOMES
FOLLOWING 60 mg/m2 DOSE

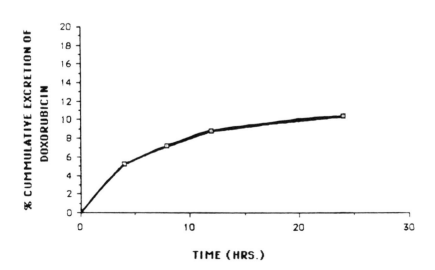

(12,14,26). The goal of using liposomes as a carrier system involves a high concentration and/or long duration of action at a target site where beneficial effects may occur while maintaining a low concentration and/or reduced duration at other sites where adverse side effects may occur. This, in essence, involves altering the pharmacokinetic and organ distribution of the drug substantially.

The present studies demonstrate that liposomal encapsulation of doxorubicin significantly alters its pharmacokinetics in plasma as compared to free drug. A markedly enhanced plasma concentration of the drug is acheived in rats when it is administered entrapped in liposomes (Fig. 1) with a terminal half-life of 69.3 h compared to 17.3 h with free doxorubicin. The area under the plasma concentration with liposomal doxorubicin is 40-fold higher than with free drug (Table 1). The enhanced drug levels in plasma with liposomal doxorubicin indicate a different rate of clearance occurring during first pass through the circulation, as well as a decrease in volume of distribution compared to free drug. The steady state volume of distribution with liposomal doxoruibcin was 23-fold less than free drug in rats following an equivalent dose of 6 mg/kg i.v. This represents a decrease in non-specific binding as well as a selective sequestration of the drug to particular tissues when administered entrapped in liposomes; however, no differences in biliary or urinary excretion were observed in rats following administration of free or liposomal doxorubicin. This may relate different localization of liposomes and the rate of release of doxorubicin from this carrier system.

The pharmacokinetic parameters of doxorubicin in tissues are greatly altered following administration in liposomes. The terminal half-life in cardiac tissue with free doxorubicin is 17.7 h compared to 12.8 h with doxorubicin entrapped in liposomes. Similarly, the C X t values of free drug in cardiac tissue are 2-fold higher than the values obtained with liposomal drug (Table 2). These results are consistent with our previous observations (16,19); furthermore, as has been shown previously by us and other workers (13,16,27), the behavior of liposomal-encapsulated drug is largely controlled in vivo by the interaction of liposomes with the reticuloendothelial system. This results in enhanced sequestration of drug in liver and spleen, with a much larger terminal half-life and higher C X t values.

As a correlation to animal studies, our Phase I studies demonstrate that liposomal encapsulation of doxorubicin significantly alters its pharmacokinetics in plasma as compared to free drug. The peak plasma concentration of drug with liposomal administration is $6.7 \pm .34$ ug/ml at 5 minutes which is about 10 fold higher than observed with free drug at this dose level. Concurrently, the AUC values with liposomal drug are 15 - 20 fold higher than observed with free drug. On the contrary, the volume of distribution is 15-20 fold decreased with liposomal doxorubicin compared to free drug (Table 3). This indicates that liposomal administration of doxorubicin effectively protected from non-specific binding of the drug and provides a selective sequestration of the drug in particular tissues. However, the urinary excretion of liposomal doxorubicin (Figure 4) with doses of 60 mg/m^2 is similar what has been observed in previous studies with free drug (24) indicating that the primary route of excretion of the drug is bile with this modality of treatment.

This Phase I study indicates that liposomal doxorubicin at doses of <90 mg/m^2 causes minimal nausea and vomiting and myelosuppression. Also the incidence of alopecia is minimal upto doses of 60 mg/m^2. The tolerance observed in man with our liposomes is extremely good with only 2/14 patients showing minor treatment-related toxicities comprising of chill and lumbar pain. Earlier clinical studies with [99mTc]-labelled liposomes by Lopez-Berestein (28) have demonstrated that liposomes are well tolerated by patients, accompanied by huge lipid doses. In a subsequent study they have established the superior therapeutic efficacy of liposomal amphotericin B for the treatment of systemic fungal infection in cancer patients suffering from leukemia and lymphoma (29). Our ongoing Phase II studies in recurrent breast cancer patients with liposomal encapsulated doxorubicin at doses of

75 mg/m^2 demonstrate that this modality of treatment is highly effective in producing complete regression of lesions and these responses are being seen in soft-tissues and visceral diseases (30). In summary, lipo-somal encapsulated doxorubicin is a novel approach in cancer chemotherapy and further clinical studies with different human neoplasms are warranted.

ACKNOWLEDGEMENT

The authors acknowledge with thanks Lympho Med Inc, Rosemont, Illinois for the support of these studies and Ms. Karen O. Bivins for typing this manuscript.

REFERENCES

1. Bonadonna G, Monfardini S, DeLena MD, Fossati-Bellani F, Beretter G (1970) Phase I and Preliminary Phase II Evaluation of Adriamycin (NSC-123127) Cancer Res 30:2572-2582.

2. Bonadonna G, Delenar MD, Monfardini S, Milani F (1975) Combination Chemotherapy with Adriamycin in Malignant Lymphoma. In: Adriamycin Review. European Press Medicon, Ghent, pp 200-215.

3. Haanen C, Hillen G (1975) Combination Chemotherapy with Doxorubicin in "Bad Risk" Leukemia Patients. In: Adriamycin Review. European Press Medicon. Ghent, pp 193-199.

4. Oldham RK, Pomeroy TC (1972) Treatment of Ewing's sarcoma with Adriamycin (NSC-123127). Cancer Chemother Rep 56:635-639.

5. Middleman E, Luce J, Frei E (1971) Clinical Trials with Adriamycin. Cancer 28:844-850.

6. Wang JJ, Cortes E, Sinks LF, Holland JF (1971) Therapeutic Effect and Toxicity of Adriamycin in Patients with Neoplastic Disease. Cancer 28:837-843.

7. Chabner BA, Myers CE (1982) Clinical Pharmacology of Cancer Chemotherapy. In: DeVita VT Jr, Hellman S, Rosenberg SA (eds) Cancer: Principles and Practice of Oncology. J.B. Lippincott Company, Philadelphia, p. 182.

8. Rinehart JJ, Louis RP, Baleerzak SP (1974) Adriamycin Cardiotoxicity in Man. Ann Intern Med 81:475-478.

9. Dana B, Jones S (1982) Doxorubicin Cardiotoxicity: Detection and Prevention Current Concepts in Use of Doxorubicin Chemotherapy ed. by S. Jones 157-163.

10. Myers CE, McGuire W, Young R (1977) Adriamycin: The Role of Lipid Peroxicdation in Cardiac Toxicity and Tumor Response. Science 165-167.

11. Juliano RL, Stamp D (1978) Pharmacokinetic of Liposome-Encapsulated antitumor drugs. Biochem Pharmacol 27:21-27.

12. Juliano RL, Stamp D, McCullough N (1978) Pharmacokinetics of Liposomes Encapsulated Anti-tumor Drug and Implications for Therapy. In: Papahadjopolous D (ed) Liposomes and Their Uses in Biology and Medicine. Ann NY Acad Sci 308:411-423.

13. Juliano RL, Lopez-Berestein G, Mehta R, Hopfer R, Mehta K, Dasi L (1983) Pharmacokinetic and Therapeutic Consequences of Liposomal Drug Delivery: Fluorodeoxyuridine and Amphotericin B as Examples. Biol Cell 47:39-46.

14. Gregoriadis G (1978) Liposomes in Therapeutic and Preventive Medicine: The Development of the Drug-Carrier Concept. Annals New York Academy Sciences 393-361.

15. Gregoriadis G, Tavill A (1974) Drug-Carrier Potential of Liposomes in Cancer Chemotherapy. The Lancet (6)29:1313-1316.

16. Rahman A, White G, More N, Schein P (1985) Pharmacological, Toxicological and Therapeutic Evaluation in Mice of Doxorubicin Entrapped in Cardiolipin Liposomes. Cancer Research 45:796-803.

17. Herman E, Rahman A, Ferrans V, Vick J, Schein P (1983) Prevention of Chronic Doxorubicin Cardiotoxicity in Beagles by Liposomal Encapsulation. Cancer Research 43:5427-5432.

18. Rahman A, Fumagalli A, Barbieri B, Schein, P, Casazza A (1986) Antitumor and Toxicity Evaluation of Free Doxorubicin and Doxorubicin Entrapped in Cardiolipin Liposomes. Cancer Chemother Pharmacol 16:22-27.

19. Rahman A, Ganje A, Neefe J (1986) Comparative Immunotoxicity of Free Doxorubicin and Doxorubicin Encapsulated in Cardiolipin Liposomes. Cancer Chemother Pharmacol 16:28-34.

20. Rahman A, Joher A, Neefe J (1986) Immunotoxicity of Multiple Dosing Regimens of Free Doxorubicin and Doxorubicin Entrapped in Cardiolipin Liposomes. Br J Cancer 54:401-408.

21. Formelli F, Pollini C, Carazza AM, DiMarco A, Mariani A (1981) Fluoroescence assays and pharmacokinetic studies of 4'deoxydoxorubicin and doxorubicin in organs of mice bearing solid tumors. Cancer Chemother Pharmacol 5:139-144.

22. Holfold NHG, Drug firm. (1982) In: Pery, HM (ed) Prophet Public Procedures Notebook. Cambridge, MA: Bolt Beranek and Newman.

23. Knot C (1979) MLAB - a mathematical modeling tool. Comput Programs Biomed 10:271-280.

24. Riggs CE, Benjamin RS, and Serpick AA (1977) Biliary disposition of Adriamycin. Clin Pharmacol Ther 22:234-241.

25. Chan KK, Chlebowski RT, Tong M, Chen H-S E, Gross JF, Bateman JR (1980) Clinical pharmacokinetics of Adriamycin in hepatoma patients with cirrhosis. Cancer Res 40:1263-1268.

26. Alving CR, Steck EA, Chapman WL, Jr, Waits VB, Hendricks LD, Swartz GM, Jr and Hanson WL (1978) Therapy of Leishmaniasis: Superior efficacies of liposomes-encapsulated drugs. Proc Natl Acad Sci, USA 75:2959-2963.

27. Alving CR (1982) Therapeutic potential of liposomes as drug carriers in leishmaniasis, malaria and vaccine, in: Targeting of Drugs, (Gregoriadis C, Senior J and Trouet A, eds). Plenum Publishing Corp. p 337.

28. Lopez-Berestein G, Kasi L, Rosenblum MG, Haymie T, Johns N, Glenn H, Mehta R, Marligit R and Hersh EM (1984) Clinical pharmacology of ^{99m}Tc-labelled liposomes in patients with cancer. Cancer Res 44:375-378.

29. Lopez-Berestein G, Fainstein V, Hopfer R, Mehta K, Sullivan MP, Keating M, Rosenblum MG, Mehta R, Luna M, Hersh EM, Reuben J, Juliano RL, Brody GP (1985) Liposomal amphotericin B for the treatment of systemic fungal infections in patients with cancer, a preliminary study. J Infect Dis 151:704-710.

30. Treat J, Frost D, Woolley P, Rahman A (1988) Liposome encapsulated doxorubicin (LED): A Phase II study in measurable recurrent breast cancer patients. Proc Am Soc Clin Oncol 7:41.

Liposomes in the Therapy of Infectious Diseases and Cancer, pages 391–402
© 1989 Alan R. Liss, Inc.

LIPOSOME-ASSOCIATED DOXORUBICIN:
PRECLINICAL PHARMACOLOGY AND EXPLORATORY CLINICAL PHASE [1,2]

A. Gabizon, A. Sulkes, T. Peretz,
S. Druckmann, D. Goren, S. Amselem, and Y. Barenholz

Departments of Oncology and Membrane Biochemistry,
Hadassah Medical Center and Hebrew University -
Hadassah Medical School, Jerusalem, Israel

ABSTRACT   An array of observations in preclinical models strongly suggests that the administration of doxorubicin (DOX) in liposome-associated form (L-DOX) offers significant potential for improving the therapeutic index in cancer therapy. We have observed in rodents marked changes in the pharmacokinetics and tissue distribution of L-DOX, and a reduction in acute and chronic toxicities. The antitumor activity appears to be influenced by the anatomic site of tumor growth, in agreement with the differences observed in tissue distribution. Optimal antitumor activity was obtained against tumors infiltrating the liver. On the basis of these preclinical findings, we have started an exploratory clinical phase of L-DOX. Preliminary results of these clinical studies indicate that L-DOX is well tolerated and that the maximal tolerated single dose (MTD) with the conventional three-weekly regimen is not less than 85 mg/msq. Various aspects related to formulation and stability may play an important role in the pharmacology of L-DOX.

---

[1]Supported by Liposome Technology, Inc., 1050 Hamilton Court, Menlo Park, California 94025

[2]Correspondence: Alberto Gabizon, Department of Oncology, Hadassah Medical Center, Jerusalem 91120, Israel

INTRODUCTION

One of the most encouraging areas of research in the field of liposome applications is the delivery of anthracyclines. Several groups of investigators have pointed at a reduction in systemic toxicity and cardiotoxicity when doxorubicin (DOX) is administered in the liposome-associated form (1-4). In various tumor models, the therapeutic activity of liposome-associated DOX (L-DOX) has been found to be equal or superior to that of free DOX (5-7). Several clinical trials have recently been started to examine whether the preclinical observations can be extended to humans (8-9). In this report, we will present a summary of the most relevant pharmacological aspects of our preclinical work, together with our preliminary observations after administration of L-DOX in humans.

RESULTS AND DISCUSSION

1. Preclinical Pharmacology.

1.1 Changes in tissue distribution and pharmacokinetics in mice. The tissue distribution of DOX in mice is profoundly altered by administration of the drug in liposome-associated form. In the experiment presented in Figure 1, the drug levels achieved with L-DOX were higher in liver and spleen, and lower in heart, kidneys, lungs and small intestine, when compared to the same dose of free DOX. When expressed as AUC (area under the curve) values for the period of 24 hours after injection, the differences are in the range of two- to three-fold (data not shown). Of note, peak tissue concentrations are obtained within the first hour after injection for both free and L-DOX, indicating that drug distribution is a relatively fast process.

The plasma clearance of L-DOX, as that of free DOX, follows a biexponential decay (Figure 2), although its pharmacokinetics parameters are markedly different from those of free drug (Table 1). During the initial phase, L-DOX is cleared with a much longer half-life than free DOX. Plasma levels at 1 minute and 15 minutes post-injection were 4-fold and 16-fold greater, respectively, when L-DOX is compared to free DOX. Terminal half-lives are similar in both cases although plasma drug levels are 2- to 3-fold higher for L-DOX. The end-result is an increased AUC, decreased clearance, and decreased volume of distribution for L-DOX as

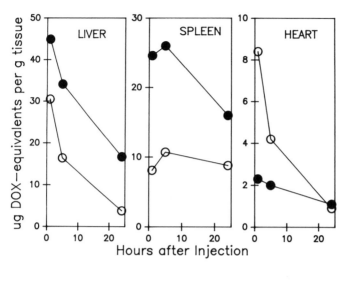

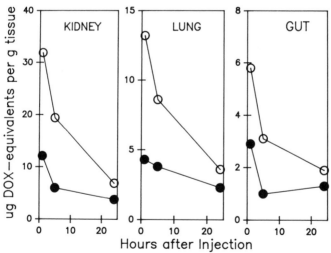

<u>Figure 1</u>: Tissue distribution of L-DOX and free DOX in mice.   Sonicated PG-PC-Chol liposomes were used in this study. BALB/c male mice received IV 10 mg/kg DOX in free or liposome-associated form. DOX was extracted from tissues and quantitated fluorometrically as described previously (17). Each time point is the average of three mice. -●-, L-DOX; -o-, free DOX.

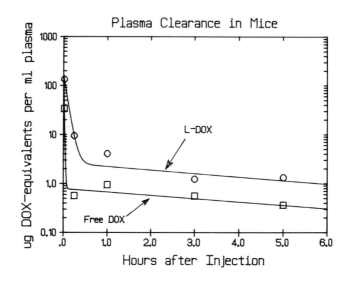

Figure 2: Plasma clearance of L-DOX and free DOX in mice. Experimental details are as in Figure 1.

TABLE 1
PHARMACOKINETIC PARAMETERS OF L-DOX AND
FREE DOX IN MICE

	Dose (mg/kg)	$t_{1/2\alpha}$ (min)	$t_{1/2\,\beta}$ (hr)	AUC (ug·hr/ml)	Clearance[2] (ml/hr)	VDss[3] (ml)	Co (ug/ml)
Free DOX	10	0.8	3.5	5.8	34.5	127.8	80.5
L-DOX	10	3.3	4.2	28.4	7.0	23.6	165.2

1. Based on total fluorescence of Dox and metabolites in BALB/c male mice. Plasma concentration data were analyzed using a polyexponential curve stripping/nonlinear least squares data fitting program (Rstrip, MicroMath Inc., Salt Lake City, UT).
2. Clearance = Dose/AUC.
3. Volume of Distribution at steady state (VDss) = Dose · area under the moment curve/$(AUC)^2$.
4. Extrapolated concentration at time 0 (Co) = $C_1 + C_2$.

compared to free DOX.   These observations suggest that liposomes restrict the distribution of drug to the extravascular compartment.

The present findings on plasma and tissue distribution of L-DOX are compatible with two simultaneous processes affecting the circulation of liposome-associated drug. One process is the leakage of drug from the liposomes, which would be followed by the extensive and fast distribution that characterizes the free drug (10). The other one is the uptake of liposome-associated drug following liposome clearance rates, which are mainly determined by liver and spleen (11). The plasma clearance curve of L-DOX during the initial phase is probably a hybrid of these two processes, although it remains unclear what is the respective contribution of each of them.

1.2 Toxicity and anti-tumor efficacy in mice.   In rodents, bone marrow is generally not a dose-limiting factor for DOX therapy. Acute toxicity is mainly related to the gastro-intestinal tract, while chronic toxicity is characterized by cachexia, nephrotoxicity, and cardiotoxicity (3). If the increased drug concentrations in liver and spleen are well tolerated, then one may expect that the reduced distribution of L-DOX to sensitive tissues such as small intestine, heart, and kidneys, will result in decreased toxicity. Indeed, as shown in Table 2, L-DOX is less toxic than free DOX by approximately twofold as assessed by the LD50 (median lethal dose). The degree of toxicity reduction is in close agreement with the two- to threefold reduction in drug exposure that was monitored in small intestine, heart, and kidneys (Figure 2). Table 2 also points at the need for long periods of follow-up (~90 days) after single injection in order to detect the chronic toxicity death wave, and establish an accurate LD50.

The therapeutic efficacy of L-DOX against the J6456 tumor is summarized in Table 3. In this tumor model, death generally results from internal bleeding. There is minimal involvement of the liver when tumor cell are injected IP or SC. In contrast, massive hepatomegaly follows IV tumor cell inoculation.   Clearly, the antitumor effect of L-DOX is influenced by the site of tumor inoculation. Thus, while the experimental conditions remain the same, more than a four-fold difference in the percent increase in median survival was observed when the tumor was inoculated IV (131.6%) instead of SC (30.4%). In contrast, only a negligible difference was seen when treatment consisted of free DOX (57.9% for IV tumor vs. 60.9% for SC tumor). When L-DOX and

TABLE 2
MOUSE LD50 OF L-DOX AND FREE DOX[1]

	SINGLE INJECTION LD50-MG/KG-(R COEFFICIENT)			
	TIME OF OBSERVATION (DAYS)			
	14	30	60	90
Free Dox	17.2 (0.99)	15.3 (0.99)	13.1 (0.96)	12.8 (0.87)
L-Dox (sonicated)[2]	25.9 (0.94)	20.9 (0.94)	20.9 (0.94)	20.3 (0.99)
L-Dox (0.2um-extruded)[2]	26.3 (0.98)	25.3 (0.99)	25.3 (0.99)	21.0 (0.99)

1. Escalated doses (10 to 35 mg/kg with increments of 5 mg/kg of free DOX and L-DOX were injected IV into groups of 5 to 6 BALB/c male mice. The medium lethal dose (LD50) was calculated by linear regression between the two closest dose levels causing 100% survival and 100% mortality.
2. Liposome composition: PG-PC-Chol (3-7-4).

TABLE 3
COMPARATIVE ANTI-TUMOR ACTIVITY OF IV-ADMINISTERED FREE DOX AND L-DOX[1]

Tumor Inoculation Route	Dominant Site of Tumor Growth	% Increase in Median Survival[2]	
		Free DOX	L-DOX
IV	Liver	57.9	131.6
IP	Ascites	88.9	50.0
SC	Limb	60.9	30.4

1. BALB/c male mice inoculated with 10^6 J6456 tumor cells and treated IV with either free DOX or L-DOX (8 mg/kg) on days 3, 10 and 17. For each inoculation route, differences between free DOX and L-DOX treatment groups were statistically significant (p < 0.05). Liposome composition: PG-PC-Chol (3-7-4).
2. Calculated as (T x 100/C) - 100, where T and C are respectively the median survival in days of treated and control-untreated animals.

free DOX are compared, the former was more effective when the tumor was inoculated IV, but less effective when the tumor was inoculated SC or IP. These results correlate well with the increased hepatosplenic uptake of L-DOX, and the concomitant reduction of the fraction of drug reaching other tissues described above. Therefore, site-specificity is an important feature of the antitumor activity of L-DOX. Tumors infiltrating the liver and spleen are the most logical targets for free DOX. In the case of bone-marrow infiltrating leukemic cells, the activity of L-DOX appears to be equivalent to that of free DOX (12). L-DOX may be less efficacious than free DOX against tumors growing in other body sites. It is possible, however, that increasing the dose of L-DOX above the MTD of free DOX will ultimately result in an equal or superior therapeutic efficacy in all instances.

2. Exploratory Clinical Phase.

      Based on the preclinical observations, a clinical study was designed to examine the tolerance to L-DOX in humans and study its pharmacokinetics.
      2.1 Formulation. During the course of our preclinical work, the relevance of several factors affecting the formulation became evident. In the course of our studies, we have prepared DOX-containing liposomes using the standard technique of thin lipid film hydration. When DOX is added to the hydration solution at pH 5 to 7, the resulting drug capture depends primarily on the molar fraction of negatively-charged lipid. Optimal results were obtained using a 3:7, PG to PC ratio. The percent of drug capture is variable but usually ranges between 70 to 90%. Cholesterol was included in the formulation based on preclinical work pointing at higher stability in plasma when cholesterol was present (12). Sonication used in the initial preclinical studies was replaced with extrusion through 0.2 um-membranes, resulting in an ultrafiltrable preparation with improved size homogeneity. To reduce iron-induced chemical changes and DOX-mediated lipid peroxidation during storage, small amounts of deferoxamine and alpha-tocopherol succinate were added to the formulation (Goren D., Gabizon A., and Barenholz Y., submitted). For preclinical testing, free DOX was removed from the L-DOX preparation by gel filtration. This procedure could not be used with the clinical material in our facility due to problems of endotoxin contamination. However, in the last part of this clinical study, we applied a method of free drug removal using a cation-exchange resin. These resins

have been shown to bind avidly free DOX, by a combination of electrostatic and hydrophobic interactions (13).

2.2 Clinical observations. Twenty-five patients with primary or secondary neoplastic liver involvement have been entered to the study. The number of patients evaluable for acute toxicity, subacute toxicity, and antitumor activity are 25, 21, and 13 respectively. The dose of L-DOX has been escalated from 20 to 85 mg/msq. The maximal cumulative dose administered has reached 340 mg/msq (4 courses of 85 mg/msq) without any decreased tolerance. Two instances of grade 3 toxicity (leukopenia and stomatitis) were noticed in a group of 5 patients receiving a total of 9 courses of 85 mg/msq. The median white blood cells nadir at this dose level was 3,200 cells per ul. The study is being continued to achieve a precise estimate of the MTD. It should be stressed that DOX-induced myelosuppression is generally more severe in patients with liver involvement (14) and, therefore, these results may not be directly extrapolated to other patient populations.

Nausea and vomiting were mild and infrequent (6/47 courses) following administration of L-DOX. Transient pyrexia was observed in 6 instances. It was usually accompanied by chills and developed several hours after injection. Partial or complete alopecia was seen in 12 out of 17 patients receiving 50 mg/msq or higher doses.

We have observed 4 minor responses among 13 valuable patients, lasting between 3 to 7 months. The responses occurred in 2 hepatoma patients, one patient with metastatic leiomyosarcoma, and one patient with metastatic carcinoma of pancreas. In the last two cases, the response was confined to the liver, with primary tumors not responding.

2.3 Pharmacokinetic study. Figure 3 shows the total plasma DOX-equivalents measured in a group of patients receiving L-DOX. Plasma clearance follows a biexponential curve with a rapid and extensive distribution phase and a relatively long terminal phase. A similar pattern has been observed following determination of intact DOX in plasma by high pressure liquid chromatography. These features are very similar to those reported for free DOX (10) although quantitative differences may exist.

Of note, the AUC obtained in patient 1 was significantly greater than in the other patients receiving the same or higher doses of L-DOX (Figure 3). Patient 1 developed severe subacute toxicity in the form of grade 4 myelosuppression with fever.

It should be noted that the results presented in Figure 3 were obtained with resin-untreated liposome preparations. Pharmacokinetic analysis of patients injected with resin-treated L-DOX is in progress.

The pharmacokinetics of liposome-encapsulated drugs are complicated by the fact that most of the conventional methods of drug determination in plasma do not discriminate between liposome-associated drug and non-liposome-associated drug. This has important implications for the following reasons.

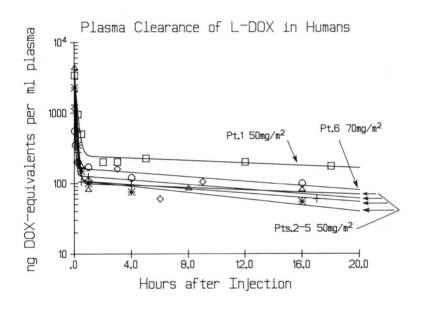

Figure 3: Plasma clearance of L-DOX in humans. DOX was extracted from plasma as described previously. Plasma data were analyzed as described in footnote 1 in Table 1.

The fraction of drug circulating in liposome-associated form is not bioavailable as such. Therefore, in the case of L-DOX, high peak levels are not necessarily correlated with toxicity as proposed for the free drug (15). In addition, the distribution of L-DOX to peripheral tissues is limited by extravasation problems (16) and, unlike protein-bound DOX, L-DOX is not in equilibrium with free DOX. Currently, we are developing a technique to separate liposome-associated drug from protein-bound and free drug in plasma using the same resin applied to remove free drug from the liposome preparation. Preliminary results indicate that some cation-exchange resins can remove free and protein-bound DOX, but not liposome-associated DOX from plasma (authors' unpublished results).

CONCLUDING REMARKS

The differences in toxicity and anti-tumor activity between L-DOX and free DOX are probably the result of changes in tissue distribution. To allow for such changes to occur, the L-DOX formulation must be reasonably stable in circulation. Namely, liposomes should be able to retain a sizable fraction of the drug until they are removed from the circulation by the RES. Obviously, the presence of free drug and of a pool of rapidly exchangeable drug in the liposomes will decrease in vivo stability. In this regard, the use of a resin-cleaning step has represented an important technological improvement to reduce the fraction of free drug and standardize a critical parameter of the formulation.

Tumors infiltrating the liver and sharing its vascularization appear to be the optimal therapeutic targets for L-DOX, since local drug concentration may be increased and systemic toxicity decreased using conventional doses. However, since cancer is usually a disease with widespread dissemination, a therapeutic strategy based on L-DOX should result in preserved systemic antitumor activity in addition to control of hepatic metastases and reduction of toxicity. To achieve this, it is likely that L-DOX will have to be administered at higher than conventional doses. Therefore, establishing whether the MTD of L-DOX is significantly higher than that of free DOX will be a critical aspect of the early clinical trials.

REFERENCES

1.   Olson F, Mayhew E, Maslow D, Rustum Y, Szoka F (1982). Characterization, Toxicity and Therapeutic Efficacy of Adriamycin Encapsulated in Liposomes. Eur J Cancer Clin Oncol 18:167.

2. Herman EH, Rahman A, Ferrans VJ, Vick JA, Schein PS (1983). Prevention of Chronic Doxorubicin Cardiotoxicity in Beagles by Liposomal Encapsulation. Cancer Res. 43:5427.

3. Gabizon A, Meshorer A, Barenholz Y (1986). Comparative Long-Term Study of the Toxicities of Free and Liposome-Associated Doxorubicin in Mice After Intravenous Administration. J Natl Cancer Inst. 77:459.

4. Van Hoesel QG, Steerenberg PA, Crommelin DJ, Van Dijk A, Van Oort W, Klein S, Douze JM, de Wildt DJ, Hillen FC (1984). Reduced Cardiotoxicity and Nephrotoxicity with Preservation of Anti-Tumor Activity of Doxorubicin Entrapped in Stable Liposomes in the Lou/M Wsl Rat. Cancer Res. 44:3698.

5. Gabizon A, Goren D, Fuks Z, Meshorer A, Barenholz Y (1985). Superior Therapeutic Activity of Liposome-Associated Adriamycin in a Murine Metastatic Tumor Model. Br. J. Cancer, 51:681.

6. Rahman A, Fumagally A, Barbieri B, Schein PS, Casazza AM (1986). Anti-Tumor and Toxicity Evaluation of Free Doxorubicin and Doxorubicin Entrapped in Cardiolipin Liposomes. Cancer Chemother Pharmacol. 16:22.

7. Mayhew EG, Goldrosen MH, Vaage J, Rustum YM (1987). Effects of Liposome-Entrapped Doxorubicin on Liver Metastases of Mouse Colon Carcinomas 26 and 38. J Natl Cancer Inst. 783:707.

8. Gabizon A, Peretz T, Ben-Yosef R, Catane R, Biran S, Barenholz Y (1986). Phase I Study with Liposome-Associated Adriamycin: Preliminary Report. Proc Am Soc Clin Oncol. 5:43 (Abstract).

9. Treat J, Roh JK, Woolley PV, Neefe J, Schein PS , Rahman A (2987). A Phase I Study: Liposome-Encapsulated Doxorubicin. Proc Am Soc Clin Oncol. 6:31 (Abstract).

10. Greene RF, Collins JM, Jenkins JF, Speyer JL, Myers CE (1983). Plasma Pharmacokinetics of Adriamycin and Adriamycinol: Implications for the Design of In Vitro Experiments and Treatment Protocols. Cancer Res. 43:3417.

11. Gabizon A, Papahadjopoulos D (in press). New Liposome Formulations with Prolonged Circulation Time in Blood and Enhanced Uptake by Tumors. Proc Natl Acad Sci USA.

12. Gabizon A, Goren D, Ramu A, Barenholz Y (1986). Design, Characterization and Anti-Tumor Activity of Adriamycin-Containing Phospholipid Vesicles. In Gregoriadis G, Senior J, Poste G (eds): "Targeting of Drugs with Synthetic Systems," New York: Plenum Press, p. 229.

13. Storm G, Van Bloois L, Brouwer M, Crommelin DJ (1985). The Interaction of Cytostatic Drugs with Adsorbents in Aqueous Media. The Potential Implications for Liposome Preparation. Biochim Biophys Acta. 818:343.
14. McKelvey EM, Gottlieb JA, Wilson HE, et al (1976). Hydroxyldaunomycin (Adriamycin) Combination Chemotherapy in Malignant Lymphoma. Cancer. 38:1484.
15. Legha SS, Benjamin RS, Mackay B, et al (1982). Reduction of Doxorubicin Cardiotoxicity by Prolonged Continuous Intravenous Infusion. Ann Intern Med. 96:133.
16. Poste G (1983). Liposome Targeting In Vivo: Problems and Opportunities. Biol Cell. 47:19.
17. Gabizon A, Dagan A, Goren D, Barenholz Y, Fuks Z (1982). Liposomes as In Vivo Carriers of Adriamycin: Reduced Cardiac Uptake and Preserved Anti-Tumor Activity in Mice. Cancer Res. 42:4734.

VI. NOVEL APPROACHES IN LIPOSOME DEVELOPMENT

Liposomes in the Therapy of Infectious Diseases and Cancer, pages 405–415
© 1989 Alan R. Liss, Inc.

STEALTH^{TM} LIPOSOMES: AVOIDING RETICULOENDOTHELIAL UPTAKE

T.M. Allen

Department of Pharmacology, University of Alberta,
Edmonton, Alberta   T6G 2H7

ABSTRACT   We have examined some of the factors
involved in the ability of liposomes to avoid uptake
by the reticuloendothelial (RE) system. We have
achieved liposomal formulations which substantially
avoid RE uptake and have called these 'stealth'
liposomes for their ability to avoid detection by the
cells of the RE system. Ganglioside GM_1, but not
other gangliosides or glycolipids, incorporated into
the liposomes allows them to circulate for prolonged
periods of time.   The effect of G_{M1} is concentration dependent, with optimum G_{M1} concentrations in
the range of 7 to 15 mol%.   Bilayer rigidity, for
example in sphingomyelin-containing liposomes, acted
synergistically with GM_1 in decreasing RE uptake. RE
uptake increased with increasing liposome size and
also with age of the mice. Removal of sialic acid
from GM_1 increased liposomal uptake into the RE
system, as did incorporation of other negatively
charged phospholipids, in particular phosphatidylserine, into liposomes.   The ability of stealth
liposomes to circulate for prolonged periods of time
significantly improves their therapeutic potential
for a variety of applications e.g. drug targeting or
slow release systems within the vasculature.

INTRODUCTION

The search for improved ways of administering drugs
to patients in order to achieve maximum efficacy with
minimal toxicity has been a major occupation of the
medical community for decades. Particulate drug delivery
systems, which result in altered drug pharmacokinetics,

are being explored as a means of achieving this end (1). The best studied of the particulate systems are the liposomal drug delivery systems which have the advantage of high drug to carrier ratios, of low inherent toxicity and immunogenicity, and of biodegradability (1,2).

Liposomes, when administered in vivo by a variety of routes, rapidly accumulate in the reticuloendothelial (RE) system, also termed the mononuclear phagocyte system. The major sites of accumulation of liposomes are liver and spleen (3). This can be an advantage if one is attempting to treat diseases involving the RE system or using therapies which require drug delivery to macrophages (2,4). However, in many therapeutic applications of liposomal drug delivery systems, rapid and extensive uptake of liposomes by the RE system is a significant disadvantage. Accumulation of liposomes in the RE system, with repeated dosings can lead to RE blockade and impairment of an important host defense system (5). In addition, rapid removal of liposomes from circulation significantly impairs our ability to target liposome-associated drugs to non-RE tissues and prevents, to a large degree, the use of liposomes as a depot system for slow release of drugs within the vasculature.

We have recently formulated liposomes which sub-stantially avoid RE uptake and therefore circulate for extended periods of time (6). These new liposomal formu-lations, termed "stealth" liposomes for their ability to substantially avoid detection and uptake by the cells of the RE system, makes possible a number of therapeutic applications which were severely limited by traditional liposomal formulations. The factors involved in the avoidance of RE uptake of liposomes are discussed in this manuscript.

EXPERIMENTAL

Egg phosphatidylcholine (PC), distearoylphosphati-dylcholine (DSPC), bovine brain sphingomyelin (SM), phosphatidic acid (PA), phosphatidylserine (PS), and phosphatidylethanolamine (PE), were purchased from Avanti Polar Lipids, Inc. (Birmingham, AL). Globosides (GLOB), asialiogangliosides ($ASGM_1$) and bovine brain sulfatides (SO_4^-) were purchased from Supelco (Bellefonte, PA). Glucocerebrosides (GLU) and cholesterol (CH) were purchased from Sigma Chemical Co., St. Louis, MO).

Gangliosides (Makor Chemicals Ltd., Jerusalem; Calbiochem, La Jolla, CA; or Supelco, Bellefonte, PA) were dissolved in chloroform: methanol, 2:1 and aliquots at the appropriate concentrations were added to mixtures of phospholipids with or without cholesterol as desired. Large unilamellar liposomes (LUV) were prepared according to Szoka and Papahadjopoulos (7), and extruded through Nucleopore filters of defined pore size (8). For liposomes containing SM, the organic solvent was chloroform:ether, 1:1. Many of the preparations were sized by laser light scattering (Nicomp Instruments). Different liposome preparations extruded through similar sized filters were very similar in size, and sizes were in agreement with published data on extruded liposome preparations (9,10).

ICR female mice (University of Alberta Breeding Unit) averaging 20-25 g in weight, 3 per group, were injected in the tail vein with 0.5 mg liposomes containing entrapped ^{125}I-tyraminylinulin (11) in 0.2 ml sterile phosphate-buffered saline. At appropriate times post-injection the mice were sacrificed and whole organs (liver, spleen lungs, heart, thymus, kidneys), carcass and 100 μl blood were excised and counted for ^{125}I in a Beckmann 8000 gamma counter. Blood volume was determined from ^{111}In-labelled red blood cells (12) to be 7.7% of body weight. Blood correction factors were determined for each organ using ^{111}In-labelled red blood cells and individual organs and carcass were corrected for ^{125}I counts present in blood.

Ganglioside incorporation was measured as sialic by the resourcinal method (13) and phospholipid was determined by the Bartlett method (14).

Results were sometimes expressed as blood/RES ratios which are determined according to the formula % injected dose in blood $\div$ % injected dose in liver plus spleen.

RESULTS

Blood correction factors for individual organs and for carcass, as determined 10 minutes post-injection of ^{111}In-labelled red blood cells, are given in Table 1. Total blood volume was determined to be 7.7% of body weight and was not significantly different between young and old mice.

TABLE 1
BLOOD CONTENT OF TISSUES IN ICR MICE

Tissue	% Total blood volume (n=9)
liver	5.9 ± 0.1
spleen	1.1 ± 0.3
lung	1.9 ± 0.3
heart	0.4 ± 0.07
kidney	2.0 ± 0.3
thyroid	0.4 ± 0.1
brain	0.1 ± 0.05
stomach	0.3 ± 0.6
carcass[a]	58.5 ± 7.6

[a] carcass is remainder of animal including remaining blood

TABLE 2
EFFECT OF GANGLIOSIDES OR GLYCOLIPIDS
ON BLOOD/RES RATIOS

Liposome Composition[a]	Blood/RES Ratio(n=3)	% remaining in vivo[c]
SM:PC:ASG$_{M1}$, 4:1:0.35	0.9 ± 0.5	77.8 ± 3.1
SM:PC:G$_{M1}$, 4:1:0.35	3.5 ± 0.4	57.0 ± 1.6
SM:PC:G$_{M2}$, 4:1:0.35	0.6 ± 0.3	54.3 ± 2.1
SM:PC:G$_{M3}$, 4:1:0.35	0.3 ± 0.2	77.9 ± 8.7
SM:PC:GD$_{1a}$, 4:1:0.35	0.6 ± 0.3	72.3 ± 5.0
SM:PC:G$_{T1b}$, 4:1:0.35	0.2 ± 0.2	80.1 ± 4.9
SM:PC:G$_{T1b}$, 4:1:0.5	0.1 ± 0.1	64.9 ± 1.6
SM:PC:G$_{T1b}$, 4:1:0.25	0.2 ± 0.2	53.1 ± 2.2
SM:PC:G$_{T1b}$, 4:1:0.15	0.03 ± 0.01	69.0 ± 2.7
SM:PC:GLOB, 4:1:0.4	0.1 ± 0.0	80.4 ± 2.4
SM:PC:GLOB, 4:1:1	0.0 ± 0.0	87.1 ± 1.4
SM:PC:GLU, 4:1:0.25 (0.1μ)[d]	1.1 ± 0.3	51.1 ± 4.6
SM:PC:GLU, 4:1:0.5 (0.1μ)[d]	1.2 ± 0.3	66.3 ± 6.8
SM:PC:GLU, 4:1:0.75 (0.1μ)[d]	2.4 ± 0.8	48.6 ± 2.9

[a] liposomes were LUV extruded through a 0.2μ filter except where indicated

[b] ratio determined in ICR mice 2 hours post-injection

[c] % of injected cpm remaining in vivo 2 hours post-injection (mean±S.D., n=3)

[d] liposomes were MLV extruded through a $0.1\ \mu$ filter

We have screened a variety of gangliosides and glycolipids for their ability to prolong circulation times of liposomes. Of the many compounds screened, only monosialylganglioside GM_1 was capable of providing significant prolongation of circulation times i.e. increased blood/RES ratios (Table 2). Removal of sialic acid from GM_1 ($ASGM_1$) abolished the effect on prolongation of circulation time.

Determination of sialic acid in the liposomes containing gangliosides after passage over Sepharose 4-B columns demonstrated that the gangliosides were 100% incorporated into the liposomes at the ganglioside concentrations examined (5-15 mol %). The ganglioside incorporation was symmetrical across the bilayer as determined from measurements of sialic acid before and after treatment of the liposomes with 0.1% TX-100.

We have compared a more rigid liposomal formulation (SM:PC,4:1) with a fluid liposomal formulation (PC:CH,2:1) as previous experiments in our laboratory have demonstrated that bilayer rigidity acts synergistically with ganglioside to decrease RE uptake of liposomes (6). Increasing GM_1 concentration led to decreased uptake into liver and spleen and increased concentrations of liposomal-entrapped contents in blood (Fig. 1). These results were more dramatic for rigid liposomes (left panel) than for fluid liposomes (right panel). At 2 hours post-injection there was no evidence of increased uptake into carcass (Fig.1) or other sampled tissues (not shown). The percentage of injected counts remaining in vivo tended to decrease with increasing ganglioside concentration, but a significant portion of liposome contents remained liposome associated even at the highest ganglioside concentration (Fig.1). The entrapped label, when released from liposomes, is rapidly eliminated from the body with a half-time of a few minutes (6,11).

Tissue distribution of ganglioside-containing liposomes for a period of 24 hours post-injection is shown in Figure 2. There is a gradual increase in the percentage of liposome contents in liver, carcass and spleen (Fig.2) but not other sampled organs (not shown). Blood values slowly decrease over 24 hours, but there are still significant levels of liposomes (0.2μ LUV) in blood 24 hours post-injection as well as a significant

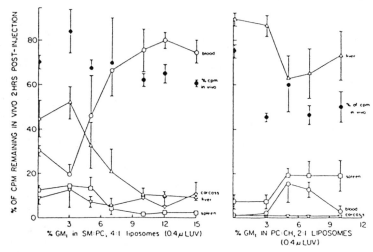

FIGURE 1. Effect of GM_1 concentration on tissue distribution of liposome-entrapped [^{125}I]-tyraminylinulin
(0.2 μ LUV), 2 hours post-injection (mean ± S.D., n = 3)

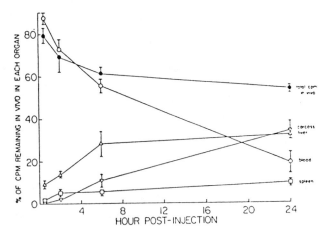

FIGURE 2. Tissues distribution for 24 hours
post-injection of liposomes composed of SM:PC:GM_1,
1:1:0.14 (0.2μ LUV) containing entrapped [^{125}I]
tyraminylinulin (mean ± S.D., n = 3).

percentage of the injected counts remaining in vivo at the same time point (Fig.2).

Because ganglioside GM_1 imparts negative charge to the surface of membranes, we explored the effect on RE uptake of surface negative charge added in the form of other membrane constituents. The results are given in Table 3. GM_1 was clearly superior to other negatively charged phospholipid headgroups. Addition of phosphatidylserine to the liposomes dramatically increased their uptake by RE cells.

TABLE 3

EFFECT OF NEGATIVE CHARGE ON BLOOD/RES RATIOS IN MICE 2 HOURS POST-INJECTION

Liposome Composition[a]	Blood/RES Ratio[b]	% remaining in vivo[b]
SM:PC,1:1	2.2 ± 1.5	67.1 ± 3.1
SM:PC:GM_1,1:1:0.35	4.4 ± 2.4	64.0 ± 8.2
SM:PC:PA, 1:1:0.5	1.2 ± 0.3	70.2 ± 2.0
SM:PC:SO_4, 1:1:0.5	1.1 ± 0.0	75.8 ± 12.6
SM:PC:PS, 1:1:0.5	0.02 ± 0.00	81.2 ± 1.7

[a] 0.2μ LUV
[b]   mean ± S.D., n = 3

The uptake of ganglioside-containing liposomes by the RE system was also a function of liposome size. As liposome sizes decreased, their uptake into liver and spleen decreased i.e. blood/RES ratios increased (Table 4). However, liposomes of 70nm average diameter showed decreased blood/RES ratios compared to larger liposomes (Table 4). Increased liver uptake of very small liposomes has been a consistent finding in our laboratory. A possible explanation may lie in the ability of the smaller liposomes to pass through liver fenestrations and gain access to hepatocytes.

We have also examined the uptake of long-circulating liposomes in mice as a function of age. There was a tendency for young mice (6-8 week females) to have higher blood/RES ratios than older mice (retired breeders of approximately 1 year), but the differences were not statistically significant (Table 5).

TABLE 4

EFFECT OF SIZE ON BLOOD/RES RATIOS IN MICE 2 HOURS
POST-INJECTION

Liposome Composition	Filter Size(μ)	Measured size (nm)	Blood/RES Ratio[a]
SM:PC:GM$_1$,1:1:0.14	0.4	180 ± 67	5.1 ± 1.3
	0.2	159 ± 45	5.2 ± 1.8
	0.1	106 ± 22	7.0 ± 0.7
	0.08	98 ± 20	8.3 ± 1.0
	0.05	70 ± 19	3.6 ± 0.4

[a]   mean ± S.D., n = 3

TABLE 5

EFFECT OF AGE ON BLOOD/RES IN MICE

Time (hrs) Post-injection[a]	Blood/RES ratio[b]	
0.5	7.7 ± 1.7	3.0 ± 2.5
2	3.8 ± 0.5	2.5 ± 0.8
6	1.7 ± 0.1	1.1 ± 0.4
24	0.44 ± 0.17	0.18 ± 0.08

[a]   SM:PC:G$_{M1}$, 1:1:0.14 (0.2μ LUV)
[b]   mean ± S.D., n = 3
[c]   female ICR mice, 6 – 8 weeks
[d]   female ICR retired breeders, 1 year

DISCUSSION

The ability of liposomes to avoid uptake by the RE
system appears to be related to a number of factors
including glycolipid type and concentration, surface
negative charge, bilayer rigidity, liposome size and age
of the animals.

Of the many glycolipids screened to date, only
GM$_1$-containing liposomes showed substantial decrease in RE
uptake.   Other glycolipids either increased RE uptake
relative to control liposomes or had little or no effect,
e.g. glucosylcerebrosides.   The sialic acid of GM$_1$ was

important in the non-recognition effect, as removal of the
sialic acid increased RE uptake substantially.   The
position of the sialic acid relative to the carbohydrates
in GM_1 and relative to the membrane surface appears also
to be important, as sialic acid is present in all of the
other gangliosides which were screened (Table 2) and yet
all of the others, when incorporated into liposomes,
resulted in increased RE uptake of the liposomes.   There
is also an important contribution of bilayer rigidity to
the phenomenon.   Fluid liposomes containing gangliosides
were removed from circulation much more rapidly than
ganglioside-containing liposomes composed of more rigid
components like sphingomyelin or distearoylphosphatidylcholine (DSPC), or containing cholesterol (6).   Rigidity
imparted by intramolecular hydrogen bonding in the
headgroup region (e.g. SM) resulted in less RE uptake than
rigidity in the tail region (e.g. DSPC).   This phenomenon
may be related to the ease of opsonization of the various
liposome compositions by plasma proteins.

Surface negative charge imparted by molecules other
than sialic acid tended to increase RE uptake.   This was
particularly pronounced in the case of PS which may be
serving as a specific recognition signal for removal of
scenescent erythrocytes and other cells from circulation
(15).

As liposome size decreases liposomes containing GM_1
circulate for longer periods of time, but even large
liposomes (0.2 - 0.4μ LUV) containing bilayer rigidifying
lipids and GM_1 in optimum concentrations are capable of
circulating for prolonged periods of time.   It has been
our experience that the size dependence of the
GM_1-containing liposomes is not as steep as for other
liposome formulations.   For example, for liposomes
composed of PC:CH:GM_1, 2:1:0.14 LUV (0.4μ) there was a
12-fold increase in blood/RES ratios as the liposomes
decreased in size from 0.4 to 0.1 μ.   By comparison for
liposomes composed of SM:PC:GM_1, 1:1:0.14 there was only a
1.4-fold increase in blood/RES ratios for similar
decreases in liposome size.   The lack of a pronounced size
dependence of the GM_1-containing liposomes suggests that
we have succeeded, to a significant degree, in disguising
them as "self", probably by mimicking important properties
of the outer monolayer of red blood cells (16).

In summary, we have succeeded in formulating
liposomes with dramatically reduced RE uptake, especially

for large liposomes. The extended circulation times achieved by these liposomes have a number of important therapeutic applications. These include their use as a slow release system within the circulation for rapidly degraded drugs like peptides, etc. Another application is in the area of drug targeting where the ability of these liposomes to circulate for several hours provides us with the opportunity to direct liposomes to specific target cells by means of surface antibodies to cell-associated antigens.

ACKNOWLEDGEMENTS

Chris Hansen provided excellent technical assistance and Karen O'Donnell provided excellent secretarial assistance. This work was supported by grants from the Medical Research Council of Canada (MA-9127) and from Liposome Technology Inc.

REFERENCES

1. Poznansky MJ, Juliano, RL (1984). Biological approaches to the controlled delivery of drugs: A critical review. Pharmacol Rev 36:277.
2. Ostro MJ (1987). Liposomes. Sc Am 256:102.
3. Gregoriadis G, Ryman BE (1972). Fate of protein-containing liposomes injected into rats. An approach to the treatment of storage diseases. Eur J Biochem 24:485.
4. Poste G (1983). Liposome targeting in vivo: Problems and opportunities. Biol Cell 47:19.
5. Allen TM, Murray L, MacKeigan S, Shah M (1984). Chronic liposome administration in mice: Effects on reticuloendothelial function and tissue distribution. J Pharmacol Exp Therap 229:267.
6. Allen TM, Chonn A (1987). Large unilamellar liposomes with low uptake into the reticuloendothelial system. FEBS Lett 223:42.
7. Szoka F, Papahadjopoulos D (1978). Procedure for the preparation of liposomes with large internal aqueous space and high capture by reverse-phase evaporation. Proc Natl Acad Sci 75:4194.

8. Olson F, Hunt CA, Szoka FC, Vail WJ, Papahadjopoulos D (1979). Preparation of liposomes of defined size distribution by extrusion through polycarbonate filters. Biochim Biophys Acta 557:9.

9. Mayer LD, Hope MJ, Cullis PR (1986). Vesicles of variable sizes produced by a rapid extrusion procedure. Biochim Biophys Acta 858:161.

10. Jousma H, Talsma H, Spies F, Joosten JGH, Junginger HE, Crommelin DJA (1987). Characterization of liposomes. The influence of extrusion of multilamellar vesicles through polycarbonate membranes on particle size, particle distribution and number of bilayers. Int J Pharmaceutics 35:263.

11. Sommerman EF, Pritchard PH, Cullis PR (1984). ^{125}I labelled inulin: a convenient marker for deposition of liposomal contents in vivo. Biochem Biophys Res Commun 122:319.

12. Scheffel V, Tsan MF, McIntyre PA (1979). Labelling of human platelets with [^{111}In] 8-hydroxyquinoline. N Nucl Med 20:524.

13. Svennerholm L (1957). Quantitative estimation of sialic acids II. A colorimetric resorcinal-hydrochloric acid method. Biochim Biophys Acta 24:604.

14. Bartlett GR (1959). Phosphorus assay in column chromatography. J Biol Chem 234:466.

15. Tanaka Y, Schroit AJ (1983). Insertion of fluorescent phosphatidylserine into the plasma membrane of red blood cells: Recognition by autologous macrophages. J Biol Chem 258:11335.

16. Op den Kamp JAF (1979). Lipid assymetry in membranes. Ann Rev Biochem 48:47.

Liposomes in the Therapy of Infectious Diseases and Cancer, pages 417–426
© 1989 Alan R. Liss, Inc.

LIPOSOMES AS CARRIER SYSTEMS FOR PROTEINS:
FACTORS AFFECTING PROTEIN ENCAPSULATION

M.E.Cruz, M.L.Corvo, J.S.Jorge and F.Lopes[1]

Departamento de Tecnologia de Industrias Químicas (LNETI)
Estrada das Palmeiras, 2745 Queluz - Portugal

ABSTRACT Proteins were incorporated into different types
of liposomes and the effect of incorporation method,pro-
tein concentration, lipid composition, ionic strength,
osmolarity, pH and molecular weight of proteins was
investigated. It was found that, within a similar class
of liposomes (multilamellar made of the same lipids) hydration and lyophilization are crucial steps to obtain
high protein concentration into liposomes with high
recoveries. Lyophilizable systems (LMLV and SDRV) were
selected as the most appropriate for protein
encapsulation. Protein concentration at the hydration
phase affects protein encapsulation until saturation is
reached. Further, for a low protein concentration at the
hydration phase, the M.W. of proteins ranging from 40 to
480 Kdalton, does not affect protein encapsulation. The
increase of ionic strength at the hydration phase
decreases protein encapsulation while increasing osmolarity up to 300 mOSM does not significantly affect encapsulation. Proteins with enzymatic activity were also
incorporated into liposomes. The specific activity of
the encapsulated forms varies from 50 % to 85 % of the
free forms, according to the incorporation conditions
used. The stability of liposomal system containing en -
zyme in the presence of human plasma was tested. The
decrease of encapsulated enzyme with time might be due
to disruption of liposomes after interaction with plasma
components.

This work was supported by Fundação Luso Americana Para
o Desenvolvimento and by Junta Nacional de Investigação
Científica e Tecnológica (Contr. nº 836.86.212).
1- Fac.Farmácia - Univ.Lisboa- Av.Forças Armadas, Lisboa

INTRODUCTION

Peptides and proteins seem attractive as potential therapeutic agents due to the number of diseases   which theoretically can be cured by their action (1,2). But, long term treatment with free proteins has been limited by their adverse reactions and behaviour in the living organisms and also by the high cost. In recent years, the increasing availability of pure recombinant proteins and the development of a new generation of liposomes and the improved technologies for correct evaluation of liposome behaviour, seem to open new perspectives for the use of proteins as therapeutic agents.

The application of liposome encapsulated proteins for therapy requires the knowledge of the factors that define their physical and chemical properties either in buffers, in vitro, in vivo and on storage. In spite of the significant amount of related work, basic questions remain mostly unans - wered as comparison of studies concerning protein encapsula - tion into liposomes and factors governing it are difficult due to the wide range of encapsulated proteins, lipid composi tion and methodology used (2,3,4). For further understanding of the effect of several parameters on protein encapsulation we have undertaken systematic studies using standard proteins and multilamellar vesicles.

METHODS

Multilamellar vesicles (MLV) were prepared as described elsewhere (5); lyophilized multilamellar vesicles (LMLV) according to (3) with some modifications (6); simplified dehydration - rehydration vesicles (SDRV) were prepared by lyophilization and rehydration of MLV containing intra and extra liposomal protein, alternatively to fusion of preformed empty MLV or SUV in the presence of external protein, as described elsewhere (4). Intra and extra liposomal protein is separated by three cycles of 30 fold dilution and centrifugation at 38,000 x g for 30 min. The parameters used   to estimate protein encapsulation are: protein to lipid (P/L) ratio, meaning protein encapsulated into liposomes (μg/μmol) and specific encapsulation efficiency (E.E.) defined as the percentage of final to intial P/L ratio.

RESULTS

Table 1 shows the encapsulation of bovine serum albumin
(BSA), into different types of liposomes. Using PC:Chol(4:1),
the P/L ratio of 2 ug/umol obtained with MLV increased to 4
and 27 µg/µmol for LMLV and SDRV, respectively. The encapsula
tion efficiency increased around 4 fold   for   SDRV. When
stearylamine (SA) was added to the lipid, a 4 and 10 fold
increase was observed for E.E. and P/L ratio respectively, in
LMLV system.For the SDRV system smaller changes were observed.

TABLE 1
PROTEIN ENCAPSULATION INTO LIPOSOMES

TYPE OF LIPOSOMES	APPARENT INTERNAL SPACE (µl/µmol)	DIAMETER (µm) (%)	PROTEIN/LIPID (µg/µmol)	SPECIFIC ENCAPSULATION EFFICIENCY (%)
M LV	1.9	0.2−0.6 (55)	2	8
LM LV	3	0.2−0.6 (52)	4 [40]	8 [35]
SDRV	2.8	0.2−0.6 (54)	27 [32]	30 [45]

PROTEIN− Bovine serum albumin (1mg/ml)

LIPID   − PC:Chol (4:1); PC:Chol:SA (7:1:2)(into parenthesis)

The vesicles diameter was determined by exclusion
through policarbonate filters.The values in brack
ets represent the percentage of vesicles popula -
tion with diameters ranging from 0.2 to 0.6 µm
(adapted from ref. 6).

The behaviour of protein encapsulation into LMLV as a
function of initial protein concentration is shown in   Fig -
ure 1. The P/L ratio of liposomes increases with the initial
protein concentration until saturation is   reached. Starting
with P/L ratio of 1300 µg/µmol, the E.E. reaches a maximum of
about 80%. For higher ratios, the E.E. drops to smaller
values: 20% for P/L ratio of 4000 µg/µmol. Initial P/L ratio

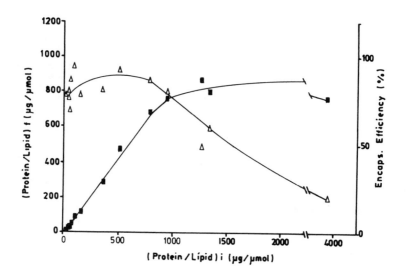

Figure 1. Effect of initial P/L on final P/L ratio (■)
and on E.E. (Δ) (From ref. 7).

higher than 1400 µg/µmol results in a constant final ratio
of 800 µg/µmol. Similar behaviour was found for protein
encapsulation into MLV (7) and for DRV (Lopes,F.and Cruz,M.E.
unpublished data).
      For   a low protein concentration (1mg/ml) at   the
hydration phase, the protein molecular weight, ranging from
40 to 480 Kdalton does not affect protein encapsulation (7).
      Figure 2 shows the effect of ionic strength on protein
encapsulation for SDRV. Increasing the ionic strength with
0.154 M NaCl instead of water at rehydration step systemati -
cally decreases P/L ratio and E.E. (up to 30%) irrespective
of the lipid composition of liposomes.
      Figure 3 shoes the effect of osmolarity on protein encap
sulation. The P/L ratio and E.E. of liposomes rehydrated in
the presence of water or 0.300 M mannitol are not significantly different for the lipid mixtures tested. Fluctuations of
about 6 to 15% on encapsulation parameters were observed.
      The pH effect on protein encapsulation is strongly depen
dent on protein, lipid composition and encapsulation method.
Figure 4 shows the effect of pH on encapsulation of BSA into
LMLV with different lipid composition. For a neutral lipidic

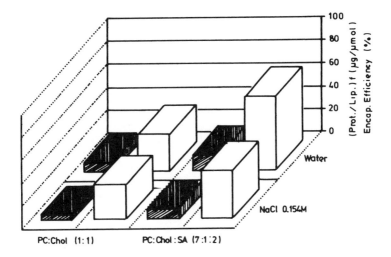

Figure 2. Effect of ionic strength on P/L ratio (▨) and on E.E. (□). SDRV were rehydrated in the presence of either water or 0.154 M NaCl.

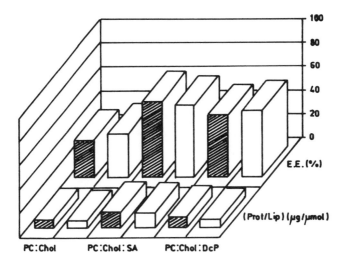

Figure 3. Effect of osmolarity on protein encapsulation into SDRV. Liposomes were rehydrated in the presence of either water (▨) or 0.300 M mannitol (□).

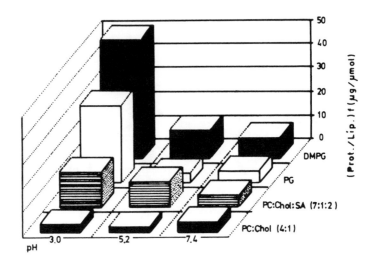

Figure 4. Effect of pH on the protein encapsulation into LMLV made from different lipids. BSA at initial concentration of 2.0 mg/ml was used. (From ref. 6).

mixture as PC:Chol, no significant change is found for pH above (7.4), equal (5.2) and below (3.0) the isoelectric point of protein. The mixture of PC:Chol with SA, which renders positive charge to vesicles, increases the E.E. from 4 to 7% at pH 7.4 and to 11 or 24% for pH of 5.2 or 3.0,respectively. Pure negatively charged lipids at neutral pH, as PG and DMPG, allows much higher encapsulation efficiencies and P/L ratios. Acidic pH (3.0) favors encapsulation into these vesicles, as E.E. increases to 50% and 80% and P/L ratios to 33 and 50 µg/µmol respectively for PG and DMPG:

Figure 5 shows parameters of protein encapsulation into LMLV, at pH 3.0, as a function of lipid composition. Neutral lipids such as PC:Chol and DMPC showed very low values for P/L ratio (about 3 µg/µmol) and E.E. (smaller than 10%). Also low values were found for PC:Chol:DcP which might be neutralized by protonation at low pH.

The encapsulation of BSA into SDRV is less affected by pH and lipid composition (Jorge,J.S. and Cruz,M.E.M. unpublished data).

Figure 6 shows the stability of urease encapsulated into multilamellar vesicles in the presence of human plasma. The

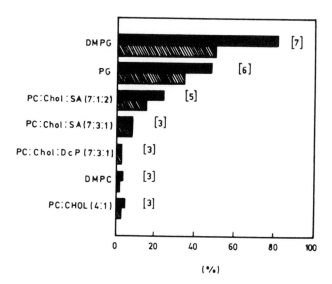

Figure 5. Effect of lipid composition on protein encap - sulation into LMLV. BSA at initial concentration of 2.0 mg/ml was used. Hydration was performed at pH 3.0. Final P/L ratio (▨); E.E. (■); [number of determinations]. (From ref. 6).

activity of encapsulated enzyme decreases with time. The maximal decrease (5 to 10%) was observed after 2 to 6 hours of incubation. This decreasing rate is smaller for longer time periods and after 84 hours 70% of the initial activity is still present. This decrease is followed by the amount of lipid in liposomal form, which decreases to 60% after the same time period. By analysing the extraliposomal fluid (upper part of the curve) we see that, concomitantly with the decrease of lipid and enzyme in liposomes, an increase of the free forms is observed. These data indicate that a disruption of liposomes, due to the interaction with plasma components, might occur with a consequent release of the entrapped material (2).

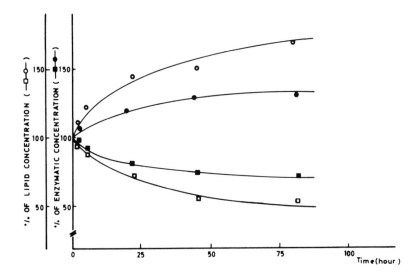

Figure 6. Stability of MLV in human plasma at 37º. Urease at 1 mg/ml initial concentration was encapsulated into liposomes prepared with PC:Chol (2:1). Stability was estimated by determining the enzymatic (■,●) and lipidic (□,○) concentration either in pellet(lower curves) or supernatant (upper curves) after 15,000xg for 10 min. centrifugation. (From Ref. 7).

DISCUSSION

From the results it is clear that the efficient encapsulation of water soluble proteins into liposomes is dependent on a variety of factors. Convenient control of these factors is required to obtain high encapsulation efficiencies without protein denaturation, particularly in the case of expensive proteins, and to obtain liposome formulations easy to prepare, to scale up and with high stability.

Within a given type of liposomes (multilamellar, made from the same lipids,with similar apparent internal space and similar size distribution), hydration and lyophilization are crucial steps to obtain high protein encapsulation (7). In a classical MLV preparation when the dry film of lipid is hydrated, a bilayer structure is formed on the outer surface of the lipid, encapsulating solvent and solutes (5). This layer which acts as a semipermeable membrane excludes solutes, but

not water, to the inner layers,is responsible for small pro -
tein encapsulation (Table 1). Much higher encapsulation parameters were observed either hydrating lyophilized lipid with
aqueous phase containing protein (LMLV) or liposomes previ -
ously lyophilized in the presence of protein (SDRV). The
higher values obtained for LMLV system are intimately   related to the kind of structure built at lyophilization being
for this reason strongly dependent on lipid composition (6).
For SDRV system less dependency was found on lipid composition, probably due to the fact that enhanced protein encapsulation occurs after rehydration of a fused lipid - protein
structure (Jorge,J.S. and Cruz, M.E., unpublished results).

The pH effect on protein encapsulation is correlated with
protein, lipid composition of liposomes and with incorporation method. The surprisingly high parameters obtained for
BSA encapsulation into LMLV made from PG and DMPG, at pH 3.0,
is due to the lipidic structure achieved after lyophilization.
Near the pK value (2.9)of PG phosphate group(8),neutralization
occurs with a reduction of the repulsive forces and a
stabilization of the structure by the establishment of intermolecular lipid-lipid hydrogen bonding. This hypothesis is
supported by the progressive reduction of encapsulation parameters observed for pH 5.2 and 7.4. An increase in protein
encapsulation can also be achieved by the enlargement of
aqueous space through the incorporation of positively charged
lipids (SA) into neutral liposomes (PC:Chol) (Fig. 4). This
effect is proportional to the charge density of liposomes,
created either by the introduction of different proportions
of positively charged lipids or by lowering the pH (6).

Ionic strength is another important factor which influ-
ences protein encapsulation (Fig. 2). The increase in encap
sulation parameters observed after reduction of ionic
strength might be due to reinforcement of electrostatic pro -
tein-lipid interactions,which are inhibited at high ionic
strength (9). In spite of the effect of different intra and
extra liposomal osmolarity on the characteristics of liposo -
mes little attention has been, so far, given to this problem
(10). As demonstrated (Fig. 3), increasing osmolarity (up to
0.30 OSM) does not significantly affect protein encapsulation.
These results seem valuable in the light of therapeutic
applications. The use of liposomes isosmolar with human plasma avoids changes in volume and shape while diminishing the
release of permeant contents by a solvent drag mechanism. The
mode of action of liposomes can be envisaged either by a slow
release process or by degradation of external permeant subs -
trates by encapsulated enzyme. As shown in Figure 6,the first

mechanism is closely related with the stability of liposomes in human plasma (7) and so with lipid composition of liposo - mes (2). Lipid composition and in particular charged lipids also determine the possibility of the second mechanism occur- ring, since the latter depends on the permeability of liposo- mes to external substrates. The optimization of the two mecha nisms must be taken into account in designing appropriate carrier system for proteins.

The necessity of optimizing encapsulation conditions for individual proteins is well established. However, the similarities in physico-chemical properties and behaviour of water soluble proteins should allow extrapolation of results obtained with model proteins. We think that, this report will contribute to the establishment of methodologies and the search for factors regulating protein encapsulation.

REFERENCES

1. Boivon P, Boisse J, Lestradet H, Gajdos A (1987). "Enzymopathies".Paris:Masson.
2. Gregoriadis G (1983)."Liposome Technology:Incorporation of Drugs,Proteins and Genetics Materials"Boca Raton:CRS Press.
3. Eppstein DA, Marsh YV, Van der Pas M, Felgner PL (1985). Biological activity of liposomes-encapsulated murine inter feron is mediated by a cell membrane receptor. Proc Natl Acad Sci 82:3688.
4. Kirby C, Gregoriadis G (1984). Dehydration-rehydration vesicles; a simple method for high yield drug entrapment in liposomes. Biotechnology 2:979.
5. Hope MG, Bally MB, Mayer LD, Janoff AS, Cullis PR (1986). Generation of multilamellar and unilamellar phospholipid vesicles. Chemistry and Physics of Lipids 40:89.
6. Corvo ML, Cruz ME (1988). Factors affecting the encapsula tion of hydrophilic protein into liposomes (submited).
7. Cruz ME , Lopes F (1988). Liposomes as carrier systems for Proteins. Actas do Instituto de Bioquímica (in press).
8. Boggs JM (1987). Lipid intermolecular hydrogen bonding: Influence on structural organization and membrane function. Biochim Biophys Acta 906:353.
9. Carrier D, Pezolet M (1986). Investigation of polylisine - dipalmitoylphosphatidylglycerol interactions in model membranes. Biochemistry 25:4167.
10.Cruner SM (1987). Materials properties of liposomal bilayers.In Ostro MY (ed): "Liposomes, from Biophysics to Therapeutics."New York: Marcel Dekker, Inc,Chap 1.

Liposomes in the Therapy of Infectious Diseases and Cancer, pages 427–439
© 1989 Alan R. Liss, Inc.

pH-SENSITIVE LIPOSOMES FOR THE DELIVERY OF IMMUNOMODULATORS[1]

Rajiv Nayar[2] and Alan J. Schroit[3]

[2]The Canadian Liposome Co. and [3]M.D. Anderson Hospital and Tumor Institute

ABSTRACT   We have designed pH-sensitive liposomes for the delivery of immunomodulators for macrophage activation. The liposomes are generated by incorporating the pH-sensitive lipid, N-Succinyl-dioleoylphosphatidlyethanolamine (SOPE), in dioleoylphosphatidlyethanolamine (DOPE) liposomes. The in vitro characteristics of these liposomes are described and the potential use of these liposomes for rapid delivery of soluble immunomodulators such and muramyl dipeptide and gamma interferon (IFN) to macrophages in situ is discussed.

INTRODUCTION

The therapeutic potential of liposomes as drug delivery vehicles is dependant upon the efficient delivery of liposome-entrapped compounds to target cells. Although significant advances have been made in the ability to direct liposomes to various cell types in vitro, attempts to direct liposomes to cells in vivo other than those of the mononuclear phagocytic system have been met with frustration due to the natural phagocytic function of the reticuloendothelial system (RES) (1). To take advantage of this natural in vivo localization of liposomes, efforts have been made towards generating liposomes that would release their entrapped aqueous contents following their uptake by the RES. As a result, specific lipid systems have been designed

---

[1]This work was supported in part by Developmental Fund Grant 175416 from the University of Texas M.D. Anderson Hospital and Tumor Institute at Houston and by National Institutes of Health Grant CA-40149.

which result in enhanced particle uptake by cells
and/or rapid breakdown of their membrane barrier
when exposed to specific intracellular pH
environments which results in the release of
entrapped therapeutic compounds.

In this chapter, we review the properties of
SOPE-containing liposomes which preferentially
release their entrapped aqueous contents when
exposed to acidic endosomal compartments. In
addition, these liposomes are stable at neutral pH
and interact strongly with cells of the macrophage-
monocyte lineage due to the negative charge of the
particles. The potential of these liposomes is for
rapid delivery of soluble immunomodulators to the
RES for activating macrophages to the tumoricidal
state.

RESULTS

The general strategy used in the construction
of pH-sensitive liposomes has been to incorporate
lipids containing pH-sensitive groups, which have a
pK_a between 4 and 5, into liposomal membranes.
Examples of these lipids are the carboxyl-containing
lipids, N-palmitoyl homocysteine (PHC), cholesteryl
hemisuccinate (CHEMS), oleic acid (OA), and N-
succinyl-PE (SOPE) (Figure 1). The pH-sensitive
liposomes generated from PHC, CHEMS, and OA in
combination with PE as an obligatory phospholipid
constituent have been recently described (2-6). In
vitro studies with cultured cell lines have
indicated that they are indeed effective in
enhancing the cytoplasmic delivery of encapsulated
compounds (4, 6). It should be noted, however, that
the stability of these liposomes in vivo could be
hampered by the potential exchange/transfer of the
pH-sensitive amphiphiles by serum components. This
could result in destabilization of the liposomes
before they reach their destination. In this
context, CHEMS has been shown to be rapidly
incorporated by adsorption into acceptor lipid
bilayers (7) and PE/OA liposomes have been shown to
leak their contents upon exposure to the mouse serum
following intravenous injection (8). Therefore, the
in vivo applicability of using pH-sensitive
amphiphiles appears to be somewhat restricted.

In order to reduce the potential problem of lipid transfer, we synthesized a pH-sensitive phospholipid by carboxylating phosphatidylethanolamine with succinic anhydride (9). By generating liposomes containing SOPE alone or in combination with dioleoylphosphatidylethanolamine (DOPE), liposomes with a wide range of pH-induced leakage properties have been produced (9).

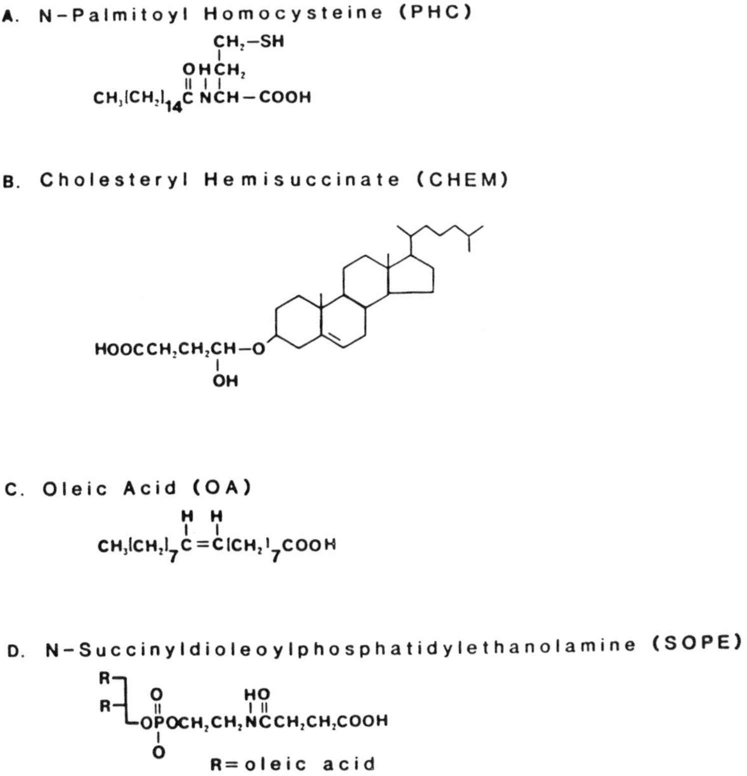

A. N-Palmitoyl Homocysteine (PHC)

$$CH_2-SH$$
$$OH CH_2$$
$$CH_3(CH_2)_{14}C\ \overset{\shortmid}{N}CH-COOH$$

B. Cholesteryl Hemisuccinate (CHEM)

$$HOOCCH_2CH_2CH-O$$
$$OH$$

C. Oleic Acid (OA)

$$CH_3(CH_2)_7\overset{H}{C}=\overset{H}{C}(CH_2)_7COOH$$

D. N-Succinyldioleoylphosphatidylethanolamine (SOPE)

$$R$$
$$R$$
$$O\qquad HO$$
$$OPOCH_2CH_2NCCH_2CH_2COOH$$
$$O$$
$$R = oleic\ acid$$

FIGURE 1. Structures of pH-sensitive lipids

Liposomes composed exclusively of SOPE release encapsulated ANTS/DPX at pH 7.4 but not at pH 4.0 (Figure 2a). Leakage of these vesicles appeared to be due to the electrostatic interactions between the negatively charged SOPE molecules. A dramatic reversal of the leakage properties was observed in

the mixed-lipid vesicles composed of SOPE and DOPE.
Unlike pure SOPE vesicles, the DOPE/SOPE (7:3 mol
ratio) vesicles preferentially released their
aqueous contents (ANTS/DPX) under acidic (pH 4.0)
conditions (Fig. 2b). The leakage from the

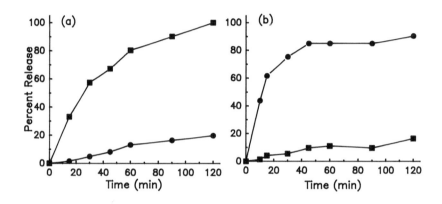

FIGURE 2. Release of ANTS/DPX from SOPE (a)
and DOPE/SOPE (7:3,b) vesicles.

DOPE/SOPE liposomes was attributed to fusion of the
DOPE/SOPE vesicles induced by the nonbilayer
properties of DOPE upon protonation of the SOPE
(10). This has been shown to be significantly
enhanced in the presence of physiological calcium
concentrations.

DOPE/SOPE Liposome-Macrophage Interactions

    We have characterized the interaction of
DOPE/SOPE liposomes with cultured macrophages with
the goal of exploiting the passive localization of
i.v. administered liposomes to mononuclear
phagocytes as a means of stimulating macrophage-
mediated host defense mechanisms The therapeutic
potential of soluble immunomodulators, such as gamma
interferon (IFN) and muramyl dipeptide (MDP), in
cancer therapy has been limited by their short
plasma half-life in vivo and/or undesirable side
effects. One approach of prolonging the half-life

of these agents while directing them towards cells of the RES has been to associate them with liposomes. This approach has been used by several groups and has facilitated macrophage "activation" in vivo which resulted in the eradication of experimental metastasis (11-13). It has been shown, for example, that the systemic administration of multilamellar vesicles (MLVs) containing lipophilic derivatives of muramyl dipeptide can activate macrophages in situ to become cytotoxic against virus-infected cells (review, 14) and tumor cells (review, 15).

In order to enhanced delivery of soluble immunomodulators by liposomes to cells of the RES, certain criteria need to be fulfilled: (i) liposomes should be avidly taken up by the cells before the serum components induce leakage of the liposome contents, (ii) efficient cytoplasmic delivery of the encapsulated compounds in their active form should occur, and (iii) the liposomes should be non-toxic. As indicated below, SOPE-containing liposomes fulfull these criteria.

Phagocytosis of DOPE/SOPE MLV

Early in vitro studies on liposome-macrophage interactions have shown that the majority of liposomes that became cell associated are rapidly internalized by the cells (13, 16, 17). However, the extent of liposome binding and subsequent ingestion by macrophages is greatly influenced by the type of liposomes employed. For example, MLVs are better phagocytosed than SUVs of identical lipid composition (18). In addition, liposomes containing negatively charged phospholipids are better bound to and phagocytosed by macrophages. As shown in Figure 3, liposomes containing SOPE fulfill the general requirement of negative charge. It can be seen that DOPE/SOPE and PC/PS MLVs are more avidly phagocytosed by the macrophages than are MLVs composed exclusively of PC.

Cytoplasmic Delivery of Calcein by DOPE/SOPE MLVs

Macrophages were incubated with calcein-containing liposomes to compare the efficiency of DOPE/SOPE with that of PC/PS liposomes to deliver entrapped compounds into the cell cytoplasm. Fluorescence microscopy of macrophages incubated with DOPE/SOPE vesicles containing entrapped calcein, revealed a diffuse distribution of

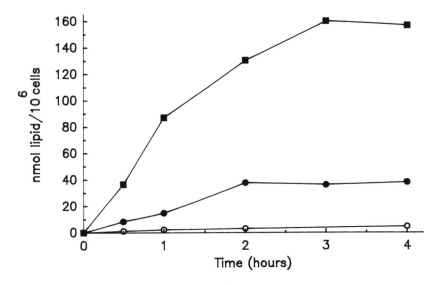

FIGURE 3.   Phagocytosis of PC (O), PC/PS (7:3, ●), and DOPE/SOPE (7:3, ■) MLV by peritoneal macrophages.

fluorescence, which suggests that these liposomes released their encapsulated contents to the cytoplasm while still sequestered in the endosomes (21). In contrast, only punctate fluorescence was observed when calcein-containing PC/PS vesicles were phagocytosed by the macrophages, corresponding to surface-bound liposomes and liposomes sequestered in intracellular endocytic vesicles. These observations are consistent with the results from previous studies which showed efficient cytoplasmic

delivery of entrapped calcein by PE/PHC (4) and
PE/OA (6) liposomes.

In Vitro Activation of Macrophages by pH-Sensitive Liposomes containing Immunomodulators

Previous studies from our laboratory have shown
that liposome containing immunomodulators such as
MAF, IFN, MDP, and MTP-PE can render cells of the
monocyte-macrophage lineage tumoricidal more
effectively than can free unencapsulated compounds
(12, 19, 20). We have extended these observations
by employing two types of pH-sensitive liposomes-
pure SOPE MLV and DOPE/SOPE (7/3 mol ratio) MLV,
which preferentially release their encapsulated
contents at pH 7.4 and pH 4, respectively (9).
Table 1 summarizes the results obtained from
experiments using these MLVs for the induction of
macrophage tumoricidal properties. It can be seen
that control SOPE and DOPE/SOPE MLVs (containing
buffer alone) did not induce macrophage toxicity.
On the other hand, only immunomodulators associated
with DOPE/SOPE liposomes were effective in rendering
the macrophages tumoricidal (Table 1). Pure SOPE
vesicles were ineffective presumably because the
immunomodulators leaked from the liposomes (at the
neutral pH of the media) before they were
internalized by the macrophages. In contrast,
DOPE/SOPE liposomes probably retained their contents
until sequestered in the macrophage endosomes, where
the acidic environment induced release of the
immunomodulators into the cytoplasm. These results
suggest that pH-sensitive DOPE/SOPE liposomes
effectively deliver encapsulated immunomodulators to
the macrophages in active form.

Biodistribution and In Situ Activation of Alveolar Macrophages by DOPE/SOPE Liposomes.

The biodistribution of PC, PC/PS, and DOPE/SOPE
MLV was determined by using a non-exchangeable
biodegradable lipid marker, ^{125}I-phenylpropionyl-PE.
This lipid is a convenient marker for vesicle
integrity and is degraded and released when the

TABLE 1
IN VITRO ACTIVATION OF MACROPHAGES TO THE
TUMORICIDAL STATE BY LIPOSOMES CONTAINING   IFN AND
MDP

==

Treatment of Macrophages[a]	Radioactivity in viable cells on day 3
Tumor cells alone	2117±166
SOPE (100 nmol)	2017±154
SOPE [IFN+MDP][b]	2506±143
DOPE/SOPE (100 nmol)	1622±104
DOPE/SOPE [IFN+MDP][b]	773±224 (63%)[c]

==

[a]Peritoneal macrophages were activated for 24 hr
with the indicated agents. B16-BL6 melanoma target
cells (10^4) labeled with [^{125}I]-IUdR were plated
onto the macrophage monolayers (10^5). Target cell-
associated radioactivity was monitored after 72 hr
of cocultivation.
[b]MLVs were made in media containing 24,000 U/mL IFN
and 800 ng/mL MDP. The unassociated IFN and MDP
were removed by repeated centrifugation of MLVs.
[c]Percentage of cytotoxicity as compared with taht of
control macrophage cultures. $\underline{P}$<0.005.

labelled-liposomes are metabolized. Mice (C57/BL6,
20 g) were injected with 2.5 umol of MLV and the
radioactivity determined in various organs at 15
min, 1 and 4 hours following i.v. injection. As
shown in Table 2, both PC/PS and DOPE/SOPE MLV are
rapidly cleared by the major organs of the RES
(liver and spleen). At 1 and 4 hours, significant
amount of radioactivity was found in the G.I tract
persumably due to the degradation of the lipid
label. The total recovery of the PC/PS and
DOPE/SOPE MLV was 31 and 20 %, respectively,
compared to 74 % for the PC MLV. These results
suggest that the PC/PS and DOPE/SOPE MLV are rapidly
taken up and broken down by the RES.

In the next series of experiments, we determined
whether alveolar macrophages (AM) can be activated
to the tumoricidal state following intravenous
injection of PC/PS and PE/SOPE MLV containing MDP
and IFN. MLV were prepared in media alone and media
containing 24,000 U/mL of IFN and 800 ng/mL MDP.

TABLE 2
BIODISTRIBUTION OF EGG PC, PC/PS (7:3), AND
DOPE/SOPE (7:3) MLV IN MICE.

===
Percent Injected Dose[a]

	Blood	Lung	Liver	Spleen	GI Tract	Total[b]
10 min.						
EPC	52.8	20.0	17.5	2.6	1.4	97.4
PC/PS	50.9	18.7	15.0	10.4	3.0	101
PE/SOPE	51.0	6.5	26.7	7.8	2.7	96.8
1 HR						
EPC	1.7	20.4	45.1	12.4	3.8	85.4
PC/PS	4.1	3.6	29.4	9.9	12.7	61.2
PE/SOPE	5.1	0.5	28.6	6.0	19.5	60.7
4 HR						
EPC	1.6	13.9	39.1	9.9	7.4	73.6
PC/PS	2.8	1.4	5.5	1.7	19.0	31.1
PE/SOPE	2.6	0.4	4.6	0.6	11.6	20.3

===

[a] Results are expressed as percent of total injected
dose (0.1 uCi). Groups of five C57/BL6 mice (20 g)
were used and were injected intravenously with 2.5
umol lipid in 0.2 mL. The liposome marker was ^{125}I-
phenylpropionyl-PE.
[b] Total represents all the above organs and kidneys.

The non-associated immunomodulators were removed by
centrifugating the MLV three times at 12,000g for 10
min. Mice were injected intravenously with 2.5 umol
of MLV and AM were isolated by pulmonary lavage
24hours later. Tumoricidal activity of the AM was
assessed against B16 melanoma target cells. Results
from two separate experiments are shown in Table 3.

TABLE 3
IN SITU ACTIVATION OF MACROPHAGES TO THE TUMORICIDAL
STATE BY LIPOSOMES CONTAINING IFN AND MDP

==

Treatment of macrophages	Radioactivity in viable cells on day 3	
	Expt. I	Expt. II
Tumor cells alone	1301±60	3880±279
PC/PS (2.5 umol)	1328±48	3968±67
PC/PC [IFN+MDP]	1241±189 (5%)[b]	3392±148 (13%)[b]
DOPE/SOPE(2.5 umol)	1209±72 (7%)[b]	4162±10
DOPE/SOPE [IFN+MDP]	625±66 (52%)[b]	2779±173 (28%)[b]

==

[a]AM were isolated and adhered onto plastic tissue
culture wells. B16-BL6 melanoma target cells (10^4)
labeled with [^{125}I]-IUdR were plated onto the AM
monolayers (10^5).Target cell-associated
radioactivity was monitored after 72 hr of
cocultivation.
[b]Percentage of cytotoxicity as compared with that of
control AM cultures.

Both empty preparations of PC/PS and DOPE/SOPE
MLV failed to activate the AM to the tumoricidal
state, whereas, the immunomodulator-containing
DOPE/SOPE MLV were more effective than the PC/PS MLV
in activating the AM in situ. These results clearly
show that although equivalent amounts of immunomodulators were associated with both types of MLV,

the pH-sensitive DOPE/SOPE MLV were more effective
than the pH-insensitive PC/PS MLV in macrophage
activation under in vivo conditions.

DISCUSSION

It is conceivable that pH-sensitive liposomes
can be therapeutically effective in delivering
biologically active molecules to cells of RES. The
major advantages of utilizing such liposomes are
that they are avidly taken up by the phagocytes and
that they remain stable (i.e. nonleaky) until an
acidified environment is encountered. The in vitro
and in vivo results presented above indicate that
DOPE/SOPE liposomes are effective in rendering
macrophages cytotoxic towards tumor cells and
suggest that they may be useful for the delivery of
pharmaceutically active agents to macrophages in
situ for the eradication of metastasis.

ACKNOWLEDGMENTS

Rajiv Nayar is a fellow of the Medical Research
Council of Canada.

REFERENCES

1.   Poste G (1980). Liposome targeting in vivo:
      Problems and opportunities. Biol Cell 47:19.
2.   Yatvin MB, Kreutz W, Horwitz M, Shinitzky M
      (1980). pH-sensitive liposomes: Possible
      clinical implications. Science 210:1253.
3.   Connor J, Yatvin MB, Huang L (1984). pH-
      sensitive liposomes: acid-induced liposome
      fusion. Proc Natl Acad Sci (USA) 81:1715.
4.   Connor J, Huang L (1985). Efficient cytoplasmic
      delivery of a fluorescent dye by pH-sensitive
      immunoliposomes. J Cell Biol 101:582.
5.   Ellens H, Bentz J, Szoka FC (1984). pH-induced
      destabilization of phosphatidylethanolamine-
      containing liposomes: Roles of bilayer contact.
      Biochemistry 23:1532.
6.   Straubinger RM, Duzgunes N, Papahadjopoulos D
      (1985). pH- sensitive liposomes mediate

cytoplasmic delivery of encapsulated
macromolecules. FEBS Lett 179:148.

7. Fugler L, Clejan S, Bittman R (1985). Movement
    of cholesterol between vesicles prepared with
    different phospholipids or sizes. J Biol Chem
    260:4098.

8. Connor J, Morley N, Huang L (1986).
    Biodistribution of pH-sensitive liposomes.
    Biochim Biophys Acta 884:474.

9. Nayar R, Schroit AJ (1985). Generation of pH-
    sensitive liposomes: Use of large unilamellar
    vesicles containing N-succinyldioleoylphos-
    phatidylethanolamine. Biochemistry 24:5967.

10. Nayar R, Tilcock CPS, Hope MJ, Cullis PR,
    Schroit AJ (1988). N-succinyldioleoylphos-
    phatidylethanolamine: structural preferences in
    pure and mixed model membranes. Biochim Biophys
    Acta 937:31.

11. Fidler IJ, Poste G (1982). Macrophage-mediated
    destruction of malignant tumor cells and new
    strategies for the therapy of metastatic
    disease. Springer Semin Immunopath 5:161.

12. Fidler IJ, Sone S, Fogler WE, Barnes Z (1981).
    Eradication of spontaneous metastases and
    activation of alveolar macrophages by
    intravenous injection of liposomes containing
    muramyl dipeptide. Proc Natl Acad Sci (USA)
    78:1680.

13. Poste G, Kirsh R, Fogler WE, Fidler IJ (1979).
    Activation of tumoricidal properties in mouse
    macrophages by lymphokines encapsulated in
    liposomes. Cancer Res 39:881.

14. Koff WC, Fidler IJ (1985). The potential use of
    liposome-mediated antiviral therapy. Antiviral
    Res 5:179.

15. Nayar R and Fidler IJ (1985). The systemic
    activation of macrophages by liposomes
    containing immunomodulators. Springer Semin
    Immunopathol. 8:413.

16. Gregoriadis G, Buckland RA (1973). Enzyme
    containing liposomes alleviate a model for
    storage disease. Nature 244:170.

17. Weissmann G, Bloomgarden D, Kaplan R, Cohen C,
    Hoffstein S, Collins T, Gotlkieb A and Nagle D
    (1975). A general method for the introduction
    of missing enzymes into the cytoplasm of

cultured mammalian cells by means of immunoglobulin-coated liposomes, into lysosomes of deficient cells. Proc. Natl. Acad. Sci. U.S.A. 72:88.

18. Schroit AJ, Fidler IJ (1982). Effects of liposome structure and lipid composition on the activation of the tumoricidal properties of macrophages by liposomes containing muramyl dipeptide. Cancer Res 42:161.

19. Saiki I, Fidler IJ (1985). Synergistic activation by recombinant mouse interferon- and muramyl dipeptide of tumoricidal properties in mouse macrophages. J Immunol 135:684.

20. Schroit AJ, Galligioni E, Fidler IJ (1983). Factors influencing the in situ activation of macrophages by liposomes containing muramyl dipeptide. Biol Cell 47:87.

21. Schroit AJ, Madsen, J, Nayar, R (1986). Liposome-cell interactions: In vitro discrimination of uptake mechanism and in vivo targeting strategies to mononuclear phagocytes. Chem. Phys. Lipids 40:373.

Liposomes in the Therapy of Infectious Diseases and Cancer, pages 441–451

SELECTIVE DEPLETION OF MACROPHAGES USING TOXINS ENCAPSULATED IN LIPOSOMES: EFFECT ON ANTIMICROBIAL RESISTANCE

Angelo J. Pinto[1], Deneen Stewart[1], Alvin Volkman[2]
Gordon Jendrasiak[2], Nico van Rooijen[3], and
Page S. Morahan[1]

[1] Department of Microbiology and Immunology,
The Medical College of Pennsylvania,
Philadelphia, PA 19129; [2] Department of Pathology,
East Carolina University School of Medicine,
Greenville, NC 27858; [3] Department of Histology,
Free University, Amsterdam, The Netherlands

ABSTRACT The current study demonstrates that selective depletion of macrophages (MO) reduces antimicrobial resistance. CD-1 mice were selectively depleted of spleen and liver MO by i.v. administration of the toxin dichlororomethylene diphosphonate (DMDP) encapsulated in liposomes and of peritoneal MO by i.p. administration of the toxin ricin encapsulated in liposomes. DMDP liposomes, when given at day-3 and day-1 before infection, significantly decreased resistance to i.v. challenge with herpes simplex virus type 2 (HSV-2). Ricin liposomes, when given at day-1 before infection, significantly decreased resistance to i.p. challenge with Listeria monocytogenes. Collectively, these results demonstrate the importance of tissue MO in host antimicrobial resistance.

INTRODUCTION

Macrophages (MO) have been well documented to be important in the resistance against pathogenic microorganisms. Evidence includes broad spectrum extrinsic and intrinsic antiviral activity (1,

2), antibacterial activity (3), and immuno-regulation of other immune system effectors (4).

TABLE 1.

APPROACHES FOR MACROPHAGE DEPLETION

Genetic: Bg/Bg (5), Sld/Sld (6, 7), PJ (8)

Toxins: silica (9), dextran sulfate (10), trypan blue (10), ricin (11), L-leucine methyl ester (12), gliotoxin (13), 2-chloroadenosine (14), vepesid (15), asbestos (16), chlorinated water (17), carrageenan (18), and frog virus 3 (19)

Toxins in liposomes: ricin, dichloro-methylene diphosphonate (20), and lipoprotein sequestered DDT (21)

Antibody: polyclonal anti-MO antibody (22), ricin-anti-MO monoclonal antibody (23)

Radiation: 89Sr (24), whole body radiation (25), and partial radiation (25)

To further explore the role of MO in antimicrobial resistance various MO depletion methods have been developed (table 1). While no single method is completely effective or selective, use of independent depletion approaches can provide overlapping data to define the role of MO in host resistance. One novel method we have used is administration of 89Sr, a bone marrow seeking isotope which depletes circulating monocytes without affecting tissue macrophages (24). Another method we have recently begun to explore is selective depletion of splenic and liver MO with liposomes encapsulating the toxin DMDP. This agent, when inoculated i.v., has profound depleting effects on spleen and liver MO without affecting other tissue MO compartments (26, 27). As a counterpoint to i.v. DMDP treatment we have also used i.p. inoculation

of the toxin ricin in liposomes, to selectively
deplete the peritoneal M0 compartment. Using such
methods, we demonstrate that depletion of tissue
macrophages markedly reduces resistance to
infection with HSV-2 and L. monocytogenes.

RESULTS AND DISCUSSION

Depletion of Peritoneal Macrophages With Ricin.

Ricin is a toxic plant lectin isolated from
castor beans (28). Isolation procedures have
yielded two major forms, ricin RCA I and the more
toxic ricin, RCA II. RCA II is a heterodimer
composed of two chains, A and B (28). When tested
separately, only the A (RAC) chain proved toxic
(29), while the B chain appears to be involved in
binding to the cell surface (29). The mechanism
of ricin toxicity is thought to be inhibition of
protein synthesis (30).
Our toxicity studies showed that only whole
ricin, and not RAC was toxic in mice when given
i.p. at doses of 10 ug/ml. Only 2.5 ug/ml i.p. of
whole ricin was needed to eliminate peritoneal M0
(data not shown), but there was a problem in that
there was also a strong granulocyte (PMN) influx
to the peritoneal cavity at ricin doses of < 4
ug/ml. This was not present at higher doses,
suggesting ricin receptors may be present on
PMNs, but possibly the binding affinity is low.

Depletion of Peritoneal Macrophages with Ricin in
Liposomes.

To minimize the inflamatory effects and
systemic toxicity of free ricin in the peritoneal
cavity, and to target the toxin exclusively to
M0, liposomal delivery of ricin was studied.
Ricin and RAC were incorporated into negatively
charged multilamellar liposomes (prepared from
phosphatidyl choline, phosphatidic acid and
cholesterol in a molar ratio of 7:1:3) and
inoculated i.p. in CD-1 mice. Mice were

sacrificed 24 hours later, peritoneal cells obtained by lavage, and differential cell counts made. Whole ricin in liposomes caused a 74% reduction in peritoneal MO when compared with control mice, whereas RAC in liposomes had no

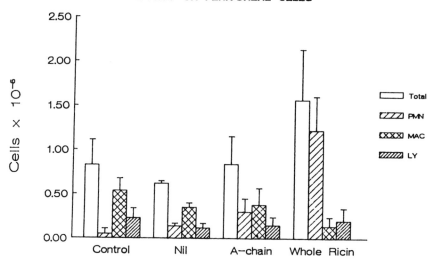

RICIN AND RICIN A-CHAIN LIPOSOMES
EFFECT ON PERITONEAL CELLS

FIGURE 1.   Effects of liposome-encapsulated ricin and ricin A-chain on peritoneal cells 24 hours after i.p. administration of each agent. PMN, polymorphonuclear leukocytes; MAC, macrophages; Ly, lymphocytes. Each group represents the mean of 3- 5 mice.

more effect on peritoneal MO than did empty liposomes (figure 1). There was no effect on peritoneal lymphocyte numbers presumably because lymphocytes have no receptors for ricin. The influx of PMNs in the ricin liposome treated mice may be associated with leakage of a small amount of ricin from liposomes or release of ricin from dead cells before its biological inactivation. Kinetic studies indicated peritoneal M0 in mice treated with ricin liposomes were depleted for 3 days (data not shown). Thus, administration of ricin liposomes may provide depletion of M0 for a slightly longer time than does administration of agents such as silica, where M0 are depleted for less than 24 hours (9, 23).

Effect of I.P. Ricin Liposomes on Resistance to Infection with L. monocytogenes.

A comparative study was performed of the effects of i.p. ricin liposomes in control mice and in mice depleted of blood monocytes and bone

TABLE 2.

Effect of i.p. Administration of Ricin-Liposomes on Resistance of Mice to i.p. Infection with L. monocytogenes.

Treatment		Log 10 CFU Listeria in		
89Sr	Ricin-L	Spleen	Liver	Peritoneum
−	−	1.6	< 1.0	< 0.7
−	+	3.2	2.9	2.7
+	−	1.5	1.7	0.9
+	+	4.4	4.3	3.3

Mice were injected i.v. with 89Sr, and i.p. with ricin liposomes (ricin-L) 13 days later. The next day mice were challenged with approximately an LD50 dose of L. monocytogenes, and were sacrificed 28 hours later. The titer of listeria per organ was determined by colony forming units (CFU) on blood agar. Each group represents the mean of 3-5 mice.

marrow by i.v. administration of 89Sr, 2 uCi per gram body weight, 13 days before liposome injection. Control mice received 88Sr equivalent

to amounts of carrier in the radioactive inoculum. Control values for the effectiveness of 89Sr indicated 87% depletion of blood monocytes at the time of liposome inoculation.

Consistent with our previous findings (24), there was no significant difference in resistance to i.p. infection with L. monocytogenes between 88Sr and 89Sr treated mice (table 2). Such data suggest that resistance to L. monocytogenes does not require normal levels of circulating monocytes, but that tissue MO may be very important. In support of this concept, treatment i.p. with ricin liposomes caused a profound decrease in resistance to i.p. infection with L. monocytogenes whether the mice were treated with 88Sr or 89Sr (table 2). There was increased

TABLE 3.

Effects of i.v. DMDP Liposomes

- Decrease in spleen and liver MO (20, 27)

- Decrease in liver uptake of liposomes containing methotrexate (31)

- Decrease in antibody response to TI-2 antigen (TNP-Ficoll) (26)

- No decrease in antibody response to TI-1 antigen (TNP-LPS) or TD antigen (TNP-KLH) (26)

- Decrease in resistance to i.v. infection with HSV-2 and L. monocytogenes (32)

-No effect on peritoneal MO number or ectoenzyme phenotype (32)

-Transient decrease in natural killer activity for 1 day (32)

growth of L̲. monocytogenes in the organs of all
mice treated with ricin liposomes (table 2) as
well as increased mortality (data not shown).

Effect of I.V. DMDP Liposomes on Resistance to
Infection with HSV-2.

In addition to evaluating the effect of
selective depletion of peritoneal MO on host
resistance, we also evaluated the effect of
depletion of splenic and liver MO by i.v.
treatment of CD-1 mice with liposomes (prepared
without phosphatidic acid, and hence carrying
little or no charge) encapsulating the toxin
DMDP. DMDP, when administered i.v. in liposomes,
has a variety of effects on host resistance
including a profound depleting effect on splenic
and liver MO (table 3).
        Double i.v. treatment with DMDP liposomes on
days -3 and -1 before infection caused a profound

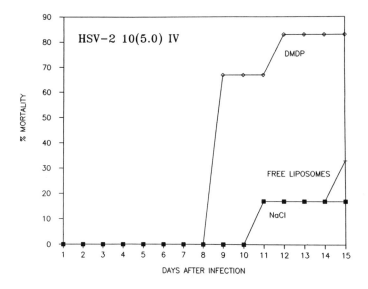

FIGURE 2.   Effect of i.v. DMDP liposomes on
resistance to HSV-2 infection in CD-1 mice. n = 6
mice/group

decrease in resistance to i.v. challenge with HSV-2. Most mice died down through the 10^{-5} dose which contained only 28 plaque forming units (figure 2).

ACKNOWLEDGEMENTS

This work was supported by ONR N00014-82-K-0069 and DMAD 17-86-6-6117. The DMDP was a gift from Dr. Nico van Rooijen, Free University, The Netherlands; and Dr. Edelberto Cabrero, Norwich-Easton Pharmaceutical Company.

REFERENCES

1. Morahan PS, Connor JR, Leary KR (1985). Viruses and the versital macrophage. Brit Med Bult 41:15.
2. Morahan, PS (1983). Interactions of herpesviruses with mononuclear phagocytes. In Rouse B, Lopez C (eds): "Immunology of Herpes Simplex Virus Infections," Boca Raton: CRC, p 71.
3. Kimball JW (1983). "Introduction to Immunology." New York: Macmillan, p 231.
4. Gordon S. (1986). Biology of the macrophage. J Cell Sci Suppl 4: 267.
5. Mahoney KM, Morse SS, Morahan PS (1980). Macrophages from beige (Chediak-Higashi Syndrome) mice show delayed antitumor activity. Cancer Res 40:3934.
6. Shibata Y, Volkman A (1985). The effect of hemopoietic microenviornment on suppressor macrophages in the congenitally anemic mice of the genotype Sl/Sld. J Immunol 135:3905.
7. Hackett J, Bennett M, Kumar V (1985). Origin and differentiation of natural killer cells. I. Characteristics of a natural killer cell precursor. J Immunol 134:3731.
8. Vogel SN, Weinblatt AC, Rosenstreich DL (1981). Inherent macrophage defects in mice. In Gershwin ME, Merchant B (eds): "Immunologic Defects in Laboratory Animals," New York: Plenum, p 327.

9. Morahan PS, Kern ER, Glasgow, LA (1977). Immunomodulator induced resistance against herpes simplex virus. Proc Soc Exp Biol Med 154:615.

10. McGeorge MB, Morahan PS (1978). Comparison of effects of various macrophage inhibiting agents on systemic or vaginal herpes simplex virus type 2 infection. Infect Immnu 22:623.

11. Simmons BM, Stahl PD, Russell JH (1986). Mannose receptor-mediated uptake of ricin toxin and ricin A chain by macrophages. Multiple intracellular pathways for a chain translocation. J Biol Chem 17:7912.

12. Thiele DW, Lipsky PE (1986). The immuno-suppressive activity of L-Leucyl-Leucine methyl ester: selective ablation of cytotoxic lymphocytes and monocytes. J Immunol 136:1038.

13. Eichner RD, Al Salami M, Wood PR Mullbacher A (1986). The effect of gliotoxin upon macrophage function. Int J Immunopharm 8:789.

14. Schultz RM, Tang JC, DeLong DC, Ades EW, Altom MG (1986). Inability of anti-asialo-GM1 and 2-chloroadenosine to abrogate maleic anhydride divinyl ether-induced resistance against experimental murine lung carcinoma metastases. Cancer Res 46:5624.

15. Meddens MJM, Thompson J, Mattie H, van Furth R (1985). Role of granulocytes and monocytes in the prevention and therapy of experimental Staphylococcus epidermidis endocarditis in rabbits. J Infect 11:41.

16. Dean JH, Boorman GA, Luster MI, Adkins BJr, Lauer LD, Adams DO (1984). Effect of agents of enviornmental concern on macrophage functions: In Volkman, A (ed): "Mononuclear Phagocyte Biology," New York: Marcel Dekker, p 473.

17. Fidler IJ (1977). Depression of macrophages in mice drinking hyperchlorinated water. Nature 270:735.

18. Keller R (1976). Promotion of tumor growth in vivo by antimacrophage agents. J Natl Cancer Inst 57:1355.

19. Mccuskey RS, Mccuskey PA, Gendrault JL, Ditter B, Becker K, Stefan AM, Kirn A (1986). In vivo and electron microscopic stydy of dynamic events occurring in hepatic sinusoids

following frog virus 3 infection. In Kirn A, Knook DL, Wisse E (eds): "Cells of the Hepatic Sinusoid Vol I," New York: Marcel   Dekker   p 351.

20. van Rooijen R, van Nieuwmegen R, Kamperdiijk EWA (1985). Elimination of phagocytic cells in the spleen after intravenous injection of liposome-encapsulated   dichloromethylene diphosphonate.   Ultrastructural   aspects of elimination of   marginal zone macrophages. Virchows Arch (Cell Pathol) 49:375.

21. Kaminski NE, Wells DS, Dauterman WC, Roberts JF, Guthrie FE (1986). Macrophage uptake of lipoprotein-sequestered toxicant: A potential route of immunotoxicity. Toxic and Appl Pharm 82:474.

22. Kaminski NE, Roberts JF, Guthrie FE (1986). Target ricin by coupling to an anti-macrophage monoclonal antibody. J Immunopharm 8:15.

23. Zisman B, Hirsch MS, Allison AC (1970). Selective effects of antimacrophage serum, silica and antilymphocyte serum on the pathogenesis of herpes virus infection of young adult mice. J Immunol 104:1155.

24. Morahan PS, Dempsey WL, Volkman A, Connor J (1986). Antimicrobial   activity of various immunomodulators: Independence from normal levels of circulating monocytes and NK cells. Infect and Immun 51:87.

25. Zarling JM, Tevethia SS (1973). Transplanta- tion immunity to simian virus 40 transformed cells in tumor bearing mice. II. Evidence for macrophage participation at the effector level of tumor cell rejection. J Natl Cancer Inst 50:149.

26. Claassen E, Kors N, van Rooijen N (1986). Influence of carriers on the development and localization   of   anti-2,4,6-trinitrophenyl (TNP) antibody-forming cells in the murine spleen. II. Suppressed antibody response to TNP-ficoll after elimination of marginal zone cells. Eur J Immunol 16:492.

27. van Rooijen N, van Nieuwmegen R (1984). Elimination of phagocytic cells in the spleen after intravenous injection of liposome encapsulated dichloromethylene diphosphonate.

Cell and Tissue Res 238:355.
28. Ishiguro M, Takahashi T, Funatsu G, Hayashi K, Funatsu M (1964). Biochemical studies on ricin. I. Purification of ricin. J Biochem (Tokyo) 55:587.
29. Olsnes S, Pihl A (1973). Different biological properties of the two constituent peptide chains of ricin, a toxic protein inhibiting protein synthesis. Biochemistry 12:3121.
30. Benson S, Olsnes S, Pihl A, Skorve J, Abraham KA (1975). On the mechanism of protein-synthesis inhibition by abrin and ricin. Inhibition of the GTP-hydrolysis site on the 60-S ribosomal subunit. Eur J Biochem 59:573.
31. Claassen E, van Rooijen N (1984). The effect of elimination of macrophages on the tissue distribution of liposomes containing [3H] methotrexate. Biochimica et Biophysica Acta 802:428.
32. Pinto AJ, Morahan PS, Volkman A, van Rooijen N, Stewart D, Jendrasiak G (1988). Effect of intravenous injection of liposomes encapsulting dichloromethylene diphosphonate on host antimicrobial resistance. In preparation.

Liposomes in the Therapy of Infectious Diseases and Cancer, pages 453–466
© 1989 Alan R. Liss, Inc.

AN INDUSTRIAL LIPOSOMAL DOSAGE FORM FOR
MURAMYL-TRIPEPTIDE-PHOSPHATIDYLETHANOLAMINE
(MTP-PE)

Peter van Hoogevest and Peter Fankhauser

CIBA-GEIGY Limited, Research and Development
Basle, Switzerland

ABSTRACT

The characteristics of a liposomal dosage form of
the immunomodulator MTP-PE for i.v. administration are
described. The liposomes can be constituted in the
clinic from a dry lyophilisate advantageous in storage
and shipment, using a simple standard constitution
procedure. Using the synthetic phospholipids OOPS and
POPC as bulk phospholipids this concept results in a
stable dry lyophilisate, from which multilamellar
liposomes can be reproducibly prepared.
It may be concluded that for specific use with
lipophilic drugs, the technological difficulties
hindering commercial pharmaceutical use of liposomes
have been overcome.

INTRODUCTION

Since the publication of the discovery of the
liposomal structure by Bangham in 1963 (1), a wealth
of promising applications of liposomes as drug
carriers has been suggested and evaluated (for a
review see ref. 2). Even 25 years after this
discovery, however, no single commercial drug product
has as yet been launched by the pharmaceutical
industry. A major reason for this is the existence

of several technological hurdles on the way to an
industrial product. To ensure its therapeutic
properties a liposomal dosage form must be stable and
reproducible with respect to its key characteristics.
To achieve this, reproducible quality of phospholipids
and a reproducible production process are mandatory.

In this paper we report the characteristics of
the liposomes containing MTP-PE. The pharmacological
properties are reported separately (3).

MATERIALS AND METHODS

Materials

N-acetylmuramyl-L-alanyl-D-isoglutaminyl-
L-alanine-2-[1,2-dipalmitoyl-sn-glycero-3-(hydroxyphosphoryloxy)] ethylamide, mono-sodium salt (=
MTP-PE) and 1,2-dioleoyl-sn-glycero-3-phospho-L-serine
mono-sodium salt (OOPS) were synthesized at CIBA-GEIGY
Ltd. by patented procederes. POPC (1-palmitoyl-2-
oleoyl- sn-glycero-3-phosphocholine) (POPC) was
purchased from Avanti Polar Chemicals. All other
chemicals were of pharmaceutical analytical reagent
grade.

Preparation of Dry Lyophilisate of Liposomal Components

The phospholipids and MTP-PE are dissolved under
nitrogen in t-butanol at 50° C. The clear solution is
sterile filtered through a Gelman-TF-200 (0.2 μm
filter). Aliquots (1 ml containing 175 mg POPC, 75 mg
OOPS and 1 mg MTP-PE) are lyophilised in standard
vials (15 ml) using a Lyovac GT 4 lyophilisor. The
resulting dry lyophilisates are sealed and stored
under argon.

Standardized in-Situ Preparation of Liposomes

The liposomes are prepared in-situ at room temperature
from the dry lyophilisate by addition of 2.5 ml of

suspension medium (0.2 mg disodium salt of EDTA, 0.2 mg potassium chloride, 8.0 mg sodium chloride, 0.2 mg monobasic potassium phosphate and 1.2 mg dibasic sodium phosphate per ml water for injection) followed by hydration for 15 seconds and shaking during 1 minute, using a Vortex lab shaker (model K-550-GE) at dial setting 7.

Characterisation of Dry Lyophilisate and Liposomes

Physical The mass size distribution and average size of liposomal suspensions is measured using a Coulter TA II particle sizer with a capillary of 50 μm aperture (after 400000 fold dilution of the original liposomal suspension of 100 mg phospholipid/ml with suspension medium (sterile filtered). Mass distribution is derived from the number distribution assuming identical specific density of the liposomes in every electronic measurement channel.

The absence of liposomes or aggregates having diameters larger than 50 μm is checked by light microscopy using interference contrast (Reichert-Jung, Polyvar MET microscope).

The presence of multilamellar liposomes is confirmed by observation of birefringent structures with crossed polarisors (Polyvar MET, Reichert, Wien) and Freeze Fracture Electron Microscopy according to established procedures (4).

The encapsulated buffer volume of the constituted liposomes is determined using a conductivity method. The measurement is based on the following principle: When a known volume of liposomal suspension in a buffer solution is diluted with an isotonic nonionic solution (5 % glucose), the volume of buffer entrapped in the liposomes is not diluted and does not contribute to the conductivity.

Details of this method will be published elsewhere (5).

Chemical Residual t-Butanol in dry lyophilisate is analysed by standard head-space gaschromatography.

Residual water in the dry-lyophilisate is determined by titration with Karl Fischer reagent.

HPLC analysis of liposomal components in dry lyophilisate and suspension: The dry lyophilisate is dissolved in 10.0 ml mobile phase. The aqueous liposomal suspension is dissolved in mobile phase without water added (15/985, v/v). 25 µl of this solution, containing about 3 µg MTP-PE, are injected and quantified against a reference solution. Mobile phase: 10^{-2}M Tetramethylammonium fluoride, 5×10^{-3}M Tricaprylylmethylammonium chloride in 985/15 v/v methanol/water. (Column: Stainless steel 10 cm x 4.8 mm, Nucleosil -5 C18, 60 bar, room temperature, 1 ml/min flow rate, UV detection at 214 nm).

Homogeneity of composition and incorporation of MTP-PE. In-situ constituted liposomes are sequentially ultrafiltered at low pressure (40-150 mBAR) through Nucleopore filters of 5 and 1 µm at room temperature with a 10 ml Amicon stirred filtration cell with continuous replacement of the buffer (dialysis mode). Fractions are analysed by HPLC (see above) for MTP-PE and phospholipid content. In addition the liposomal suspension is centrifuged (60 min, 50'000 x g, room temperature, Beckman Model J 2-21 M induction drive centrifuge, JA 20.1 rotor). Sediment and supernatant are analysed by HPLC for MTP-PE and phospholipid content.

Sterility of the dry lyophilisate. The liposomes are removed from a vial using aseptic technique and incubated with 100 ml caseinpeptone-soyflour nutrition medium (14 days, 20-25° C).

Phase transition temperature: Liposomes are constituted from a dry lyophilisate as described but with 2.5 ml of a mixture of equal volumes of aqueous buffer (100 mM NaCl, 40 mM Tris Hcl, pH = 7.0) and ethyleneglycol. Calorimetric scans are performed with 25 mg of this liposomal suspension on a Mettler TA 3000 Differential Scanning Calorimeter in the temperature range of -40° C to +40° C (heating rate: 10° C/min).

RESULTS

Using POPC and OOPS as bulk phospholipids, the lyophilisation from t-butanol results in a white, porous cake. Following sterile filtration and aseptic processing, the lyophilisate was found to be sterile. In 8 separately manufactured batches the residual water content ranged from 0.2 - 0.9 mg per 250 mg phospholipids and the residual t-butanol content was always lower than 50 ppm.

Chemical stability data for the lyophilisate are given in Table 1. The amounts of POPC, OOPS and MTP-PE per vial were unchanged during two years at 4° C and during 1 year at 23° C storage. After 2 years 23° the OOPS content and at 35° C the OOPS and MTP-PE content per vial had clearly decreased.

TABLE 1

CHEMICAL STABILITY OF DRY LYOPHILISATE COMPOSED OF POPC, OOPS AND MTP-PE

	storage time (months)	storage temperature		
		5° C	23° C	35°C
Percentage of	3	100	99	94
original	6	104	100	83
MTP-PE per vial	12	99	100	50
	24	100	101	15
Percentage of	3	100	98	85
original	6	99	101	83
OOPS per vial	12	99	97	65
	24	101	88	25
Percentage of	3	100	100	99
original	6	100	101	99
POPC per vial	12	99	100	97
	24	100	98	90

As determined by quality control of 8 separately manufactured batches at the time of manufacture, the constituted liposomes have an average mass size diameter ranging from 2.0 to 3.5 μm and an encapsulated buffer volume of 2.3 - 3.2 1/mol phospholipid. The latter value signifies that 30 - 40 % of the added buffer is encapsulated in the liposomes.

A typical example of the size distribution of the resulting liposomes is depicted in Fig. 1.

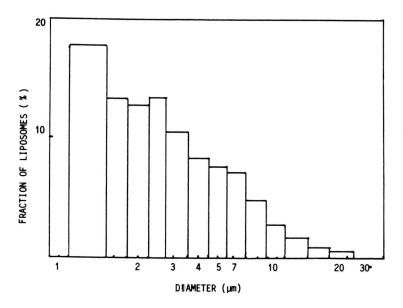

FIGURE 1. Size distribution of liposomes

To illustrate the reproducibility of the constitution procedure within and between batches Fig. 2 gives the data obtained with 10 vials of each of two different batches.

The (mass) average diameter (n = 10; ± S.D.) was 2.5 ± 0.1 μm for the first and 2.8 ± 0.1 μm for the second batch. The fraction of liposomes having a diameter equal to or larger than 1.4 μm was 86 ± 2 % and 88 ± 1 % respectively. The fraction of liposomes equal to larger than 11.0 μm was 4 ± 2 % and 5 ± 2 %.

After 2 years storage of the lyophilisates at 4° C, 23° C or 35° C the constituted liposomal suspensions did not differ in average liposome size and size distribution from suspensions prepared from fresh lyophilisates.

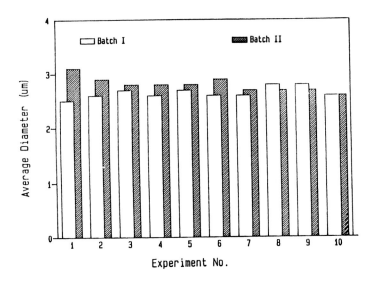

FIGURE 2. Inter and intrabatch reproducibility of average size of liposomes containing MTP-PE

The resulting liposomes were mostly of multilamellar character as observed by freeze fracture electron microscopy (Fig. 3a) and microscopy with polarized light, where the presence of typical birefringence patterns (Maltese crosses), indicates the presence of several lamellae per liposome (Fig. 3b, 3c). Liposomes larger than 20 μm are very rare, liposomes larger than 50 μm have never been observed.

The gel to liquid crystalline phase transition temperature of the liposomes was found to be - 9.3° C with an transition enthalpy of 31.9 J/g phospholipid. The phospholipid mixture started melting at about -20° C and the transition to the liquid crystalline state was complete at +10° C (Fig. 4).

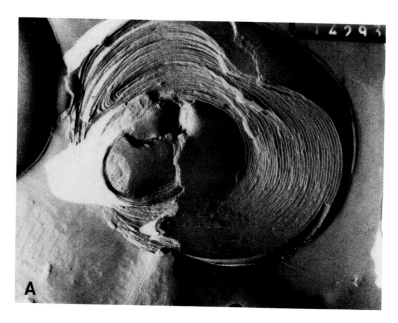

FIGURE 3A. Freeze fracture electron microscopical picture of liposome containing MTP-PE (1 cm = 0.25 um)

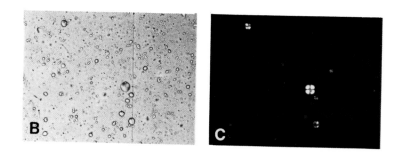

FIGURE 3B and 3C. Light microscopical picture of liposomes containing MTP-PE. Interference contrast (left), polarised light (right)

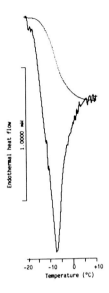

FIGURE 4.   Calorimetric scan on liposomal suspension.

The constituted liposomes are stable for at least
1 year at 4°C, physically with respect to changes of
average size (Table 2) and chemically (Table 3).

TABLE 2
PHYSICAL STABILITY OF LIPOSOMES
CONTAINING MTP-PE

Average Diameter in µm:

storage time (month)	storage temperature		
	5° C	23° C	35° C
1	2.8	3.3	3.1
3	2.7	2.9	2.8
6	2.7	n.d.	n.d.
12	2.8	n.d.	n.d.

n.d. = not determined

TABLE 3
CHEMICAL STABILITY OF LIPOSOMES
CONTAINING MTP-PE

temperature	storage time (months)	storage		
		5° C	23° C	35°C
Percentage of	1	101	102	99
original	3	99	95	80
MTP-PE per vial	6	103	n.d.	n.d.
	12	101	n.d.	n.d.
Percentage of	1	100	102	100
original	3	99	98	91
OOPS per vial	6	101	n.d.	n.d.
	12	100	n.d.	n.d.
Percentage of	1	102	101	100
original	3	98	98	97
POPC per vial	6	100	n.d.	n.d.
	12	99	n.d.	n.d.

n.d. = not determined

Separation of the constituted liposomes into size-fractions showed similar ratios of MTP-PE to POPC to OOPS in all fractions as in the original lyophilisate (Table 4) proving homogeneity of composition for all sizes and complete incorporation. HPLC analysis after centrifugation showed that 95 % of the phospholipid and active substance could be sedimented simultaneously, confirming the complete incorporation of MTP into the liposomes.

TABLE 4
HOMOGENEITY OF COMPOSITION OF LIPOSOMES
CONTAINING MTP-PE

		CGP 19835 weight %	POPC weight %	OOPS weight %
	> 5	0.4	71	29
Filter	< 5	0.4	71	28
fractions	1-5	0.4	70	29
(μm)	< 1	0.4	70	28
Total unfractioned suspension		0.4	70	29
Dry Lyophilisate		0.4	70	30

The standardised constitution procedure for the clinic is characterized by a fixed hydration period of 15 seconds, a fixed shaking time period of 1 minute using a specific lab-vortex shaker at a fixed dial setting. In order to evaluate the sensitivity of the process to these parameters experiments were performed with systematic change of individual parameters, observing the effect on the average diameter and size fraction equal to or larger than 1.4 μm. The effects are depicted in Fig. 5a for the hydration time period. in Fig. 5b for the shaking time period and in Fig. 5c for the shaking speed. It can be seen that within the tested ranges only the shaking speed could slightly influence the size of the resulting liposomes.

DISCUSSION

The use of a sterile dry lyophilisate of liposomal components for storage and shipment, an idea originally proposed by an ICI group (7), combined with a convenient constitution procedure for the liposomes in the clinic avoids the enormous technological hurdles which would have to be overcome for aseptic

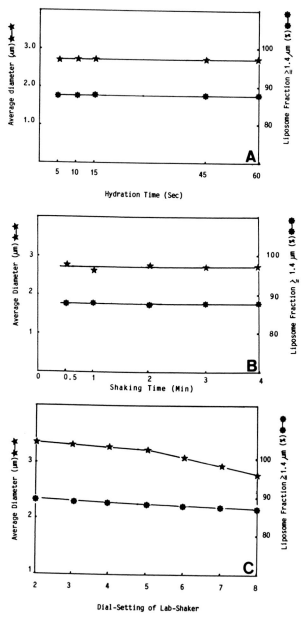

FIGURE 5A,B,C. Influence of hydration time (A),
shaking time period (B) and
shaking speed (C) on the
characteristics of the liposomes.

production of aqueous liposomal suspensions on a large scale. All that is required is conversion of common large scale lyophilisation processes for vials to removal of organic solvents rather than water and a constitution procedure, proven to be reproducible. The results obtained prove that this simple concept indeed works: The drug is incorporated completely and homogeneously, the liposome characteristics between and within batches are reproducible, the properties are largely unaffected by variations of the in-situ constitution procedure, the dry lyophilisate is stable for prolonged storage and even the constituted liposomes are stable for a reasonably long time. The handling of these liposomes in the clinic is therefore simple and safe.

This concept, however, is dependent on the selection of the appropriate mixture of the bulk lipids: POPC and OOPS in a ratio of 7:3 (8). This mixture provides the following advantages:

- the synthetic phospholipids have a constant fatty acid composition. The excellent reproducibility of their physicochemical properties would be hard to match by natural phospholipids even from standardised sources.
- lipids with mono-unsaturated acyl chains are more stable towards oxydation than the poly-unsaturated analogs isolated from natural sources
- the low phase-transition temperature of -9° C allows the in-situ preparation of the liposomes at room temperature. Since proper liposome formation occurs only above the phase transition temperature, saturated synthetic phospholipids would not be suitable.
- The selected synthetic phospholipids form a stable, porous lipid cake after lyophilisation from organic solvents , which allows reproducible hydration. Most phospholipids and especially egg PC and soy PC have oily, waxy appearance and do not form physically stable lyophilisates.
- the solubility of the selected phospholipids and of the active agent MTP-PE (which also contains a phospholipid group (9)). in t-butanol allows co-lyophilisation which results in complete incorporation of the MTP-PE in the liposomal structure.

Due to their composition, structure and size, the resulting liposomes meet all the requirements for the desired therapeutic effect after i.v. administration: Size and PS content lead to increased uptake by macrophages and increased lung localisation, the multilamellar structure results in prolonged action of the drug (10). The concomitant change of the body distribution pattern explains the improvement of the therapeutic index as compared to free MTP (3, 11).

The liposomal dosage form of MTP-PE presented in this paper is the first parenteral liposomal drug product meeting the combined criteria of satisfactory pharmacological activity, sufficient stability, reproducible characteristics and suitability for large scale industrial production.

It can therefore be concluded that for specific use with lipophilic drugs the difficulties hindering commercial pharmaceutical use of liposomes have been overcome.

REFERENCES

1. Bangham AD (1963) Physical structure and behaviour of lipids and lipid enzymes. Adv Lipid Res 1:65
2. Gregoriadis G (1984). Liposome Technology, Volumes I,II and III. CRC Press Inc., Boca Ralon.
3. Schumann G, Comparison of free and liposomal MTP-PE: Pharmacological, toxicological and pharmacokinetic aspects; this book
4. Müller M, Meister N, Moor H (1980). Freezing in a propane jet and its application in freeze-fracturing, Mikroskopie (Wien) 36:129.
5. Van Hoogevest P, Arnold L, and Fankhauser P (1988) in preparation.
6. Fidler I.J. (1986) Immunomodulation of macrophages for cancer and antiviral therapy. In Tomlinson E, Davis SS (eds): "Site specific drug delivery", Chichester, New York, Brisbane, Toronto Singapore: John Wiley and Sons, p. 111
7. US Patent specification 4, 370, 349
8. European published patent application 178624
9. UK Patent 1570625.
10. Schroit AJ, Galligioni E, and Fidler IJ (1985). Factors influencing the in-situ activation of macrophages by liposomes containing muramyl dipeptide. Biol Cell 47:87
11. Schumann G (1987). Immunostimulants: Now and Tomorrow. In Azuma I and Jolies G: Japan Sci. Soc. Press, Tokyo/Springer-Verlag, Berlin, p 71.

Index